Psychiatry

First and second edition authors:

Darran Bloye

Simon Davies

Alisdair D Cameron

Third edition authors:

Julius Bourke

Matthew Castle

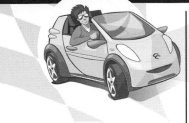

4th Edition
CRASH COURSE

SERIES EDITOR:
Dan Horton-Szar
BSc(Hons) MBBS(Hons) MRCGP
Northgate Medical Practice,
Canterbury,
Kent, UK

FACULTY ADVISOR:
Jeremy Hall
MA MB BChir MPhil PhD MRCPsych
Professor of Psychiatry and Neuroscience,
University of Cardiff,
Cardiff, UK

Psychiatry

Katie Marwick
MA(Hons) MB ChB (Hons) MRCPsych
Core Trainee (CT3) in Psychiatry, South-East Scotland Deanery;
ECAT Clinical Lecturer in Psychiatry, University of Edinburgh, UK

Steven Birrell
MB ChB MRCPsych
Clinical Teaching Fellow in Medical Education and Honorary
Specialty Registrar in General Adult Psychiatry, NHS Lothian;
Honorary Fellow, College of Medicine and Veterinary Medicine,
University of Edinburgh, UK

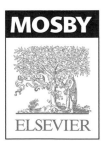

MOSBY

ELSEVIER

Edinburgh London New York Oxford Philadelphia St Louis Sydney Toronto 2013

MOSBY
ELSEVIER

Commissioning Editor: Jeremy Bowes
Development Editor: Sheila Black
Project Manager: Andrew Riley
Designer: Christian Bilbow
Illustration Manager: Jennifer Rose

First edition 1999

Second edition 2004

Third edition 2008

Reprinted 2010

Fourth edition 2013

ISBN: 978-0-7234-3636-2

British Library Cataloguing in Publication Data
A catalogue record for this book is available from the British Library

Library of Congress Cataloging in Publication Data
A catalog record for this book is available from the Library of Congress

ELSEVIER your source for books, journals and multimedia in the health sciences
www.elsevierhealth.com

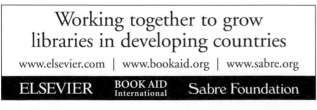

Working together to grow libraries in developing countries

www.elsevier.com | www.bookaid.org | www.sabre.org

ELSEVIER   BOOK AID International   Sabre Foundation

The Publisher's policy is to use **paper manufactured from sustainable forests**

Printed in China

Series editor foreword

The *Crash Course* series was first published in 1997 and now, 16 years on, we are still going strong. Medicine never stands still, and the work of keeping this series relevant for today's students is an ongoing process. These fourth editions build on the success of the previous titles and incorporate new and revised material, to keep the series up-to-date with current guidelines for best practice, and recent developments in medical research and pharmacology.

We always listen to feedback from our readers, through focus groups and student reviews of the *Crash Course* titles. For the fourth editions we have completely re-written our self-assessment material to keep up with today's 'single-best answer' and 'extended matching question' formats. The artwork and layout of the titles has also been largely re-worked to make it easier on the eye during long sessions of revision.

Despite fully revising the books with each edition, we hold fast to the principles on which we first developed the series. *Crash Course* will always bring you all the information you need to revise in compact, manageable volumes that integrate basic medical science and clinical practice. The books still maintain the balance between clarity and conciseness, and provide sufficient depth for those aiming at distinction. The authors are medical students and junior doctors who have recent experience of the exams you are now facing, and the accuracy of the material is checked by a team of faculty advisors from across the UK.

I wish you all the best for your future careers!

Dr Dan Horton-Szar
Series Editor

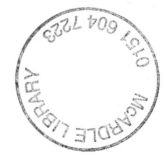

Authors

Just starting psychiatry? What are all these weird symptoms and wacky questions? Why isn't there a blood test for schizophrenia? Why is it ever acceptable to give patients treatment they don't want? As junior doctors who qualified four and six years ago we well remember how difficult and confusing psychiatry felt as medical students. Your hard-won knowledge of blood tests, ECGs and X-rays is still required but not sufficient to do psychiatry. Instead, what you yourself discover through observing and communicating with patients is what matters, and for that you need to enhance your clinical skills. You have to learn about bizarre symptoms which are hard for you to describe, let alone your patients. You have to train your observation skills to include a patient's mental state, not just their physical signs. You have to learn how to comfortably ask deeply personal questions and learn to tolerate hearing about the seemingly infinite capacity of humans to hurt each other.

We hope this book will bring clarity to this confusion by guiding you down paths of systematic assessments, rational diagnoses and evidence based management plans. We've worked hard to always get down to the 'clinical bottom line', with lots of practical tips, but we hope also to spark your interest in some of the new neuroscientific findings in psychiatry.

If you choose a speciality with any patient contact, the communication skills and knowledge you gain from studying psychiatry will help you be a better doctor. We wish you the best of luck!

Dr Katie Marwick and Dr Steven Birrell

Faculty Advisor

If you are looking for an accessible yet comprehensive introduction to psychiatry, this book has no rivals. The previous editions have received well-deserved places on medical student bookshelves throughout the country, but the current authors have substantially revised this edition to make it even better. In particular, the self-assessment questions offer a range of carefully constructed, realistic, clinical vignettes that focus on key diagnostic and management decisions to help you make good decisions when you come to work in A&E, the wards, clinics and GP surgeries. Reading this book will prepare you well for both upcoming exams and a career in psychiatry – enjoy!

Professor Jeremy Hall

Acknowledgements

We are very grateful to the many people who have helped us with this book. In particular, the Edinburgh University medical students who were guinea-pigs for the new self-assessment questions: Mark Cairns, Elouise Donaldson, Kathryn Fleming, Naomi Howard, Gordon McKinnon, Claudette Phillips, Katy Robinson and Liana Romaniuk. Dr Pearce Cusack, FY2, kindly added commenting on his SHO's book to his job list. Dr Katie Beck, CT2 Psychiatry, provided a view from the south on aspects of the book to do with practice in England. Expert opinions were provided by Dr Nick Hughes (ST5 in Forensic Psychiatry), Dr Lindsay Mizen (ST4 in Psychiatry of Intellectual Disability), Dr Fiona Murray (Consultant Perinatal Psychiatrist), Dr Adam Polnay (Speciality Registrar in Psychotherapy) and Dr Gary Stevenson (Consultant Older Adult Psychiatrist). We thank Dr Susan Shenkin (Consultant Geriatrician) for permission to include tables she co-authored with us. Finally, we would like to thank our partners and families, particularly Shona, for accepting gracious defeat by The Book over the last few months, and for having us back afterwards.

Katie Marwick and Steven Birrell

Contents

Series editor foreword v

Prefaces vii

Acknowledgements ix

1. **Psychiatric assessment and diagnosis** **1**
   Interview technique 1
   Psychiatric history 2
   Mental state examination 5
   Risk assessment 8
   Physical examination 8
   The formulation: presenting the case 8
   Classification in psychiatry 10

2. **Pharmacological therapy and electroconvulsive therapy** **13**
   Antidepressants 13
   Mood stabilizers 17
   Antipsychotics 19
   Anxiolytic and hypnotic drugs 22
   Other drugs used in psychiatry 24
   Electroconvulsive therapy 24

3. **Psychological therapy** **25**
   Psychotherapeutic approaches 25
   Indications for psychotherapy 30

4. **Mental health and the law** **33**
   Mental Health Act 1983 as amended by
   Mental Health Act 2007 33
   Mental Health (Care & Treatment)
   (Scotland) Act 2003 37
   Mental Health (Northern Ireland)
   Order 1986 37
   Capacity to consent to treatment 38
   Common law 39
   Human rights legislation 39
   Fitness to drive 40

5. **Mental health service provision** **41**
   History 41
   Primary care 41
   Secondary care 41

6. **The patient with thoughts of suicide or self-harm** **45**
   Definitions and clinical features 45
   Assessment of patients who have
   inflicted harm upon themselves 45
   Patient management following self-harm or
   attempted suicide 48
   Discussion of case study 48

7. **The patient with low mood** **49**
   Definitions and clinical
   features 49
   Differential diagnosis 51
   Assessment 53
   Discussion of case study 54

8. **The patient with elevated or irritable mood** **57**
   Definitions and clinical
   features 57
   Differential diagnosis 59
   Assessment 62
   Algorithm for the diagnosis of mood
   disorders 62
   Discussion of case study 63

9. **The psychotic patient** **65**
   Definitions and clinical
   features 65
   Differential diagnosis 71
   Algorithm for the diagnosis of psychotic
   disorders 74
   Assessment 74
   Discussion of case study 75

10. **The patient with anxiety, fear or avoidance** **77**
    Definitions and clinical
    features 77
    Differential diagnosis 78
    Algorithm for the diagnosis of anxiety
    disorders 80
    Assessment 82
    Discussion of case study 82

Contents

11. **The patient with obsessions and compulsions**. 85

    Definitions and clinical features 85

    Differential diagnosis. 86

    Discussion of case study 88

12. **The patient with a reaction to a stressful event or bereavement** 91

    Definitions and clinical features 91

    Bereavement 94

    Differential diagnosis. 95

    Discussion of case study 95

13. **The patient with medically unexplained physical symptoms** 97

    Definitions and clinical features 98

    Differential diagnosis. 100

    Assessment 100

    Discussion of case study 101

14. **The patient with impairment of consciousness, memory or cognition** . . . 103

    Definitions and clinical features 103

    Common cognitive disorders 106

    Differential diagnosis. 110

    Assessment 112

    Discussion of case study 114

15. **The patient with alcohol or substance use problems** 115

    Definitions and clinical features 115

    Alcohol-related disorders 116

    Other substance-related disorders 120

    Differential diagnosis. 120

    Assessment 121

    Discussion of case study 122

16. **The patient with personality problems** 123

    Definitions and clinical features 123

    Classification. 124

    Assessment 124

    Differential diagnosis. 126

    Discussion of case study 126

17. **The patient with eating or weight problems** 127

    Definitions and clinical features 127

    Assessment 128

    Differential diagnosis of patients with low weight 129

    Discussion of case study 131

18. **The mood (affective) disorders** 133

    Depressive disorders 133

    Bipolar affective disorder 137

    Dysthymia and cyclothymia. 138

19. **The psychotic disorders: schizophrenia** 141

    Schizophrenia 141

20. **The anxiety and somatoform disorders** 147

    Anxiety disorders. 147

    Somatoform disorders 151

21. **Alcohol and substance-related disorders** 153

    Alcohol disorders. 153

    Other psychoactive substances 156

22. **The personality disorders**. 159

    The personality disorders 159

23. **Eating disorders** 163

    Anorexia and bulimia nervosa. 163

24. **Disorders relating to the menstrual cycle, pregnancy and the puerperium** . . . 167

    Premenstrual syndrome. 167

    Menopause 167

    Psychiatric considerations in pregnancy . . 167

    Puerperal disorders. 169

25. **Dementia and delirium**. 173

    Dementia 173

    Delirium. 178

26. **Older adult psychiatry** 181

    Mental illness in older adults 181

    Assessment considerations in older adults. 182

    Treatment considerations in older adults. 183

27. **Child and adolescent psychiatry** 185

    Considerations in the assessment of children 185

    Classification. 186

    Intellectual disability 186

    Developmental disorders 187

Acquired disorders 188

Child abuse 192

28. Intellectual disability 193

Intellectual disability (mental retardation/
learning disability) 193

29. Forensic psychiatry 197

Mental disorder and crime 197

Assessing and managing risk of
violence 198

Considerations in court proceedings . . . 199

30. The sleep disorders 201

Definitions and classification 201

31. The psychosexual disorders 207

Sexual dysfunction 207

Disorders of sexual preference
(paraphilias) 210

Gender identity 211

Self-assessment 213

Best of fives questions (BOFs) 215

Extended-matching questions (EMQs) 233

BOF answers 255

EMQ answers 271

Glossary 285

Index 287

Psychiatric assessment and diagnosis

1

The psychiatric assessment is different from a medical or surgical assessment in that: (1) the history taking is often longer and is aimed at understanding psychological problems that develop in patients, each with a unique background and social environment; (2) a mental state examination is performed; and (3) the assessment can in itself be therapeutic. Figure 1.1 provides an outline of the psychiatric assessment, which includes a psychiatric history, mental state examination, risk assessment, physical examination and formulation.

INTERVIEW TECHNIQUE

- Whenever possible, patients should be interviewed in settings where privacy can be ensured – a patient who is distressed will be more at ease in a quiet office than in an accident and emergency cubicle.
- Chairs should be at the same level and arranged at an angle, so that you are not sitting directly opposite the patient.
- Establishing rapport is an immediate priority and requires the display of empathy and sensitivity by the interviewer.
- Notes may be taken during the interview; however, explain to patients that you will be doing so. Make sure that you still maintain good eye contact.
- Ensure that you are seated closer to the door than the patient to allow you an unobstructed exit should it be required.
- Carry a personal alarm and/or know where the alarm in the consulting room is, and check you know how to work the alarms.
- Introduce yourself to the patient and ask them how they would like to be addressed. Explain how long

the interview will last. In examination situations it may prove helpful to explain to patients that you may need to interrupt them due to time constraints.
- Keep track of, and ration, your time appropriately.
- Flexibility is essential, e.g. it may be helpful to put a very anxious patient at ease by talking about their background before focusing in on the presenting complaint.

Make use of both open and closed questions when appropriate:

Closed questions limit the scope of the response to one or two word answers. They are used to gain specific information, and can be used to control the length of the interview when patients are being over-inclusive. For example:

- Do you feel low in mood? (Yes or no answer)
- What time do you wake up in the morning? (Specific answer)

Note that closed questions can be used at the very beginning of the interview as they are easier to answer and help to put patients at ease, e.g. 'Do you live locally?'; 'Are you married?' (see 'identifying information' below).

Open questions encourage the patient to answer freely with a wide range of responses and should be used to

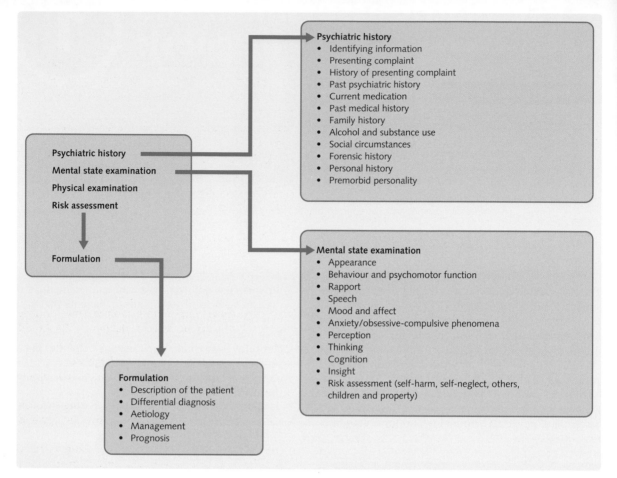

Fig. 1.1 Outline of the psychiatric assessment

elicit the presenting complaint, as well as feelings and attitudes. For example:

- How have you been feeling lately?
- What has caused you to feel this way?

PSYCHIATRIC HISTORY

The order in which you take the history is not as important as being systematic, making sure you cover all the essential subsections. A typical format for taking a psychiatric history is outlined in Figure 1.1 and is described in detail below.

Identifying information

- Name.
- Age.
- Marital status and children.
- Occupation.
- Reason for the patient's presence in a psychiatric setting (e.g. referral to out-patient clinic by family doctor, admitted to ward informally having presented at casualty).
- Legal status (i.e. if detained under mental health legislation).

For example:

   Mrs LM is a 32-year-old married housewife with two children aged 4 and 6 years. She was referred by her family doctor to a psychiatric out-patient clinic.

Presenting complaint

Open questions are used to elicit the presenting complaint. Whenever possible, record the main problems in the patient's own words, in one or two sentences, instead of using technical psychiatric terms, e.g.:

Mrs LM complains of 'feeling as though I don't know who I am, like I'm living in an empty shell'.

Patients frequently have more than one complaint, some of which may be related. It is helpful to organize multiple presenting complaints into groups of symptoms that are related; for instance, 'low mood', 'poor concentration' and 'lack of energy' are common features of depression, e.g.:

Mrs LM complains firstly of 'low mood', 'difficulty sleeping' and 'poor self-esteem', and secondly of 'increased alcohol consumption' associated with withdrawal symptoms of 'shaking, sweating and jitteriness' in the morning.

It is not always easy to organize patients' difficulties into a simple presenting complaint in psychiatry. In this case, give the chief complaint(s) as the presenting complaint and cover the rest of the symptoms or problems in the history of presenting complaint.

History of presenting complaint

This section is concerned with eliciting the nature and development of each of the presenting complaints. The following headings may be helpful in structuring your questioning:

- *Duration*: when did the problems start?
- *Development*: how did the problems develop?
- *Mode of onset*: suddenly or over a period of time?
- *Course*: are symptoms constant, progressively worsening or intermittent?
- *Severity*: how much is the patient suffering? To what extent are symptoms affecting the patient's social and occupational functioning?
- *Associated symptoms*: certain complaints are associated with clusters of other symptoms that should be enquired about if patients do not mention them spontaneously, e.g. when 'feeling low' is a presenting complaint, biological, cognitive and psychotic features of depression as well as suicidal ideation should be asked about. You can also ask about symptom clusters for psychosis, anxiety, eating problems, substance use and cognitive problems, among others. Also, certain symptoms are common to many psychiatric conditions and these should be screened for, e.g. a primary complaint of insomnia may be a sign of depression, mania, psychosis or a primary sleep disorder.
- *Precipitating factors*: psychosocial stress frequently precipitates episodes of mental illness, e.g. bereavement, moving house, relationship difficulties.

Past psychiatric history

This is an extremely important section as it may provide clues to the patient's current diagnosis. It should include:

- Previous or ongoing psychiatric diagnoses.
- Dates and duration of previous mental illness episodes.
- Details of previous treatments, including medication, psychotherapy, electroconvulsive therapy and hospitalization.
- Details of previous contact with psychiatric services.
- Details of previous assessment or treatment under mental health legislation.

Past medical history

Enquire about medical illnesses or surgical procedures. Past head injury or surgery, neurological conditions (e.g. epilepsy) and endocrine abnormalities (e.g. thyroid problems) are especially relevant to psychiatry.

Current medication

Note all the medication patients are using, including psychiatric, non-psychiatric and over-the-counter drugs. Also enquire how long patients have been on specific medication and whether it has been effective. Non-concordance as well as reactions and allergies should be recorded.

Family history

- Enquire about the presence of psychiatric illness (including suicide and substance abuse) in family members, remembering that genetic factors are implicated in the aetiology of many psychiatric conditions. A family tree may be useful to summarize information.

- Enquire whether parents are still alive and if not, causes of death. Also ask about significant physical illnesses in the family.
- Ask whether the patient has any siblings and, if so, where they are in the birth order.
- Enquire about the quality of the patient's relationships with close family members.

Personal history

The personal history consists of a brief description of the patient's life. Time constraints will not allow an exhaustive biographical account, but you should attempt to include significant events, perhaps under the following useful headings:

Infancy and early childhood (until age 5)

- Pregnancy and birth complications (e.g. prematurity, fetal distress, caesarean section).
- Developmental milestones (age of crawling, walking, speaking, bladder and bowel control).
- Childhood illnesses.
- Unusually aggressive behaviour or impaired social interaction.

Later childhood and adolescence (until completion of higher education)

- History of physical, sexual or emotional abuse (if appropriate to circumstances).
- School record (academic performance, number and type of schools attended, age on leaving, and final qualifications).
- Relationships with parents, teachers and peers. Victim or perpetrator of bullying.
- Behavioural problems, including antisocial behaviour, drug use or truancy.
- Higher education and training.

Occupational record

- Details of types and duration of jobs.
- Details of and reasons for unemployment and/or dismissal.

Relationship, marital and sexual history

- Puberty: significant early relationships and experiences as well as sexual orientation (if appropriate).
- Details and duration of significant relationships. Reasons for break-ups.
- Marriage/divorce details. Children.

- Ability to engage in satisfactory sexual relationships. Sexual dysfunction, fetishes or gender identity problems (only enquire if problem is suspected).

COMMUNICATION

A history of sexual abuse is important to detect. This can be awkward. Tact and discretion are vital. You may find it useful to grade your questions, e.g.: When was your first relationship? When was your first sexual experience? Have you ever had an unpleasant sexual experience? Sometimes such experiences are unpleasant because they are unwanted or because the person is too young to understand . . .? Leaving the question open allows the patient room to answer freely rather than 'yes' or 'no'.

Social circumstances

This includes accommodation, social supports and relationships, employment and financial circumstances, and hobbies or leisure activities. It is important to identify if the patient has current frequent contact with children, in case their presentation raises any child protection concerns. This section is important in order to understand the social context in which the patient's problems developed.

Alcohol and substance use

This section should never be overlooked, as alcohol/substance-related psychiatric conditions are very common.

The CAGE questionnaire (see p. 122) is a useful tool to screen for alcohol dependence. If a patient answers affirmatively to two or more questions, regard the screen as positive and go on to check if they meet criteria for alcohol dependence syndrome (see p. 117). Try to elicit a patient's typical drinking day including daily intake of alcohol in units, type of alcohol used, time of first drink of the day and places where drinking occurs (e.g. at home alone or in a pub).

If illicit drugs have been or are being used, record the drug names, routes of administration (intravenous, inhaled, oral ingestion) and the years and frequency of use. Also enquire about possible dependence (see p. 116, Ch. 15).

Forensic history

Enquire about the details and dates of previous offences and antisocial behaviour, including prosecutions, convictions and prison sentences. It is important to ask specifically about violent crime and the age of the patient's first violent offence.

Premorbid personality

The premorbid personality is an indication of the patient's personality and character before the onset of mental illness. It can be difficult to ascertain retrospectively. Indirect evidence of it can be provided from the personal history (e.g. have they ever been able to hold down a job or been in a long-term relationship? Have their interests changed?). Patients may be asked directly about their personality before they became ill, or it may be useful to ask a close family member or friend about a patient's premorbid personality.

For example:

A young man with schizophrenia, with prominent negative symptoms of lack of motivation and interest, and poverty of thought, was described by his mother as being outgoing, intelligent and ambitious before becoming ill.

COMMUNICATION

One way to explore premorbid personality in a patient with some insight is to ask questions such as:
How would people have described you before? How about now?

MENTAL STATE EXAMINATION

The mental state examination (MSE) describes an interviewer's objective impression of many aspects of a patient's mental functioning at a certain period of time. Whereas the psychiatric history remains relatively constant, the MSE may fluctuate from day to day or hour to hour. It is useful to try and gather as much evidence as possible about the MSE while doing the psychiatric history, instead of viewing this as a separate section. In fact, the MSE begins the moment you meet the patient. In addition to noting their appearance, you should observe how patients first behave on meeting you. This includes their body language and the way that they respond to your attempts to establish rapport.

COMMUNICATION

In the mental state examination (MSE) only record what the patient demonstrates or experiences during the interview (for example, if a patient reports having had a hallucination 5 minutes before you entered the room, that would be described in the history, not the mental state).

By the time you have finished the psychiatric history, you should have completed many aspects of the MSE,

and you should just need to ask certain key questions to finish this process off. The individual aspects of the MSE, which are summarized in Figure 1.1, are discussed in more detail below.

There is some variation in the order in which the MSE is reported (e.g. speech is sometimes described before mood, and sometimes before thought form). As long as you include the information, the exact order is not important.

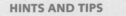

HINTS AND TIPS

Don't just ask questions and write down answers! Appearance and behaviour are vital to the mental state examination, especially with less communicative patients. Posture, facial expression, tone of voice, spontaneity of speech, state of relaxation and movements made are all important. You may find it helpful to practise with a colleague – try writing down 10 points that describe their appearance and behaviour without mentioning anything relating to questions asked.

Appearance

- *Physical state*: how old does the patient appear? Do they appear physically unwell? Are they sweating? Are they too thin or obese?
- *Clothes and accessories*: are clothes clean?
- *Do clothes match?* Are clothes appropriate to the weather and circumstances or are they bizarre? Is the patient carrying strange objects?
- *Self-care and hygiene*: does the patient appear to have been neglecting their appearance or hygiene (e.g. unshaven, dirty tangled hair, malodorous, dishevelled)? Is there any evidence of injury or self-harm (e.g. cuts to wrists or forearms)?

Behaviour and psychomotor function

This section focuses on all motor behaviour, including abnormal movements such as tremors, tics and twitches as well as displays of suspiciousness, aggression or fear, and catatonic features. Documenting patients' behaviour at the start of, and during, the interview is an integral part of the mental state examination and should be done in as much detail as possible, e.g.:

Mrs LM introduced herself appropriately, although only made fleeting eye contact. She sat rigidly throughout the first half of the interview, mostly staring at the floor and speaking very softly. She became tearful halfway through the interview when talking about her lack of self-esteem. After this her posture relaxed, her eye contact improved and there were moments when she smiled. There were no abnormal movements.

The term 'psychomotor' is used to describe a patient's motor activity as a consequence of their concurrent mental processes. Psychomotor abnormalities include *retardation* (slow, monotonous speech; slow or absent body movements) and *agitation* (inability to sit still; fidgeting, pacing or hand-wringing; rubbing or scratching skin or clothes).

Note whether you are able to establish a good rapport with patients. What is their attitude towards you? Do they make good eye contact or do they look around the room or at the floor? Patients may be described as cooperative, cordial, uninterested, aggressive, defensive, guarded, suspicious, fearful, perplexed, preoccupied, disinhibited (that is, a lowering of normal social inhibitions, e.g. being over-familiar, or making sexually inappropriate comments), etc.

Fig. 1.2 Typical questions used to elicit specific psychiatric symptoms	
Questions used to elicit ...	Chapter/page
Suicidal ideas	Ch. 6, p. 46
Depressive symptoms	Ch. 7, p. 53
Mania/hypomania	Ch. 8, p. 62
Delusions	Ch. 9, p. 75
Hallucinations	Ch. 9, p. 74
Symptoms of anxiety	Ch. 10, p. 82
Obsessions and compulsions	Ch. 11, p. 85
Somatoform disorders	Ch. 13, p. 98
Memory and cognition	Ch. 14, p. 103
Problem drinking	Ch. 15, p. 121
Symptoms of anorexia and bulimia	Ch. 17, p. 128
Symptoms of insomnia	Ch. 30, p. 203

HINTS AND TIPS

Observations of appearance and behaviour may also reveal other useful information (e.g. extrapyramidal side-effects from antipsychotic medication). It is useful to remember to look for:

- *Parkinsonism*: drug-induced signs are most commonly a reduced arm swing and unusually upright posture while walking. Tremor and rigidity are late signs, in contrast to idiopathic parkinsonism.
- *Acute dystonia*: involuntary sustained muscular contractions or spasms.
- *Akathisia*: subjective feeling of inner restlessness and muscular discomfort.
- *Tardive dyskinesia*: rhythmic, involuntary movements of head, limbs and trunk, especially chewing, grimacing of mouth and protruding, darting movements of tongue.

Mood and affect

Mood refers to a patient's sustained, subjectively experienced emotional state over a period of time. *Affect* refers to the transient ebb and flow of emotion in response to particular stimuli (e.g. smiling at a joke or crying at a sad memory).

Mood is assessed by asking patients how they are feeling. So, a patient's mood might be depressed, elated, anxious, guilty, frightened, angry, etc. It is described subjectively (what the patient says they are feeling) and objectively (what your impression of their prevailing mood is during the interview), e.g. *her mood was subjectively 'rock bottom' and objectively low.* Figure 1.2 refers

to typical questions that may be used to elicit depressed, elated or anxious moods.

Affect is assessed by observing patients' posture, facial expression, emotional reactivity and speech. There are two components to consider when assessing affect:

1. The appropriateness or congruity of the observed affect to the patient's subjectively reported mood (e.g. a woman with schizophrenia who reports feeling suicidal with a happy facial expression would be described as having an *incongruous* affect).
2. The range of affect or range of emotional expressivity. In this sense affect may be:
   - Within the normal range
   - Blunted/flat: a noticeable reduction in the normal intensity of emotional expression as evidenced by a monotonous voice and minimal facial expression.

Note that a *labile* mood refers to a fluctuating mood state that alternates between extremes (e.g. a young man with a mixed affective episode alternates between feeling overjoyed with pressure of speech and miserable with suicidal ideation).

Anxiety/obsessive-compulsive phenomena

Obsessive-compulsive and anxiety symptoms (free-floating anxiety, panic attacks, phobias, ruminatory thoughts) need not be the presenting complaint to be present to a clinically significant degree. These symptoms are common to many psychiatric disorders and, if not specifically asked patients may fail to mention them. Also record stress reactions, dissociative symptoms, and depersonalization and derealization here (see Ch. 12). Figure 1.2 can direct you to typical questions that may be used to elicit obsessive-compulsive and anxiety symptoms.

HINTS AND TIPS

Depression and obsessive-compulsive symptoms often coexist (>20%) with onset before, simultaneously or after the onset of depression. You may find it useful to have a set of screening questions ready to use.

Speech

Speech should be described in terms of:

- *Rate of production*: e.g. pressure of speech in mania; long pauses and poverty of speech in depression.
- *Quality and flow of speech*: volume, dysarthria (articulation difficulties), dysprosody (unusual speech rhythm, melody, intonation or pitch), stuttering.

Note that disorganized, incoherent or bizarre speech (e.g. flight of ideas) is usually regarded as a thought disorder and is, therefore, described under the thought section.

Thoughts

Problems with thinking are considered under two headings: thought form (abnormal patterns of thinking) and thought content (abnormal beliefs).

Thought form

Disordered thinking includes circumstantial and tangential thinking, loosening of association (derailment/knight's move thinking), neologisms and idiosyncratic word use, flight of ideas, thought blocking, perseveration, echolalia, and irrelevant answers (see p. 70, Ch. 9, for the definitions of these terms). Whenever possible, record patients' disorganized speech word for word, as it can be very difficult to label disorganized thinking with a single technical term and written language may be easier to evaluate than spoken language.

Thought content: delusions and overvalued ideas

It is diagnostically significant to classify delusions as:

- Primary or secondary.
- Mood congruent or mood incongruent.
- Bizarre or non-bizarre.
- And according to the content of the delusion (summarized in Fig. 9.2, p. 69).

See pages 67–68, Chapter 9, for a detailed discussion.

Perception

Hallucinations are often mentioned during the history However, this is not always the case, so it is important that you specifically enquire about abnormal perceptual experiences (perceptual abnormalities are defined and classified on p. 66, Ch. 9). If patients admit to problems with perception, it is important to ascertain:

- Whether the abnormal perceptions are genuine hallucinations, pseudohallucinations, illusions, or intrusive thoughts.
- From which sensory modality the hallucinations appear to arise (i.e. are they auditory, visual, olfactory, gustatory or somatic hallucinations – see p. 67).
- Whether auditory hallucinations are elementary or complex. If complex, are they experienced in the first person (audible thoughts, thought echo), second person (critical, persecutory, complimentary or command hallucinations) or third person (voices arguing or discussing the patient, or giving a running commentary)?

It is also important to note whether patients seem to be responding to hallucinations during the interview, as evidenced by them laughing inappropriately as though they are sharing a private joke, or suddenly tilting their head as though listening, or quizzically looking at hallucinatory objects around the room.

Figure 1.2 can direct you to typical questions that may be used to elicit perceptual abnormalities.

Cognition

The cognition of all patients should be screened by checking orientation to place and time. Depending on the circumstances, a more thorough cognitive assessment may be required. Cognitive tests are discussed fully in Chapter 14, including tests of generalized cognitive abilities (e.g. consciousness, attention, orientation) and specific abilities (e.g. memory, language, executive function, praxis, perception). Figures 14.1, 14.2, 14.3 and 14.12 describe methods of testing cognition.

Insight

Insight is not an all or nothing attribute. It is often described as good, partial or poor, although really patients lie somewhere on a spectrum and vary over time. The key questions to answer are:

- Does the patient believe they are unwell in any way?
- Do they believe they are mentally unwell?
- Do they think they need treatment? (pharmacological, psychological or both?)
- Do they think they need to be admitted to hospital?

RISK ASSESSMENT

Although it is extremely difficult to make an accurate assessment of risk based on a single assessment, clinicians are expected to, as far as is possible, establish some idea of a patient's risk to:

- *Self*: through self-harm, suicide, self-neglect or exploitation by others. Chapter 6 explains the assessment of suicide risk in detail.
- *Others*: includes violent or sexual crime, stalking and harassment. Chapter 29, page 198, discusses key principles in assessing dangerousness.
- *Children*: includes physical, sexual or emotional abuse as well as neglect or deprivation. Child abuse is discussed in more detail in Chapter 27, page 192.
- *Property*: includes arson and physical destruction of property.

HINTS AND TIPS

Risk assessment is a vital part of psychiatric assessment. Risk to self is one part of this and you may find it helps to also have a heading for 'risk to others'. You should try to get used to using both when presenting to examiners.

PHYSICAL EXAMINATION

The psychiatric examination includes a general physical examination, with special focus on the neurological and endocrine system. Always remember to look for signs relevant to the psychiatric history, e.g. signs of liver disease in patients who abuse alcohol, opthalmoplegia or ataxia in someone withdrawing from alcohol (indicating Wernicke's encephalopathy), signs of self-harm in patients with a personality disorder, signs of intravenous drug use (track marks) in patients who use drugs. Also, examine for side-effects of psychiatric medication (e.g. parkinsonism, tardive dyskinesia, dystonia and hypotension). In an exam situation it may not be possible to complete an examination, but you should always mention that you would do so. Always make a point of mentioning your positive physical findings when summarizing the case.

THE FORMULATION: PRESENTING THE CASE

The 'formulation' is the term psychiatrists use to describe the integrated summary and understanding of a particular patient's problems. It usually includes:

- Description of the patient.
- Differential diagnosis.
- Aetiology.
- Management.
- Prognosis.

Description of the patient

The patient may be described: (1) in detail by recounting all of the information obtained under the various headings in the psychiatric history and mental state examination; or (2) in the form of a case summary. The case summary consists of one or two paragraphs and contains only the salient features of a case, specifically:

- Identifying information.
- Main features of the presenting complaint.
- Relevant background details (e.g. past psychiatric history, positive family history).
- Positive findings in the mental state examination and physical examination.

Figure 1.3 shows a case summary in a case formulation.

HINTS AND TIPS

When presenting your differential diagnosis, remember that two or more psychiatric disorders can coexist (e.g. depression and alcohol abuse). In this event, it is important to ascertain whether the conditions are independent or related (e.g. alcohol abuse that has developed secondary to the depressive symptoms of emptiness and difficulty sleeping).

Differential diagnosis

The differential diagnosis is mentioned in order of decreasing probability. Only mention conditions that you have obtained evidence about in your assessment, as you should be able to provide reasons for and against all the alternatives on your list. Figure 1.3 provides an example of a typical differential diagnosis.

Aetiology

The exact cause of most psychiatric disorders is very often unknown and most cases seem to involve a complex interplay of biological, social and psychological factors. In clinical practice, psychiatrists are especially concerned with the question: 'What factors led to this particular patient presenting with this specific problem at this specific point in time?' That is, what factors predisposed to the problem, what factors

Fig. 1.3   Example of a case formulation (differential diagnosis, aetiology, management)

Differential diagnosis

Diagnosis	Comments
1. Schizophrenia	For: symptoms present for more than 1 month For: ICD-10 and first-rank symptoms of delusions of control or passivity (thought insertion); delusional perception; and third person, running commentary hallucinations For: clear and marked deterioration in social and work functioning
2. Schizoaffective disorder	For: typical symptoms of schizophrenia Against: no prominent mood symptoms
3. Mood disorder: either manic or depressive episode with psychotic features	Against: on mental state examination, mood was mainly suspicious as opposed to lowered or elevated, and appeared secondary to delusional beliefs Against: no other prominent features of mania or depression Against: mood-incongruent delusions and hallucinations
4. Substance-induced psychotic disorder	Against: long duration of symptoms Against: no evidence of illicit substance or alcohol use
5. Psychotic disorder secondary to a medical condition	Against: no signs of medical illness or abnormalities on physical examination

Aetiology

	Biological	Psychological	Social
Predisposing (what made the patient prone to this problem?)	Family history of schizophrenia	–	–
Precipitating (what made this problem start now?)	The peak age of onset for schizophrenia for men is between 18 and 25 years	-	Break-up of relationship Recently started college
Perpetuating (what is maintaining this problem?)	Poor concordance with medication due to lack of insight	High expressed emotion family	Lack of social support

Management

1. Investigations: social, psychological and physical

2. Management plan below

Term	Biological	Psychological	Social
Immediate to short term	Antipsychotic medication, with benzodiazepines if necessary	Establish therapeutic relationship Support for family (carers)	Admission to hospital Allocation of care coordinator (care programme approach) Help with financial, accommodation, social problems
Medium to long term	Review progress in out-patient clinic Consider another antipsychotic then clozapine for non-response Consider depot medication for concordance problems	Relapse prevention work Consider cognitive-behavioural and family therapy	Regular review under care programme approach (CPA) Consider day hospital Vocational training

Prognosis

Assuming Mr PP has a diagnosis of schizophrenia, it is likely his illness will run a chronic course, showing a relapsing and remitting pattern. Being a young man with a high level of education, Mr PP is particularly at risk for suicide, especially following discharge from hospital. Good prognostic factors include a high level of premorbid functioning and the absence of negative symptoms.

precipitated the problem and what factors are perpetuating the problem? Figure 1.3 illustrates an aetiology grid that is very helpful in structuring your answers to these questions in terms of biological, social and psychological factors – the emphasis should be on *considering* all the blocks in the grid, not necessarily on filling them.

Management

Investigations

Investigations are considered part of the management plan and are performed based on findings from the psychiatric assessment. It is useful to divide them into *physical, social* and *psychological* investigations (see p. 54, Chapter 7, for an example). Appropriate investigations relevant to specific conditions are given in the relevant chapters. Familiarize yourself with these, as you should be able to give reasons for any investigation you propose.

Case summary

Mr PP is a 23-year-old, single man in full-time education, who recently agreed to voluntary hospital admission. He presented with a 6-month history of hearing voices and bizarre beliefs that he was being subjected to government experiments. During this time his college attendance had been uncharacteristically poor, he had terminated his part-time work, and he had become increasingly socially withdrawn. He has no history of past psychiatric illness and denies the use of alcohol or illicit substances; however he did mention that his maternal uncle suffers from schizophrenia. On mental state examination he appeared unkempt and behaved suspiciously. He had delusions of persecution, reference and thought control as well as delusional perception. He also described second person command hallucinations and third person, running commentary hallucinations. He appeared to have no insight into his mental illness as he refused to consider that he might be unwell. There were no abnormalities on physical examination.

Specific management plan

It may help to structure your management plan by considering biological, social and psychological aspects of treatment (the *biopsychosocial approach*) in terms of immediate to short-term, and medium to long-term management. See Figure 1.3 for an example of this method.

Prognosis

The prognosis is dependent on two factors:

1. The natural course of the condition, which is based on studies of patient populations; these are discussed for each disorder in the relevant chapters.
2. Individual patient factors (e.g. social support, concordance with treatment, comorbid substance abuse).

See Figure 1.3 for an example.

HINTS AND TIPS

Remember that investigations do not just include physical investigations (e.g. blood tests), but also include social investigations (e.g. obtaining collateral information from the patient's GP or family, obtaining social work reports); and psychological investigations (e.g. psychometric testing, mood rating scales).

CLASSIFICATION IN PSYCHIATRY

There are two main categorical classification systems in psychiatry:

1. ICD-10: the tenth revision of the International Classification of Diseases, Chapter V (F) – Mental and behavioural disorders (published by the World Health Organization). The eleventh revision, ICD-11, is under preparation at the time of writing.
2. DSM-IV: the fourth edition of the Diagnostic and Statistical Manual of Mental Disorders (published by the American Psychiatric Association). The text of the next edition, DSM-V, is under preparation at the time of writing.

Both the ICD-10 and DSM-IV make use of a *categorical classification* system, which refers to the process of dividing mental disorders into discrete entities by means of accurate descriptions of specific categories. In contrast, a *dimensional approach* rejects the idea of separate categories, hypothesizing that mental conditions exist on a continuum that merges into normality.

The ICD-10 categorizes mental disorders according to descriptive statements and diagnostic guidelines. The DSM-IV categorizes mental disorders according to *operational definitions*, which means that mental disorders are defined by a series of precise inclusion and exclusion criteria. Note that the research version of the ICD-10 (Diagnostic criteria for research) also makes use of operational definitions.

In general, both the ICD-10 and the DSM-IV propose a *hierarchical* diagnostic system, whereby disorders higher on the hierarchical ladder tend to be given precedence. As a broad rule, organic and substance-related conditions take precedence over conditions such as schizophrenia and mood disorders, which take precedence over anxiety disorders. This does not mean that patients may not have more than one diagnosis; they may. It means that clinicians should:

- Always consider a medical, or substance-related, cause of psychological symptoms, before any other.
- Remember that certain conditions have symptoms in common. For example, schizophrenia commonly presents with features of depression and anxiety, and depression commonly presents with features of anxiety; in both cases, the treatment of the primary condition results in resolution of the symptoms – a separate diagnosis for every symptom is not needed.

The ICD-10 and the DSM-IV share similar diagnostic categories and are, for the most part, technically compatible. Figure 1.4 summarizes the main diagnostic categories in the ICD-10.

Fig. 1.4 ICD-10 categorical classification		
ICD-10 code*	**ICD-10 categories**	**Examples of included diagnoses**
F0	Organic, including symptomatic, mental disorders	Dementia Delirium Amnesic syndrome Organic mental and personality disorders
F1	Mental and behavioural disorders due to psychoactive substance use	Intoxication and withdrawal states Harmful use Dependence syndrome Psychotic disorder
F2	Schizophrenia, schizotypal and delusional disorders	Schizophrenia Schizotypal disorder Delusional disorder Acute and transient psychotic disorder Schizoaffective disorder
F3	Mood (affective) disorders	Depressive or manic episode Bipolar affective disorder Recurrent depressive disorder Cyclothymia Dysthymia
F4	Neurotic, stress-related and somatoform disorders	Phobias Panic disorder Generalized anxiety disorder Post-traumatic stress disorder Adjustment disorder Dissociative disorders Somatization and hypochondriacal disorder
F5	Behavioural syndromes associated with physiological disturbance and physical factors	Eating disorders Sleep disorders Sexual dysfunction
F6	Disorders of adult personality and behaviour	Personality disorders Gender identity disorders Disorders of sexual preference (paraphilias)
F7	Mental retardation	Mental retardation (intellectual disability)
F8	Disorders of psychological development	Specific developmental disorders Pervasive developmental disorders
F9	Behavioural and emotional disorders with onset usually occurring in childhood and adolescence	Hyperkinetic disorder (attention deficit hyperactivity disorder – ADHD) Conduct disorder Emotional disorders Elective mutism Tic disorders Non-organic enuresis and encopresis
Note that the 'F' refers to the chapter in the ICD-10 on mental and behavioural disorders, that is, Chapter V (or F).		

The DSM-IV uses a multi-axial diagnostic system with five axes. Axes I and II comprise the entire spectrum of mental disorders. Axis I includes all mental disorders except personality disorders and mental retardation, which fall under Axis II. Axis III includes any concurrent physical disorder or medical condition, whether causative of the mental condition or not. Axis IV includes any social or environmental problems that contribute to the mental condition. Axis V consists of a score from 0 to 100, obtained from a global assessment of functioning (GAF) scale.

COMMUNICATION

The term 'neurosis' is no longer used in the DSM-IV, although retained in the ICD-10 as the group heading title for the anxiety disorders: F4 – Neurotic, stress related and somatoform disorders. When first introduced, 'neurosis' was the label given to all 'diseases of the nerves'. However, in modern times, it generally refers to mental disorders:

- That do not have an identified organic or substance-related aetiology
- In which contact with reality is maintained (that is, non-psychotic disorders)
- That are characterized by symptoms within the range of normal experience (e.g. anxiety).

It is best to avoid using this vague term. Instead, use the specific term that accurately describes the condition (e.g. generalized anxiety disorder or obsessive-compulsive disorder).

Pharmacological therapy and electroconvulsive therapy

2

Objectives

After this chapter you should have an understanding of:
- The history, classification, mechanism of action, side-effects, indications and contraindications of:
  - Antidepressants
  - Mood stabilizers
  - Antipsychotics
  - Anxiolytics
  - Electroconvulsive therapy

Psychotropic (mind-altering) medication can be divided into the following groups:

- Antidepressants
- Mood stabilizers
- Antipsychotics
- Anxiolytics and hypnotics
- Other

Despite its simplicity, this arbitrary method of grouping drugs is flawed because many drugs from one class are now used to treat disorders in another class, e.g. antidepressants are first line therapies for many anxiety disorders and some antipsychotics also have mood stabilizing and antidepressant effects.

ANTIDEPRESSANTS

History

Antidepressants were first used in the late 1950s, with the appearance of the tricyclic antidepressant (TCA) imipramine and the monoamine oxidase inhibitor (MAOI) phenelzine. Research into TCAs throughout the 1960s and 1970s developed many more tricyclic agents and related compounds. A major development in the late 1980s was the arrival of the first selective serotonin reuptake inhibitor (SSRI), fluoxetine (Prozac®). There has since been considerable expansion of the SSRI class, and development of antidepressants with other mechanisms such as mirtazapine.

Classification and mechanism of action

At present we classify antidepressants according to their pharmacological actions, as we do not as yet have an adequate explanation as to what exactly makes antidepressants work. Although there are at least eight different classes of antidepressants, their common action is to elevate the levels of one or more monoamine neurotransmitters in the synaptic cleft. Figure 2.1 illustrates the mechanism of action of antidepressants at synapses. The latest research has focused on monoamine neurotransmitter activation of 'second messenger' signal transduction mechanisms. This results in the production of transcription factors that lead to the activation of genes controlling the expression of downstream targets such as 'brain-derived neurotrophic factor' (BDNF). BDNF is neuroprotective and might be one key target of antidepressant action. Figure 2.2 summarizes the classification and pharmacodynamics of the important antidepressants.

> ### HINTS AND TIPS
>
> Certain tricyclic antidepressants (e.g. clomipramine) have more potency for blocking the serotonin reuptake pump; whereas others are more selective for noradrenaline (norepinephrine) (e.g. desipramine, nortriptyline). Most, however, block both noradrenaline (norepinephrine) and serotonin reuptake.

Indications

SSRIs are used in the treatment of:

- Depression – see pages 135–136.
- Anxiety disorders – see pages 149–150.
- Obsessive-compulsive disorder – see pages 149–150.
- Bulimia nervosa (fluoxetine) – see p. 165.

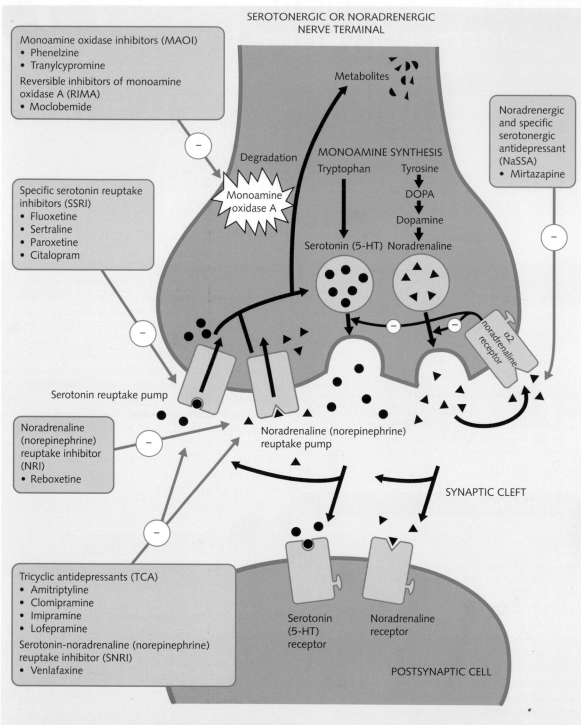

Note: the serotonin and noradrenaline (nerepinephrine) pathways are presented together for convenience; they do not occur in the same nerve terminal

Fig. 2.1 Mechanism of action of antidepressants at the synaptic cleft

Fig. 2.2 Classification and pharmacodynamics of the antidepressants

Class of antidepressant	Examples	Mechanism of action
Tricyclic antidepressant (TCA)	Amitriptyline, lofepramine, clomipramine, imipramine	Presynaptic blockade of both noradrenaline (norepinephrine) and serotonin reuptake pumps (to a lesser extent – dopamine) Also blockade of muscarinic, histaminergic and α-adrenergic receptors
Selective serotonin reuptake inhibitor (SSRI)	Fluoxetine, sertraline, paroxetine, citalopram, fluvoxamine	Selective presynaptic blockade of serotonin reuptake pumps
Serotonin-noradrenaline reuptake inhibitor (SNRI)	Venlafaxine	Presynaptic blockade of both noradrenaline (norepinephrine) and serotonin reuptake pumps (also dopamine in high doses) but with negligible effects on muscarinic, histaminergic or α-adrenergic receptors (in contrast to TCAs)
Monoamine oxidase inhibitor (MAOI)	Phenelzine, tranylcypromine, isocarboxazid	Non-selective and irreversible inhibition of monoamine oxidase A and B
Reversible inhibitor of monoamine oxidase A (RIMA)	Moclobemide	Selective and reversible inhibition of monoamine oxidase A
Noradrenergic and specific serotonergic antidepressant (NaSSA)	Mirtazapine	Presynaptic alpha 2 receptor blockade (results in increased release of noradrenaline (norepinephrine) and serotonin from presynaptic neurons)
Selective noradrenaline reuptake inhibitor (NARI)	Reboxetine	Selective presynaptic blockade of noradrenaline (norepinephrine) reuptake pumps
Serotonin 2A antagonist/serotonin reuptake inhibitor (SARI)	Trazodone	Which action is important in sedative and anxiolytic effect is unclear

Others:
Tetracyclic antidepressants: mianserin
Dopaminergic and noradrenergic antidepressants: bupropion, pramipexole

Mirtazapine is used in the treatment of:

- Depression (particularly where sedation or increased oral intake is desirable).

Tricyclic antidepressants are used in the treatment of:

- Depression – see pages 135–136.
- Anxiety disorders – see pages 149–150.
- Obsessive-compulsive disorder (clomipramine) – see pages 149–150.
- Other: chronic pain, nocturnal enuresis (see p. 191), narcolepsy (see p. 204).

MAOIs are used in the treatment of:

- Depression (especially atypical depression, characterized by hypersomnia, overeating, anxiety) – see pages 135–136.
- Anxiety disorders – see pages 149–150.
- Other: eating disorders, chronic pain, Parkinson's disease, migraine prophylaxis, tuberculosis.

Side-effects and contraindications

SSRIs

SSRIs have fewer anticholinergic effects than the TCAs, and are not sedating. The majority of patients find them alerting, so they are prescribed in the morning. Soon after initiation, or when taken at high doses, some patients can feel alerted to the point of agitation/anxiety. This may be associated with an increased risk of suicide, particularly in adolescents. The only SSRI recommended in under 18s is fluoxetine. Due to their low cardiotoxicity, SSRIs are the antidepressant of choice in patients with cardiac disease and in those who are at risk of taking an overdose. However, they do have their own side-effects that may be unacceptable to some patients. These are summarized in Figure 2.3. Venlafaxine is a selective

Fig. 2.3	Common side-effects of the SSRIs
Gastrointestinal disturbance (nausea, vomiting, diarrhoea, pain) – early*	
Anxiety and agitation – early*	
Loss of appetite and weight loss (sometimes weight gain)	
Insomnia	
Sweating	
Sexual dysfunction (anorgasmia, delayed ejaculation)	

Gastrointestinal and anxiety symptoms occur on initiation of treatment and resolve with time.

Fig. 2.4 Common side-effects of tricyclic antidepressants

Mechanism	Side-effects
Anticholinergic: muscarinic receptor blockade	Dry mouth Constipation Urinary retention Blurred vision
α-Adrenergic receptor blockade	Postural hypotension (dizziness, syncope)
Histaminergic receptor blockade	Weight gain Sedation
Cardiotoxic effects	QT interval prolongation, ST segment elevation, heart block, arrhythmias

serotonin and noradrenaline reuptake inhibitor, which has similar side-effects to SSRIs but they tend to be more severe.

Contraindications: mania.

Mirtazapine

Mirtazapine is very commonly associated with increased appetite, weight gain, and sedation (via histamine antagonism). These side-effects can be used to advantage in many patients. It is also associated with headache and a dry mouth, and less commonly dizziness, postural hypotension, tremor and peripheral oedema. It has negligible anticholinergic effects.

Contraindications: mania.

Tricyclic antidepressants

Figure 2.4 summarizes the common side-effects of the TCAs, most of which are related to the multi-receptor blocking effects of these drugs. The side-effect of sedation can be useful if patients have insomnia. TCAs with prominent sedative effects include amitriptyline and clomipramine. Those with less sedative effects include lofepramine and imipramine. Due to their cardiotoxic effects, TCAs are dangerous in overdose, although lofepramine (a newer TCA) has fewer antimuscarinic effects and so is relatively safer.

Contraindications: recent myocardial infarction, arrhythmias, severe liver disease, mania and high risk of overdose.

Trazodone is molecularly similar to tricyclics but clinically quite different. It is a relatively weak antidepressant but a good sedative. It is relatively safe in overdose and has negligible anticholinergic side-effects. It is often used as an adjunctive antidepressant in those receiving a non-sedative primary antidepressant, e.g. an SSRI.

> **HINTS AND TIPS**
>
> Antidepressants should be used with caution in patients with epilepsy, as they tend to lower the seizure threshold.

MAOIs/RIMA

Due to the risk of serious interactions with certain foods and other drugs, the MAOIs have become second line antidepressants. Their inhibition of monoamine oxidase A results in the accumulation of amine neurotransmitters and impairs the metabolism of some amines found in certain drugs (e.g. decongestants) and foodstuffs (e.g. tyramine). Because MAOIs bind irreversibly to monoamine oxidase A and B, amines may accumulate to dangerously high levels, which may precipitate a life-threatening hypertensive crisis. An example of this occurs when the ingestion of dietary tyramine results in a massive release of noradrenaline (norepinephrine) from endogenous stores. This is termed the 'cheese reaction' because some mature cheeses typically contain high levels of tyramine. Note that an early warning sign is a throbbing headache. Figure 2.5 lists the drugs and foodstuffs that should be avoided in patients taking MAOIs.

The RIMA moclobemide reversibly inhibits monoamine oxidase A. Therefore, the drug will be displaced from the enzyme as amine levels start to increase. So, although there is a small risk of developing a hypertensive crisis if high levels of tyramine are ingested, dietary restrictions are much less onerous.

When other antidepressants that have a strong serotonergic effect (e.g. SSRIs, clomipramine, imipramine)

Fig. 2.5 Drugs and food that may precipitate a hypertensive crisis in combination with MAOIs
Tyramine-rich foods
Cheese – especially mature varieties (e.g. Stilton)
Degraded protein: pickled herring, smoked fish, chicken liver, hung game
Yeast and protein extract: Bovril®, Oxo®, Marmite®
Chianti wine, beer
Broad bean pods
Soya bean extract
Overripe or unfresh food
Drugs
Adrenaline (epinephrine), noradrenaline (norepinephrine)
Amfetamines
Cocaine
Ephedrine, pseudoephedrine, phenylpropanolamine (cough mixtures, decongestants)
L-dopa, dopamine
Local anaesthetics containing adrenaline (epinephrine)

Note: the combination of MAOIs and antidepressants or opiates (especially pethidine) may result in the serotonin syndrome.

HINTS AND TIPS

The abrupt withdrawal of any antidepressant may result in a discontinuation syndrome with symptoms such as gastrointestinal disturbance, agitation, dizziness, headache, tremor and insomnia. SSRIs with short half-lives (e.g. paroxetine, sertraline) and venlafaxine are particular culprits. Therefore, all antidepressants (with the exception of fluoxetine, which has a long half-life and many active metabolites) should be gradually tapered down before being withdrawn completely. Although certain antidepressants may cause a withdrawal syndrome, they do not cause a dependence syndrome or 'addiction' in that patients do not become tolerant to them or crave them.

are administered simultaneously with an MAOI, the risk of developing the potentially lethal 'serotonin syndrome' is increased. In common with the neuroleptic malignant syndrome, it is associated with the triad of neuromuscular abnormalities, altered consciousness level and autonomic instability but the two are usually easily distinguished on the basis of the history (see Fig. 2.11). Therefore, other antidepressants should not be started for 2 weeks after an MAOI has been stopped (3 weeks in the case of clomipramine and imipramine). Conversely, an MAOI should not be started for 2 weeks after the termination of another antidepressant (3 weeks in the case of clomipramine and imipramine; 5 weeks in the case of fluoxetine, because of its long half-life). The coadministration of opiates and an MAOI can also result in the serotonin syndrome. This is because opiates (especially pethidine and tramadol) have some intrinsic serotonin reuptake inhibitory activity.

MAOIs may have further side-effects similar to the TCAs, including postural hypotension and anticholinergic effects.

Contraindications (MAOIs): phaeochromocytoma, cerebrovascular disease, hepatic impairment, mania.

MOOD STABILIZERS

These include lithium and the anticonvulsants valproate, carbamazepine and lamotrigine. Other anticonvulsants, such as gabapentin, topiramate and vigabatrin, are also being investigated for mood stabilizing properties.

History

In 1949, John Cade discovered that lithium salts caused lethargy when injected into animals, and later reported lithium's antimanic properties in humans. Trials in the 1950s and 1960s led to the drug entering mainstream practice in 1970.

Valproate was first recognized as an effective anticonvulsant in 1962. Along with carbamazepine and lamotrigine, it was later shown to be effective in bipolar affective disorder.

Mechanism of action

It is not known how any of the mood stabilizers work. Lithium appears to modulate the neurotransmitter-induced activation of second messenger systems. Valproate and carbamazepine may exert their effect via the GABA system; carbamazepine is a GABA agonist and valproate inhibits GABA transaminase. Lamotrigine reduces neural activation via inhibition of sodium channels.

Indications

Lithium is used in the treatment of:

- Acute mania – see page 137.
- Prophylaxis of bipolar affective disorder (prevention of relapse) – see page 138.

- Treatment-resistant depression (lithium augmentation) – see page 136.
- Other: adjunct to antipsychotics in schizoaffective disorder and schizophrenia; and aggression/impulsivity – see page 144 and page 161.

Valproate is used in the treatment of:

- Epilepsy.
- Acute mania – see page 137.
- Prophylaxis of bipolar of affective disorder (unlicensed indication) – see page 138.

Carbamazepine is used in the treatment of:

- Epilepsy.
- Prophylaxis of bipolar affective disorder (not first line) – see page 138.

Lamotrigine is used in the treatment of:

- Epilepsy.
- Prophylaxis of depressive episodes in bipolar affective disorder – see page 138.

HINTS AND TIPS

Valproate is available in formulations as sodium valproate, valproic acid and semisodium valproate (Depakote®), which comprises equimolar amounts of sodium valproate and valproic acid. Different formulations have different equivalent doses, so prescribe by brand.

Side-effects and contraindications

Lithium

Lithium has a narrow therapeutic window between non-therapeutic and toxic blood levels. Lower levels can be toxic in older patients.

- Therapeutic levels: 0.5–1.0 mmol/L.
- Toxic levels: >1.5 mmol/L.
- Dangerously toxic levels: >2 mmol/L.

Lithium is only taken orally and is excreted almost entirely by the kidneys. Clearance of lithium is decreased with renal impairment (e.g. in older adults, dehydration) and sodium depletion. Certain drugs such as diuretics (especially thiazides), nonsteroidal anti-inflammatory drugs (NSAIDs), and ACE-inhibitors can also increase lithium levels and should ideally be avoided or prescribed with utmost caution. Furthermore, antipsychotics may synergistically increase lithium-induced neurotoxicity; this is important as lithium and antipsychotics are often coadministered in acute mania. Figure 2.6 summarizes the side-effects and signs of toxicity of lithium.

Fig. 2.6 Side-effects and signs of toxicity of lithium	
Side-effects	**Signs of toxicity**
Thirst, polydipsia, polyuria weight gain, oedema Fine tremor Precipitates or worsens skin problems Concentration and memory problems Hypothyroidism Impaired renal function Cardiac: T-wave flattening or inversion Leucocytosis Teratogenicity	**1.5–2 mmol/L:** nausea and vomiting, apathy, coarse tremor, ataxia, muscle weakness **>2 mmol/L:** nystagmus, dysarthria, impaired consciousness, hyperactive tendon reflexes, oliguria, hypotension, convulsions, coma *Note: the treatment of lithium toxicity is supportive, ensuring adequate hydration, renal function and electrolyte balance. Anticonvulsants may be necessary for convulsions and haemodialysis may be indicated in cases of renal failure*

It follows that the following investigations are needed prior to initiating therapy:

- Full blood count.
- Renal function and electrolytes.
- Thyroid function.
- Pregnancy test (in women of childbearing age).
- Electrocardiogram (ECG) (if cardiac risk factors).

Blood levels are monitored weekly after starting treatment until a therapeutic level has been stable for 4 weeks. Lithium blood levels should then be monitored every 3 months; renal function every 6 months; and thyroid function every 12 months.

Contraindications/cautions: pregnancy, breastfeeding (see page 168), impaired renal function, thyroid disease, cardiac conditions, neurological conditions (e.g. Parkinson's or Huntington's disease).

HINTS AND TIPS

Mood stabilizers have potentially serious pharmacokinetic and pharmacodynamic interactions with many other drugs. Therefore, before prescribing new medication for patients on mood stabilizers, check a drug interactions reference (e.g. Appendix 1 in the British National Formulary (BNF)).

Sodium valproate, carbamazepine and lamotrigine

Figure 2.7 summarizes the side-effects of carbamazepine, valproate and lamotrigine. It is important to check liver and haematological functions prior to, and soon after, starting valproate or carbamazepine due to the risk

Fig. 2.7 Side-effects of valproate, carbamazepine and lamotrigine

Valproate	Carbamazepine	Lamotrigine
Increased appetite and weight gain Sedation and dizziness Ankle swelling Hair loss Nausea and vomiting Tremor Haematological abnormalities (prolongation of bleeding time, thrombocytopenia, leucopenia) Raised liver enzymes (liver damage very uncommon)	Nausea and vomiting Skin rashes Blurred or double vision (diplopia) Ataxia, drowsiness, fatigue Hyponatraemia and fluid retention Haematological abnormalities (leucopenia, thrombocytopenia, eosinophilia) Raised liver enzymes (hepatic or cholestatic jaundice rare)	Nausea and vomiting Skin rashes (consider withdrawal) Headache Aggression, irritabiity Sedation and dizziness Tremor
Note: serious blood and liver disorders do occur but are rare	*Note: serious blood and liver disorders do occur but are rare*	*Note: Stevens–Johnson syndrome can occur but it is rare*

of serious blood and hepatic disorders. Lamotrigine can, rarely, be associated with Stevens–Johnson syndrome, particularly in the first 8 weeks. Patients should be advised to stop if there is development of a rash, and reintroduction of lamotrigine at a later date considered only by a specialist.

ANTIPSYCHOTICS

History and classification

Antipsychotics or neuroleptics (originally known as 'major tranquillizers') appeared in the early 1950s with the introduction of the phenothiazine chlorpromazine. A number of antipsychotics with a similar pharmacodynamic action soon followed, e.g. the butyrophenone haloperidol in the 1960s. Their ability to treat psychotic symptoms had a profound impact on psychiatry, accelerating the movement of patients out of asylums and into the community. However, serious motor side-effects (extrapyramidal side-effects (EPSE)), soon became apparent with all these drugs.

Clozapine was the first antipsychotic with fewer EPSE, and thus was termed 'atypical'. It led to the introduction of several other atypical (or 'second generation') antipsychotics, including risperidone, olanzapine and quetiapine. The older antipsychotics such as haloperidol and chlorpromazine became known as the conventional, 'first generation', or 'typical' antipsychotics. However, this distinction is increasingly viewed as artificial – all antipsychotics can induce extrapyramidal motor side-effects if given at high enough doses. Clozapine is the only 'true' atypical antipsychotic in that it has a distinct receptor binding profile and can be effective in two-thirds of the patients for whom other antipsychotics have failed. Figure 2.8 lists common antipsychotics.

Fig. 2.8 Commonly used antipsychotics

First generation	Second generation
Chlorpromazine Haloperidol* Sulpiride Flupentixol (Depixol®)* Zuclopenthixol (Clopixol®)*	Clozapine Olanzapine Quetiapine Risperidone* Amisulpride

*Can be given in long-acting intramuscular injection (depot) form.

Mechanism of action and side-effects

The primary mechanism of action of all antipsychotics, with the possible exception of clozapine, is antagonism of dopamine D_2 receptors in the mesolimbic dopamine pathway. Clozapine is a comparatively weak D_2 antagonist but has a high affinity for serotonin type 2 receptors ($5-HT_2$) and D_4 receptors, among many other receptor targets. Most second generation antipsychotics also block $5-HT_2$ receptors.

Unfortunately, blockade of dopamine D_2 receptors occurs throughout the brain, resulting in diverse side-effects. In addition, antipsychotics also cause side-effects by blocking muscarinic, histaminergic and α-adrenergic receptors (as do TCAs). Figure 2.9 summarizes both the useful and troublesome clinical effects of D_2-receptor antagonism as well as the side-effects caused by the blockage of other receptors. Learn this table well; these effects are often asked for in exams.

The risk of metabolic syndrome (obesity, diabetes, hypertension and dyslipidaemia) is particularly high with clozapine and other second generation antipsychotics. Metabolic syndrome is associated with increased cardiovascular mortality so it is important to monitor and manage the components of this syndrome.

Fig. 2.9 The clinical effects and side-effects of conventional antipsychotics

Dopamine D_2-receptor antagonism		
Location of dopamine D_2 receptors	Function	Clinical effect of dopamine D_2-receptor antagonism
Mesolimbic pathway	Involved in delusions/hallucinations/thought disorder, euphoria and drug dependence	Treatment of psychotic symptoms
Mesocortical pathway	Mediates cognitive and negative symptoms of schizophrenia	Worsening of negative and cognitive symptoms of schizophrenia
Nigrostriatal pathway (basal ganglia/striatum)	Controls motor movement	Extrapyramidal side-effects (see Fig. 2.10): • Parkinsonian symptoms • Acute dystonia • Akathisia • Tardive dyskinesia • Neuroleptic malignant syndrome
Tuberoinfundibular pathway	Controls prolactin secretion – dopamine inhibits prolactin release	Hyperprolactinaemia • Galactorrhoea (breast milk production) • Amenorrhoea and infertility • Sexual dysfunction
Chemoreceptor trigger zone	Controls nausea and vomiting	Anti-emetic effect: some phenothiazines, e.g. prochlorperazine (Stemetil®) are very effective in treating nausea and vomiting
Other side-effects		
Anticholinergic: muscarinic receptor blockade	Dry mouth, constipation, urinary retention, blurred vision	
α-Adrenergic receptor blockade	Postural hypotension (dizziness, syncope)	
Histaminergic receptor blockade	Sedation, weight gain	
Cardiac effects	Prolongation of QT-interval, arrhythmias, myocarditis, sudden death	
Metabolic effects	Increased risk of metabolic syndrome	
Dermatological effects	Photosensitivity, skin rashes (especially chlorpromazine: blue–grey discolouration in the sun)	
Other	Lowering of seizure threshold, hepatotoxicity, cholestatic jaundice, pancytopenia, agranulocytosis	

Clozapine is associated with some rare serious side-effects such as agranulocytosis, myocarditis and cardiomyopathy which mean it is reserved for treatment-resistant cases.

Contraindications/cautions: severely reduced consciousness level (sedating), phaeochromocytoma, Parkinson's disease (can exacerbate), epilepsy (seizure threshold lowered), cardiac disease (can induce arrhythmias – consider baseline ECG) and metabolic syndrome). Clozapine should not be re-prescribed to someone with a history of agranulocytosis.

> **HINTS AND TIPS**
>
> If you can remember the side-effects of tricyclic antidepressants you can remember many of the side-effects of antipsychotics as both are multi-receptor blockers. Both groups are anticholinergic (dry mouth, constipation, blurred vision, urinary retention), anti-adrenergic (postural hypotension) and anti-histaminergic (sedation, weight gain).

> **HINTS AND TIPS**
>
> The extrapyramidal side-effects (EPSE) of parkinsonian motor symptoms and acute dystonia are due to a relative deficiency of dopamine and an excess of acetylcholine induced by dopamine antagonism in the nigrostriatal pathway. This is why anticholinergic drugs are effective treatments.

Figure 2.10 summarizes the antipsychotic-induced extrapyramidal side-effects and treatment. See also Figure 2.11.

Certain antipsychotics are available in a slow-release form, as an intramuscular depot preparation that can be administered every 1–4 weeks, e.g. flupentixol (Depixol®), zuclopenthixol (Clopixol®). They are used for patients who are poorly concordant with oral therapy.

HINTS AND TIPS

Clozapine is a very effective antipsychotic but, due to the life-threatening risk of bone marrow suppression with agranulocytosis (0.8% of patients), is only used in treatment-resistant schizophrenia. Patients should be registered with a clozapine monitoring service and have a full blood count (FBC) prior to starting treatment. This is followed by weekly FBCs for several weeks, followed by monthly FBCs for the duration of treatment. With monitoring, fatalities from agranulocytosis are very rare (less than 1 in 5000 patients on clozapine).

Indications

Psychiatric indications

- Schizophrenia, schizoaffective disorder, delusional disorder – see page 143.
- Depression or mania with psychotic features – see page 136 and page 137.
- Psychotic episodes secondary to a medical condition or psychoactive substance use.
- Delirium – see page 178 (caution in alcohol withdrawal as lowers seizure threshold).
- Behavioural disturbance in dementia – see page 177 (caution as increased risk of cerebrovascular accident).
- Severe agitation, anxiety and violent or impulsive behaviour – see page 145.

Non-psychiatric indications

- Motor tics (Gilles de la Tourette's syndrome) – see page 191.
- Nausea and vomiting, e.g. prochlorperazine.
- Intractable hiccups and pruritus, e.g. chlorpromazine, haloperidol.

Fig. 2.10 Antipsychotic-induced extrapyramidal side-effects and treatment

Extrapyramidal side-effect	Description	Treatment
Parkinsonian motor symptoms	Muscular rigidity, bradykinesia (lack of, or slowing, of movement), resting tremor. Generally occurs within a month of starting antipsychotic	Anticholinergics, e.g. procyclidine (i.v. or i.m. if unable to swallow, oral otherwise). Consider reducing dose of antipsychotic or switching to antipsychotic with fewer extrapyramidal side-effects (e.g. atypical)
Acute dystonia	Involuntary sustained muscular contractions or spasms, e.g. neck (spasmodic torticollis), clenched jaw (trismus), protruding tongue, eyes roll upwards (oculogyric crisis). More common in young men. Usually occurs within 72 hours of treatment	
Akathisia	Subjective feeling of inner restlessness and muscular discomfort. Occurs within 6–60 days	Propranolol or short-term benzodiazepines. Consider reducing dose of antipsychotic or switching to antipsychotic with fewer extrapyramidal side-effects (e.g. atypical)
Tardive dyskinesia	Rhythmic, involuntary movements of head, limbs and trunk, especially chewing, grimacing of mouth and protruding, darting movements of tongue. Develops in up to 20% of patients who receive long-term treatment with conventional antipsychotics	No effective treatment. Withdraw antipsychotic if possible. Clozapine might be helpful. Consider benzodiazepines. Do not give anticholinergics (may worsen tardive dyskinesia)
Neuroleptic malignant syndrome – see Figure 2.11.		

Fig. 2.11 Distinguishing neuroleptic malignant syndrome from serotonin syndrome

	Neuroleptic malignant syndrome	Serotonin syndrome
Defining features	Both conditions characterized by triad of neuromuscular abnormalities, altered consciousness level and autonomic dysfunction (hyperthermia, sweating, tachycardia, unstable blood pressure)	
Neuromuscular abnormalities	Reduced activity: Severe rigidity ('lead pipe'); stiff pharyngeal and thoracic muscles may lead to dysphagia and dyspnoea; bradyreflexia	Increased activity: Myoclonus or clonus, hyperreflexia, tremor, muscular rigidity (less severe than neuroleptic malignant syndrome)
Onset	Insidious	Acute
Medication history	Usually occurs within 4–11 days of initiation or dose increase of dopamine antagonist (any antipsychotic, metoclopramide)	Usually occurs after 1 or 2 doses of new serotenergic medication. Most common cause is concurrent SSRI and MAOI
Typical blood results	Elevated creatinine kinase, white cell count and hepatic transaminases; metabolic acidosis	
General treatment for all patients	Discontinue offending drugs. Cool the patient. Monitor and manage hydration and haemodynamics (e.g. intravenous fluids). Consider ITU for monitoring and/or ventilation. Monitor for complications (e.g. pneumonia, renal failure). Use benzodiazepines for sedation if agitated	
Specific treatment options to consider (depending on severity of illness)	Bromocriptine (to reverse dopamine blockade) Dantrolene (to reduce muscle spasm) ECT	Cyproheptadine (5HT-2A antagonist)
Mortality	20% untreated	Low

ANXIOLYTIC AND HYPNOTIC DRUGS

A hypnotic drug is one that induces sleep. An anxiolytic or sedative drug is one that reduces anxiety. This differentiation is not particularly helpful as anxiolytic drugs can induce sleep when given in higher doses and hypnotics can have a calming effect when given in lower doses, e.g. the benzodiazepines, which are anxiolytic in low doses and hypnotic in high doses. All of these drugs can result in tolerance, dependence and withdrawal symptoms. Furthermore, their effects, when used in combination or with alcohol, are additive. The most important drugs in this group are the benzodiazepines and 'Z drugs" (zopiclone, zolpidem and zaleplon), which have very similar actions and indications.

> **HINTS AND TIPS**
>
> In the past, the antipsychotics have been referred to as the 'major tranquillizers' and the anxiolytics as the 'minor tranquillizers'. This is misleading because: (1) these drugs are not pharmacologically related; (2) the antipsychotics do far more than just tranquillize; and (3) the effect and use of anxiolytics is in no way minor.

History

In the 1960s the benzodiazepines replaced the often abused barbiturates as the drugs of choice for the treatment of anxiety and insomnia. However, this initial enthusiasm was tempered by the observations that they were associated with serious dependence and withdrawal syndromes, and had gained a market as drugs of abuse. Z drugs were introduced in the 1990s and initially thought to be less likely to cause dependence – this is not true. Today, benzodiazepines and Z drugs are recognized as highly effective and relatively safe drugs when prescribed judiciously, for short periods, and with good patient education.

Classification

From a clinical perspective, it is important to classify benzodiazepines and Z drugs according to their strength, their length of action and their routes of administration. Figure 2.12 summarizes these qualities in some common drugs.

Mechanism of action

Benzodiazepines potentiate the action of GABA (γ-aminobutyric acid), the main inhibitory neurotransmitter in the brain. They bind to specific benzodiazepine receptors on the GABA$_A$ receptor complex, which results in an increased affinity of the complex for GABA,

Fig. 2.12 Classification of the benzodiazepines and Z drugs

Drug	Dose equivalent to 5 mg diazepam	Length of action	Half-life	Routes of administration
Benzodiazepines				
Oxazepam	15 mg	Short	8 h	Oral
Temazepam	10 mg	Short	11 h	Oral
Lorazepam	0.5 mg	Short	15 h	Oral, i.m.*, i.v.
Chlordiazepoxide	15 mg	Long	100 h	Oral
Diazepam	5 mg	Long	100 h	Oral, per rectum, i.v. Only i.m. if no alternative
Z drugs				
Zaleplon	5 mg	Very short	1 h	Oral
Zolpidem	5 mg	Short	2 h	Oral
Zopiclone	3.75 mg	Short	5 h	Oral

Note: Lorazepam is the only benzodiazepine that has predictable absorption when given intramuscularly.

and so an increased flow of chloride ions into the cell. This hyperpolarizes the post-synaptic membrane and reduces neuronal excitability. Z drugs act at a different site on the benzodiazepine receptor in the $GABA_A$ receptor complex, also potentiating chloride entry.

Indications of benzodiazepines

- Insomnia, especially short-acting benzodiazepines (short-term use) – see page 203.
- Anxiety disorders – see page 150.
- Alcohol withdrawal, especially chlordiazepoxide – see page 154.
- Akathisia – see Figure 2.10.
- Acute mania or psychosis (sedation) – see page 137, 143 and page 145.
- Other: epilepsy prophylaxis, seizures, muscle spasm (diazepam), anaesthetic premedication.

Indications of Z drugs

- Insomnia (short-term use) – see page 203.

Side-effects of benzodiazepines and Z drugs

- Risk of developing dependence, especially with prolonged use and shorter acting drugs.
- Patients should be warned about the potential dangers of driving or operating machinery due to drowsiness, ataxia and reduced motor coordination.
- Use with great caution in older adults where drowsiness, confusion and ataxia can precipitate falls or delirium.

- Use with caution in patients with chronic respiratory disease (e.g. COPD, sleep apnoea) as they may depress respiration.

HINTS AND TIPS

Benzodiazepines or Z drugs (zopiclone, zolpidem and zaleplon), are seldom fatal in overdose if taken alone, but can be when taken in combination with other sedatives. Flumazenil is an antagonist at the benzodiazepine receptor, and can reverse the effects of both benzodiazepines and Z drugs.

HINTS AND TIPS

Alcohol, opiates, barbiturates, tricyclic antidepressants, antihistamines and other sedatives may all enhance the effects of benzodiazepines and Z drugs; therefore, moderate doses of benzodiazepines in combination with some of these substances can result in respiratory depression.

Other hypnotic and anxiolytic agents

- Buspirone is a $5\text{-}HT_{1A}$ receptor agonist that is used to treat generalized anxiety disorder. It is unrelated to the benzodiazepines, does not have hypnotic, anticonvulsant or muscle relaxant properties, and is not associated with dependence or abuse. Response to treatment may take up to 2 weeks, unlike the benzodiazepines which have an immediate anxiolytic effect.

- Sedating antihistamines (e.g. diphenhydramine (Nytol®)) are available for insomnia without a prescription. Unfortunately, their long duration of action may lead to drowsiness the following day.

OTHER DRUGS USED IN PSYCHIATRY

Alcohol dependence: acamprosate, disulfiram – see page 155.

Opiate dependence: methadone, buprenorphine, lofexidine, naltrexone – see page 157.

Dementia: cholinesterase inhibitors (donepezil, rivastigmine, galantamine), memantine – see page 177.

Psychostimulants: methylphenidate, dexamfetamine – see page 189 and page 204.

Generalized anxiety disorder: pregabalin – see page 150.

ELECTROCONVULSIVE THERAPY

History

The possibility that seizures could improve psychiatric symptoms arose from the observation that convulsions appeared to lead to an improvement of psychotic symptoms in patients with comorbid epilepsy and schizophrenia. This led to seizures being induced pharmacologically with intramuscular camphor in the early 1930s. An electric stimulus was later discovered to be an effective way of inducing seizures, although it proved to be a crude and often dangerous procedure without modern-day anaesthetic induction agents and muscle relaxants. Today, ECT is a safe and often life-saving treatment for patients with serious mental illness. It is the most effective treatment known for severe depression.

Indications

ECT is predominantly used for depression, and can be particularly effective in older adults. Although antidepressants are usually tried first, ECT is considered for the following features of depression:

- Life-threatening poor fluid intake.
- Strong suicidal intent.
- Psychotic features or stupor.
- Antidepressants are ineffective or not tolerated.

Although ECT may precipitate a manic episode in patients with bipolar affective disorder, it is an effective treatment for established mania. ECT is also an effective treatment for certain types of schizophrenia, specifically catatonic states, positive psychotic symptoms and schizoaffective disorder. ECT is also used for puerperal psychosis (see Ch. 24) with prominent mood symptoms or severe postnatal depression where a rapid improvement is necessary to reunite the mother with her baby.

Administration and mechanism of action

ECT is administered 2–3 times per week. Most patients need between 4 and 12 treatments. An anaesthetist administers a short-acting induction agent and muscle relaxant that ensure about 5 minutes of general anaesthesia. During this time, a psychiatrist applies two electrodes to the patient's scalp, in a bilateral or unilateral placement, and delivers an electric current of sufficient charge to effect a generalized seizure of at least 15 seconds in duration.

It is still not clear how ECT works. It causes a release of neurotransmitters as well as hypothalamic and pituitary hormones; it also affects neurotransmitter receptors and second messenger systems, and results in a transient increase in blood–brain barrier permeability.

Side-effects

The mortality rate associated with ECT is the same as that for any minor surgical procedure under general anaesthesia (i.e. around 1 in 100 000). Loss of memory is a common complaint, particularly for events surrounding the ECT. Some patients also report some impairment of autobiographical memory. Unfortunately, studies that examine the long-term effects of ECT are difficult to perform. Memory impairment can be reduced by unilateral electrode placement (as opposed to bilateral).

Minor complaints such as confusion, headache, nausea and muscle pains are experienced by 80% of patients. Anaesthetic complications (e.g. arrhythmias, aspiration) can be reduced by good preoperative assessment. Prolonged seizures may occur, especially in patients who are on drugs that lower the seizure threshold (e.g. antidepressants and antipsychotics). In contrast, benzodiazepines increase the seizure threshold, making it more difficult to induce a seizure of adequate length.

Contraindications

There are no absolute contraindications to ECT. Relative contraindications include:

- Heart disease (recent myocardial infarction, heart failure, ischaemic heart disease).
- Raised intracranial pressure.
- Risk of cerebral bleeding (hypertension, recent stroke).
- Poor anaesthetic risk.

Psychological therapy (3)

Objectives

After this chapter you should have an understanding of:
- What is meant by 'psychological therapy'
- Which professionals deliver it
- The different approaches that may be used
- What approaches can be useful in different circumstances

Psychological therapy describes the interaction between a therapist and a client that aims to impart beneficial changes in the client's thoughts, feelings and behaviours. Psychological therapy, which is often known as 'psychotherapy' or 'talking therapy', may be useful in alleviating specific symptoms (e.g. social phobia), or in helping a client improve their overall sense of well-being.

Members of different professional disciplines, including clinical psychologists, psychiatrists, occupational therapists, mental health nurses, art and drama therapists and counsellors, may all practise psychotherapy, provided they have had adequate training and supervision.

PSYCHOTHERAPEUTIC APPROACHES

There are many different approaches to psychotherapy. Research has shown efficacy for many different types of psychotherapies for many conditions. This has led to the idea that the success of psychotherapy might be due to certain common therapeutic factors as opposed to specific theories or techniques. A comprehensive review of psychotherapy research showed that common factors (occurring in any model of therapy) account for 85% of the therapeutic effect, whereas theoretical orientation only accounts for 15%. Therefore, the use of a modality with which the patient can identify and work may be more important than the theoretical basis of the therapy itself. Common therapeutic factors include client factors (personal strengths, social supports), therapist–client relationship factors (empathy, acceptance, warmth), and the client's expectancy of change.

HINTS AND TIPS

'Self-help' is the umbrella term used to describe the process of self-guided improvement. Often, self-help resources utilize psychological techniques (especially cognitive-behavioural therapy) and educational materials. Self-help may involve books, DVDs, interactive websites and discussion groups (including Internet-based forums). Self-help materials may be provided from, and progress followed and reviewed by, healthcare professionals (known as 'facilitated' or 'guided' self-help), and can be incredibly useful for some people, either in the management of less severe psychological ailments or as an adjunct to other forms of treatment. Group-based peer support is a form of self-help delivered to groups of patients with shared symptoms, during which experiences can be shared and progress reviewed by a facilitator.

HINTS AND TIPS

The single factor most commonly associated with a good therapeutic outcome is the strength of the client–therapist relationship (therapeutic alliance), regardless of the modality of therapy. In some cases, it may be beneficial to use a mixture of modalities (e.g. psychodynamic, interpersonal, and cognitive-behavioural therapy) uniquely tailored to understanding and treating the patient (known as 'eclectic therapy').

Counselling and supportive psychotherapy

Psychotherapy is sometimes distinguished from counselling, although they exist on a continuum; from counselling and supportive psychotherapy (least complex), to psychodynamic psychotherapy and sophisticated cognitive therapy (more complex and requiring more specialist training).

Counselling is usually brief in duration and is recommended for patients with minor mental health or interpersonal difficulties, or for those experiencing stressful life circumstances (e.g. grief counselling for bereavement). Counselling helps patients utilize their own strengths, with the therapist being reflective and empathic. The provision of relevant information and advice is also considered to be counselling, which is undertaken by healthcare professionals of all specialties.

In person-centred counselling, the therapist assumes an empathic and reflective role, allowing patients to discover their own insights using the basic principle that the client ultimately knows best. Problem solving counselling is more directive and focused as patients are actively assisted in finding solutions to their problems. These types of counselling may provide some benefit for patients with mild anxiety and depression; however, they tend not to be as useful for more severe mental disorders.

Psychodynamic psychotherapy

Psychoanalysis and psychodynamic therapy have changed substantially since Sigmund Freud introduced psychoanalytic theory in the late 19th century. Figure 3.1 summarizes some of his ideas regarding personality. The contributions of many other influential theorists (e.g. Melanie Klein, Carl Jung, Alfred Adler, John Bowlby, Donald Winnicott), alongside the introduction of evidence-based practice, has meant the continued evolution of theory and technique. However, the basic assumptions of psychoanalytic theory remain consistent: namely that it is mainly unconscious thoughts, feelings and fantasies that give rise to distressing symptoms, and that these processes are kept unconscious by *defence mechanisms* (which are employed when anxiety-producing aspects of the self threaten to break through to the conscious mind, potentially giving rise to intolerable feelings (Fig. 3.2)).

The essential aim of psychoanalysis or psychodynamic psychotherapy is to facilitate conscious recognition of symptom-causing unconscious processes. It is the therapist's role to identify and interpret these

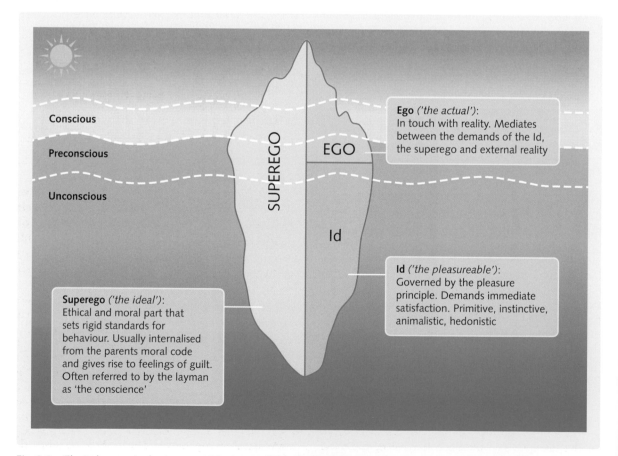

Fig. 3.1 'The iceberg metaphor', summarizing some of Freud's ideas of personality. The Iceberg itself represents the 'structural' model of the mind, while the sea represents the 'topographical model'.

Fig. 3.2   Some examples of psychoanalytic defence mechanisms

Defence mechanism	Type	Description	Example
Denial	Pathological	Failure to acknowledge the existence of an aspect of reality that is obvious to others	A man who was badly assaulted reports that it did not happen
Projection		Attribution of unconscious feelings to others	A man who strongly dislikes his neighbour states that his neighbour hates him
Splitting		Rigid separation of two extremes	A woman is convinced that her boss is an evil man after she was disciplined at work
Fantasy	Immature	Use of imagination to avoid acknowledging a difficult or distressing reality	A schoolboy thinks about killing a bully rather than taking action to stop the bullying
Somatization		The transformation of negative feelings towards others into physical symptoms	A man stuck in an unhappy marriage develops medically unexplained back pain
Repression	Neurotic	Blocking painful memories from consciousness	An adult child has no memory of being beaten by a beloved parent
Reaction-formation		The switching of unacceptable impulses into opposites	A man who hates his job works extra hard, and performs incredibly well
Intellectualization		Concentrating on intellectual aspects to avoid emotional aspects of a difficult situation	A woman diagnosed with terminal cancer develops an intense interest in the classification process of tumour staging
Humour	Mature	Using comedy to avoid provoking discomfort in self or others	A woman laughs and mocks herself after arriving at a formal dinner dressed in a casual clothes
Sublimation		Redirecting energy from unacceptable impulses into socially acceptable activities	An angry man vigorously works out at the gym
Suppression		Consciously avoiding thinking about disturbing problems	A student cleans the kitchen while waiting on exam results

processes (of which patients are unaware), and to facilitate their understanding of unconscious processes in the context of a safe, caring relationship. Historically, various methods have been used (free association; hypnosis; interpretation of dreams and fantasy material; analysis of defence mechanisms – see Fig. 3.2). However, modern psychodynamic psychotherapy mainly relies on the analysis of *transference* and *counter-transference*:

- Transference is the theoretical process by which the patient (inappropriately and unconsciously) transfers feelings or attitudes experienced in an earlier significant relationship onto the therapist (e.g. a male patient becomes angry with his therapist whom he sees as cold and uncaring, unconsciously reminding him of his mother).
- Counter-transference refers to the feelings that are evoked in the *therapist* during the course of therapy. The therapist pays attention to noticing these feelings, as these may be representative of what the patient is feeling, and so help the therapist to empathize with the patient. Often therapists have undergone therapy themselves as part of their training – this helps them to separate out what feelings belong to them, and what feelings to the patient.

Although the terms *psychoanalytic* and *psychodynamic* are often used interchangeably, they differ in the following ways:

- Psychoanalysis describes the therapy where clients see their analyst several times per week for a non-specified period of time. Psychoanalysis is conducted with clients lying on a couch with the analyst sitting behind them out of view. The analyst may be quieter than in psychodynamic therapy, and there is space for the patient to explore what comes into their mind, and for the analyst to help the client understand how they relate to the therapist (the transference) and to others.
- Psychodynamic psychotherapy is based on psychoanalytical theory; however, it tends to be more interactive, occurs once weekly for 50 minutes per session, during which time the patient and therapist

sit face to face. Duration of therapy varies depending on the patient's individual needs, but it can range from 4 months to several years. Psychodynamic psychotherapy may be conducted on an individual basis or in a group setting (p. 29).

Due to the time- and resource-intensive nature (for both the health service and the patient) of classical psychoanalysis, this is very seldom offered within the NHS, with weekly psychodynamic therapy being favoured. However, psychoanalysis is still practised within the private sector.

Mentalization-based therapy is one example of a therapy derived from psychodynamic psychotherapy, and is summarized in Figure 3.6 (p. 31).

COMMUNICATION

Transference and counter-transference are unconscious processes that often occur in settings outside psychodynamic psychotherapy. Patients may inappropriately react to healthcare professionals as if they were some significant figure from the past. An example is when patients express unwarranted anger towards doctors or nurses when they do not receive immediate attention: this may be considered anger that was initially experienced towards neglectful parents. Similarly, health workers may misplace feelings from their own earlier relationships onto patients.

Behaviour therapy

Behaviour therapy is concerned with changing maladaptive behaviour patterns that have arisen through learning (classical or operant conditioning). The premise is that if a patient changes his behaviour to make it more adaptive, this will have positive effects on how they think about things. Figure 3.3 summarizes some of the techniques used in behaviour therapy.

Cognitive-behavioural therapy

Cognitive-behavioural therapy (CBT) is based on the assumption that the way in which individuals think about things (i.e. their cognitions) subsequently determines how they feel and behave. Likewise, physical or psychological feelings can influence the way in which an individual thinks and behaves.

Automatic thoughts involuntarily enter an individual's mind in response to specific situations (e.g. 'He doesn't like me'; 'I'm such an idiot'; 'I'm so boring'). *Dysfunctional assumptions* are the faulty 'rules' that individuals live by that underlie what automatic thoughts occur. When broken (as they inevitably are), the result is normally psychological distress (e.g. 'If I don't come first, then I am completely useless'; 'If I hurt someone, then I am evil'). The rules themselves may be inherently problematic (e.g. 'If I tell people how I feel this means I'm weak'). The patient is often encouraged to keep a diary of automatic thoughts, and from this the patients

Fig. 3.3 Some techniques used in behaviour therapy

Behavioural technique	Clinical uses	Description
Exposure	Phobias and avoidance, post-traumatic stress disorder	**Graded exposure**: a hierarchy of increasingly threatening situations is created (e.g. spider in another room → spider in the same room → spider near the patient → spider on the patient's hand). Patient exposed to (or imagines) the least threatening situation and stays in the situation until their anxiety reduces towards normal levels. When anxiety relief has been achieved, patients are then exposed to increasingly threatening situations. **Flooding**: patient instantly exposed to the highest level of their anxiety hierarchy until their anxiety diminishes, (e.g. throwing patient with a fear of water in the deep end of a swimming pool) (flooding by imagination is termed *implosion therapy*)
Exposure with response prevention	Obsessive-compulsive disorder	Patients are encouraged to resist carrying out compulsions until the urge diminishes. They are then exposed to more severe compulsion-evoking situations
Relaxation	Anxiety	Progressive relaxation of muscle groups; breathing exercises; visualizing relaxing images and situations (*guided imagery*)
Modelling	Phobias and avoidance	Patients observe the therapist being exposed to the phobic stimulus, then attempt the same
Activity scheduling and target setting	Depression	Patients are encouraged to structure their day with certain activities, as reduced activity can lead to further lowering of mood due to reduced stimulation and opportunity for positive experiences

Fig. 3.4 Some examples of types of cognitive distortion

Cognitive distortion	Description	Example
All-or-nothing thinking	Evaluating experiences using extremes such as 'amazing' or 'awful'	'If I don't get this job, I'll never work again'
Mind reading	Assuming a negative response without relevant evidence	'Because she didn't reply to my text message, she hates me'
Personalization	Blaming self for an event	'It's all my fault that the relationship ended'
Over-generalization	Drawing negative conclusions on the basis of one event	'Because I spelt a word wrong in my essay, I'll get a lower grade'
Fortune telling	Assuming knowledge of the future	'Now I've been told off by my boss, he is going to be on my back forever'
Emotional reasoning	Confusing feelings with facts	'I feel so anxious: air travel must be dangerous'
Labelling	Using unhelpful labels to describe self	'I'm so horrible'
Magnification	Blowing things out of proportion	'I forgot to buy milk: my husband is going to be so angry with me'

thinking styles (technically called 'cognitive distortions') can be identified. Some examples are given in Figure 3.4.

The process of therapy draws on the principle that automatic thoughts and dysfunctional assumptions may be challenged (and changed) by *behavioural experiments* (testing dysfunctional thoughts against reality).

Using an example, Figure 3.5 illustrates the relationship between thoughts, feelings, and behaviours; how automatic thoughts and dysfunctional assumptions may affect this relationship; and how challenging these may result in change.

CBT differs from psychodynamic psychotherapy in that: it is time-limited (12–24 sessions); it is goal-oriented and predominantly focuses on present problems (less concerned with the details of how problems developed or unconscious factors); the therapeutic relationship is strongly collaborative (deciding together on the session's agenda and case formulation); it involves patients doing 'homework assignments'. Also, due to its structured format, CBT is more amenable to efficacy studies.

Some other forms of therapy that incorporate elements of CBT are summarized in Figure 3.6.

Interpersonal therapy

Interpersonal therapy (IPT) is based on the assumption that problems with interpersonal relationships and social functioning are significant contributors to the development of mental illness, as well as being a consequence of mental illness (particularly depression). IPT attempts to enable patients to evaluate their social interactions and improve their interpersonal skills in all social roles,

from close family and friendships to community and work-related roles. One of the following areas is chosen as the main focus: (1) role disputes; (2) role transitions; (3) interpersonal deficits; and (4) loss or grief. IPT tends to focus on current problems and is brief in duration (12–16 sessions).

Group therapy

Group therapy may be practised according to different theoretical orientations, from supportive to cognitive-behavioural to psychodynamic approaches. Most groups meet once weekly for an hour and consist of one or two therapists and about 5–10 patients. Therapy can run from months (CBT orientation) to years (psychodynamic orientation). Group therapy allows patients (and therapists) the opportunity to observe and analyse their psychological and behavioural responses to other members of the group in a 'safe' social setting. It is thought that group therapy owes its effectiveness to a number of 'curative factors' (e.g. universality, which describes the process of patients realizing that they are not alone in having particular problems).

Family therapy

Instead of focusing on the individual patient, this form of therapy treats the family as a whole. It may include just parents and siblings or extended family. It is hoped that improved family communication and conflict resolution will result in an improvement in the patient's symptoms. Similarly to group therapy, there are many different orientations, most notably the psychodynamic, structural and systemic approaches.

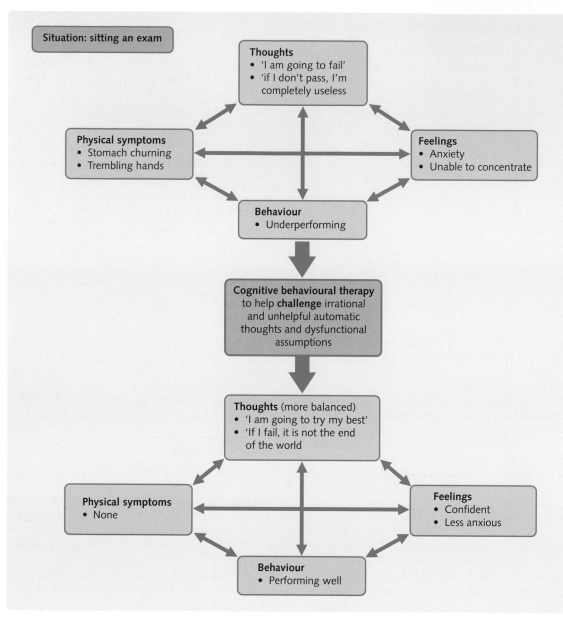

Fig. 3.5   Cognitive-behavioural formulation and the process of therapeutic change

Milieu therapy (therapeutic community)

Therapeutic communities are cohesive residential communities that consist of a group of about 30 patients who are resident for between 9 and 18 months. During this time, residents are encouraged to take responsibility for themselves and others (e.g. by allowing them to be involved in running the unit). They may be useful for patients with personality disorders (especially borderline personality disorder) and behavioural problems.

INDICATIONS FOR PSYCHOTHERAPY

The psychological treatment options for specific conditions have been discussed in each of the relevant chapters in these conditions. The main treatment options with the strongest evidence base, along with relevant cross-references, have been summarized in Figure 3.7. Note, however, that the lack of evidence for certain psychological treatments does not mean that they are not effective.

Fig. 3.6   Some therapies derived from cognitive-behavioural therapy (CBT) and psychodynamic therapy

Therapy type	Description
Dialectical behaviour therapy (DBT)	Uses a combination of cognitive and behavioural therapies, with some relaxation techniques from Zen Buddhism. It involves both individual and group therapy, and can be helpful in reducing self-harming and improving functioning
Eye movement desensitization and reprocessing (EMDR)	At the same time as giving attention to difficult (usually traumatic) memories, the therapist encourages eye movement. This is thought to utilize both sides of the brain, and aid reprocessing of memories
Mentalization-based therapy (MBT)	Developed from psychodynamic therapy, and focuses on allowing patients to better understand what is going on both in their own minds and in the minds of others. It can utilize both individual and group components
Cognitive analytic therapy (CAT)	CAT aims to help the patient understand the problematic roles that they repeatedly find themselves and others in, and the (dysfunctional) ways they cope with this. The aim is to increase the patient's flexibility in ways of relating, and to find 'exits' from dysfunctional patterns. The focus is on helping with present circumstances, while understanding from the past how things have arisen
Mindfulness-based cognitive therapy (MCBT)	Utilizes traditional CBT methods in conjunction with mindfulness and meditation. Mindfulness focuses on becoming aware of thoughts and feelings and accepting them, rather than reacting to them

Fig. 3.7   Main indications for psychological treatments

Psychiatric condition	Main psychological treatment used	Cross-reference
Stressful life events, illnesses, bereavements	Counselling	See Chapter 12
Depression	Cognitive-behavioural therapy Mindfulness-based cognitive therapy Interpersonal therapy Psychodynamic therapy Group therapy	See p. 135
Anxiety disorders	Cognitive-behavioural therapy Mindfulness-based cognitive therapy Exposure and response prevention (for obsessive-compulsive disorder) Systematic desensitization (for phobias)	See p. 148–150
Post-traumatic stress disorder	Cognitive-behavioural therapy Eye movement desensitization and reprocessing	See p. 149
Schizophrenia	Cognitive-behavioural therapy Family therapy	See p. 144–145
Eating disorders	Cognitive-behavioural therapy Cognitive analytic therapy Focused psychodynamic psychotherapy Interpersonal therapy Family therapy	See p. 164–165
Borderline personality disorder	Dialectical behaviour therapy Mentalization-based therapy Psychodynamic therapy Cognitive-behavioural therapy Cognitive analytic therapy Therapeutic communities	See p. 160–162
Alcohol dependence	Cognitive-behavioural therapy Group therapy Motivational interviewing	See p. 155–156

Mental health and the law ④ 4

4

Objectives

After this chapter you should have a basic understanding of:
- The need for mental health legislation
- The Mental Health Acts within the United Kingdom
- Common law
- Capacity and consent to treatment
- Ethical aspects of psychiatry
- The interface between mental health legislation and human rights legislation
- Fitness to drive

In some instances, mental disorders can cause patients to be at risk of self-harm, suicide, self-neglect, exploitation, or may place others at risk. The very nature of mental disorders can affect some patients' ability to make decisions regarding their care and treatment: in these instances, decisions may need to be made without the informed consent or agreement of the patient. Mental health legislation is therefore in place for the purpose of protecting patients and the public.

Differing legal systems within the UK mean that there are differences in mental health legislation across the home nations. This book will focus on mental health legislation applicable in England and Wales.

MENTAL HEALTH ACT 1983 AS AMENDED BY MENTAL HEALTH ACT 2007

In England and Wales, the Mental Health Act 1983 as amended by the Mental Health Act 2007 (MHA) provides a legal framework for the care and treatment of individuals with mental disorders. The MHA is divided into a number of parts, each of which is divided into 'Sections' (groups of paragraphs).

Part I: definitions

The term 'mental disorder' is defined as *any disorder or disability of the mind.* However, the Learning Disability Qualification states that *a person with a learning* disability (intellectual disability) *alone can only be detained for treatment or be made subject to Guardianship if that learning disability* (intellectual disability) *is associated with abnormally aggressive or seriously irresponsible conduct.*

The Appropriate Medical Treatment test stipulates that for longer term powers of compulsion (i.e. longer than 28 days) it is not possible for patients to be compulsorily detained or treated unless 'medical treatment' is available and appropriate. Medical treatment includes not only medication but psychological treatment, nursing and specialist mental health habilitation and rehabilitation.

Certain officials and bodies are designated to carry out specific duties related to implementation of the MHA. Some of these are summarized in Figure 4.1.

> **HINTS AND TIPS**
>
> Note that the Mental Health Act 1983 does not regard dependence on alcohol or drugs alone as evidence of a mental disorder. However, mental disorders which arise secondary to substance intoxication or withdrawal (e.g. delirium tremens, drug induced psychosis) are covered by the MHA.

Part II: civil Sections

Part II of the MHA relates to compulsory assessment and treatment, both in hospital and in the community. Figure 4.2 summarizes the most important Sections in this part.

Normally, the process starts because concerns are raised about an individual's mental health. Following assessment by the appropriate professionals, the patient may be admitted to hospital under Section 2 or 3 of the MHA.

In an emergency, it may not be possible to arrange review for consideration of Section 2 or 3. In these cases, there are various options available, depending on

Fig. 4.1 Mental Health Act (MHA) officials

Official or body	Description
Approved Mental Health Practitioner (AMHP)	A mental health professional (nurse, social worker, occupational therapist, clinical psychologist) with specialist training in mental health assessment and legislation, approved by the local authority. Duties of an AMHP include assessing patients, and (if appropriate) making an application for MHA detention
Section 12 approved doctor	A doctor approved under Section 12 of the MHA as having expertise in the diagnosis and treatment of mental disorder. Section 12 doctors are responsible for the assessment of patients, and to provide a recommendation for MHA detention if appropriate
Approved Clinician (AC) and Responsible Clinician (RC)	A healthcare professional (usually a doctor, but can also be a nurse, social worker, occupational therapist, clinical psychologist) who has received specialist training, and is responsible for the treatment of individuals with mental disorder detained under the MHA. An AC in charge of the care of a specific patient is known as Responsible Clinician (RC) for that patient. Their responsibility is to oversee the care and treatment of a patient detained under the MHA, and to remain responsible for administrative duties of the MHA pertinent to the patient
Second Opinion Approved Doctor (SOAD)	Appointed by the CQC (see below), the role of the SOAD is to provide an independent second medical opinion regarding treatment in patients subject to prolonged compulsory treatment who are unable to consent to their treatment, or when a patient refuses electroconvulsive therapy (ECT) (not applicable in emergency situations, see 'consent to treatment' p. 36)
Nearest Relative (NR)	The spouse, child, parent, sibling, or other relative of a patient detained under the MHA. This sometimes varies from 'next of kin'. It is the duty of the AMHP to appoint the nearest relative, although this decision can be appealed in court. AMHPs have a duty to inform the NR of the application for MHA detention. NRs can – in some instances – apply for the patient to be discharged from compulsory measures
Independent Mental Health Advocates (IMHA)	Advocacy is a process of supporting and enabling people to express their views and concerns, access information and services, defend and promote their rights and responsibilities, and explore choices and options. Most patients detained under the MHA have the right to access an independent mental health advocate
Care Quality Commission (CQC)	An independent health and social care regulatory body which oversees the use of the MHA, and ensures standards are maintained. All NHS and social care providers involved with the care of patients detained under the MHA require to be registered with the CQC
Mental Health Review Tribunal (MHRT)	MHRTs hear appeals against detention under the MHA. Their members include a lawyer, a doctor and a layperson. MHRTs have the authority to discharge patients from compulsory measures when they determine that the conditions for detention are not met
Mental Health Act Managers ('hospital managers')	Represent the hospital responsible for a detained patient. Hospital managers will hear appeals from patients against their detention and review renewals of lengthy detentions. Cases are heard in similar settings to those heard by MHRTs, and Mental Health Act Managers have the authority to discharge patients

circumstances. When any emergency measure is used to detain a patient, this should be reviewed as soon as possible by the appropriate professionals and compulsory measures either revoked, or a Section 2 or 3 granted.

Under Section 135, an Approved Mental Health Practitioner (AMHP) may apply to a magistrate for a warrant, which allows the police to enter private premises in order to remove someone with a possible mental disorder and take them to a 'place of safety' (usually a police station or hospital) for further assessment. Section 136 similarly applies when a police officer has concerns about an individual in a public place; however, the police officer need not apply for a warrant.

Patients admitted to hospital on an involuntary basis are informed of their detention and their rights. They may apply to have their case reviewed by a Mental

Fig. 4.2	Civil Sections enabling compulsory admission			
Section	**Aim**	**Duration**	**Application**	**Recommendation**
Section 2 Admission for assessment	Compulsory detention for assessment. Used when diagnosis and response to treatment are unknown. May be converted to a Section 3 if longer admission needed. Medication may be given as part of the assessment process	28 days	Approved Mental Health Professional (AMHP)	Two doctors (at least one of whom must be Section 12 approved)
Section 3 Admission for treatment	Compulsory detention for treatment. Used when diagnosis and treatment response is established. May be extended	6 months	AMHP	Two doctors (at least one of whom must be Section 12 approved)
Section 4 Emergency admission for assessment	Emergency admission to hospital for assessment when there is no time to wait for Section 2 procedures in the community	72 hours	AMHP	One doctor, with full GMC registration (usually FY2 or above)
Section 5(2) Doctor's holding power	Detention of a hospital in-patient receiving any form of treatment (not necessarily psychiatric) in order to give time to arrange review for a Section 2 or 3	72 hours	–	Doctor responsible for patient's care or other nominated doctor (with full GMC registration (usually FY2 or above))
Section 5(4) Nurse's holding power	Urgent detention of an in-patient receiving treatment for a mental disorder, to allow for review by doctor	6 hours	–	Registered Mental Health Nurse
Section 17 Community Treatment Order	Allows for supervised treatment in the community in patients liable to detention under Section 3: stipulates that patient must attend appointments. May be recalled to hospital if non-concordant with treatment or if they become unwell	6 months	Responsible Clinician (RC)	AMHP and RC
Section 135	Allows for police to enter private premises to remove someone with a suspected or known mental disorder to a place of safety for further assessment	72 hours	AMHP	Magistrate
Section 136	Allows a police officer to remove someone with a suspected or known mental disorder from a public place to a place of safety for further assessment	72 hours	–	Police officer

Health Review Tribunal, or by the Mental Health Act Manager within the hospital, both of whom have the power to remove the detention. Patients may also be discharged from their detention by the Responsible Clinician (RC), or by their nearest relative (unless the right to do this is blocked by the RC).

For patients liable to be detained under Section 3, it may be appropriate to consider the use of a Community Treatment Order (CTO) under Section 17 of the MHA.

This can be useful when treatment in the community is an option (i.e. when the associated risks of the mental disorder do not necessitate ongoing hospital admission). Conditions such as attending appointments may be enforced; however, specific treatment cannot be forcibly given. CTO allows the Responsible Clinician to recall the patient to hospital should the patient become non-concordant with treatment, or should they become unwell.

Part III: forensic Sections

Part III of the MHA incorporates Sections 35–55 and relates to mentally ill patients involved in criminal proceedings or under sentence. Figure 4.3 summarizes the most important sections in this part. It should be noted that patients who are detained under certain forensic Sections, and who are not 'restricted' patients (see Fig. 4.3) can be considered for supervised community treatment (CTO) if appropriate.

Part IV: consent to treatment

This part of the MHA clarifies the extent to which treatments can be imposed on patients subject to compulsory measures. Patients detained under Section 3 or 37 (long-term treatment orders) may be treated with standard psychiatric medication for 3 months with or without their consent. However, after 3 months and in other special cases, an extra Section from a Second Opinion Approved Doctor (SOAD) is required for treatment. These include:

- Psychosurgery and surgical implants of hormones to reduce sex drive. These require the informed consent of a patient with capacity to make such a decision, as well as the approval of a SOAD, under Section 57 of the MHA. Neither of these procedures can be carried out on a patient who lacks capacity to make these decisions.
- Administration of medical treatment in a patient who cannot provide, or refuses to provide, informed consent requires the approval of a SOAD, under Section 58 of the MHA.
- If the patient is 'capable of understanding the nature, purpose and likely effects of the treatment' then electroconvulsive therapy (ECT) cannot be given without his consent. If the patient lacks capacity, then ECT must be certified as 'appropriate' by a SOAD, under Section 58A of the MHA.

Fig. 4.3 Forensic Sections			
Section	**Aim**	**Duration**	**Application**
Section 35 Remand to hospital for report on mental condition	To prepare a report on the mental condition of an individual who is charged with an offence that could lead to imprisonment	28 days, with option to extend to 12 weeks	Crown or Magistrates' Court, on evidence of one doctor, who must be Section 12 approved
Section 36 Remand to hospital for treatment	To treat an individual who is charged with an offence that could lead to imprisonment	28 days, with option to extend to 12 weeks	Crown Court, on evidence of two medical doctors (one of whom must be Section 12 approved)
Section 37 Hospital order	Detention and treatment of an individual convicted of an imprisonable offence (similar to Section 3)	Initially 6 months, with option to extend	Crown or Magistrates' Court, on evidence of two medical doctors (one of whom must be Section 12 approved)
Section 41 Restriction order	Leave and discharge of Section 37 patients may only be granted with approval of the Home Office (recorded as 37/41) – applied to serious persistent offenders	As for Section 37	Crown Court only, on evidence of one medical doctor (who must be Section 12 approved)

In circumstances where urgent treatment is required to save the patient's life or to prevent serious suffering or deterioration, it may be appropriate to use Section 62 to waive the second opinion requirements of Sections 57 and 58 (e.g. emergency ECT for a patient who is not eating or drinking). Section 62 is only used until a second opinion can be obtained.

MENTAL HEALTH (CARE & TREATMENT) (SCOTLAND) ACT 2003

Compulsory measures in Scotland are legislated for by the Mental Health (Care & Treatment) (Scotland) Act 2003. They can be used when a patient is suffering (or thought to be suffering) from a mental disorder (mental illness, intellectual disability, personality disorder), by virtue of which the individual's ability to make decisions about treatment of their mental disorder is significantly impaired, treatment for the mental disorder (including medication, nursing and psychosocial care) is available, and without treatment there would be considerable risk to the health, safety or welfare of the individual, or to the safety of others. Also, the use of compulsory powers must be necessary and lesser restrictive options inappropriate. The use of the Act is overseen by the Mental Welfare Commission for Scotland. Under civil law, the following orders are frequently used:

Emergency Detention Order

An Emergency Detention Order (EDO) allows an individual with a mental disorder (or suspected mental disorder) to be detained in hospital for up to 72 hours, where hospital admission is required urgently for assessment, and when application for a Short Term Detention Order would cause undesirable delay. Any doctor (with full GMC registration) can implement an EDO. Wherever possible, the agreement of a mental health officer (MHO – usually a social worker specially trained in mental health) should also be obtained. Patients may not be treated against their will under an EDO, but emergency treatment is possible under common law. It should be reviewed as soon as practical by an Approved Medical Practitioner (a psychiatrist with special training and approval in the use of the Mental Health (Care & Treatment) (Scotland) Act 2003), and should either be revoked, or converted to a Short Term Detention Order.

Short Term Detention Order

A Short Term Detention Order (STDO) allows an individual with a mental disorder (or suspected mental disorder) to be detained in hospital for up to 28 days. It can only be applied by an Approved Medical Practitioner in agreement with a MHO. Patients may be given treatment for their mental disorder under a STDO. Patients have a right to appeal the STDO at any time, with their appeal being heard at a tribunal. The STDO may either be revoked, or an application for a Compulsory Treatment Order made.

Compulsory Treatment Order

A Compulsory Treatment Order (CTO) usually follows an STDO. An MHO applies to the Mental Health Tribunal for Scotland, asking them to consider granting a CTO. This requires two written medical reports, usually completed by the Responsible Medical Officer (the Approved Medical Practitioner responsible for the care of the patient) and the patient's general practitioner (GP). It also requires a proposed care plan, detailing medical treatment that would be provided if the CTO is granted. The tribunal consists of a lawyer, a doctor and a layperson, who decide whether the application is appropriate, before either granting the CTO, refusing the CTO, or suggesting an interim order while further information is gathered. A CTO lasts for 6 months initially; however, applications can be made to the Mental Health Tribunal to extend this. Patients have the right of appeal. CTOs can be used to treat patients in the community as well as in hospital.

MENTAL HEALTH (NORTHERN IRELAND) ORDER 1986

The Mental Health (Northern Ireland) Order 1986 is similar to the Mental Health Act of England and Wales, although there are some noteworthy differences:

- Unlike other UK mental health legislation, the order defines mental illness: "Mental illness" means 'a state of mind which affects a person's thinking, perceiving, emotion or judgement to the extent that he requires care or medical treatment in his own interests or the interest of other persons.'
- The various paragraphs are referred to as Articles, not Sections.
- The order does not allow for the detention of individuals with personality disorder, although individuals may be detained when a personality disorder coexists with mental illness or severe mental impairment.
- There is only one procedure for admission to hospital: All patients compulsorily admitted to hospital will be held for a period of assessment lasting up to 14 days. Following this, they may be detained under Article 12, which allows detention for treatment for up to 6 months beginning with the date of

admission. The application for assessment is made by the nearest relative or an approved social worker, and is followed by a medical recommendation, usually by the patient's GP. The order stipulates that a patient admitted for assessment should be examined by a consultant psychiatrist within 48 hours after admission, and, if detained under Article 12, examined by a consultant psychiatrist during both the first and second 7 days of the assessment period.

CAPACITY TO CONSENT TO TREATMENT

Mental capacity is defined as the ability of an individual to make their own decisions, and is defined by the Mental Capacity Act 2005 (MCA). An individual (aged 16 years or older) has capacity to make a specific decision if they can:

- Understand information given to them to make a particular decision.
- Retain that information.
- Use or weigh up the information to make the decision.
- Communicate their decision.

If an individual is unable to do one or more of the above, they lack the capacity to make the particular decision in question.

It should be noted that 'capacity' is not a blanket term, and that it should be considered on a decision-by-decision basis. For example, a lady with a moderate intellectual disability may have capacity to decide to buy a CD by her favourite singer; however, at the same time she may lack capacity to make a decision to take out a mortgage to buy a house.

Under the MCA, an individual:

- Must be assumed to have capacity until it is established that they lack capacity.
- Should not be treated as incapable until all practical steps to help them have been taken without success.
- Must not be treated as incapable merely on the basis of wishing to make an unwise decision.

Any act done, or decision made under the MCA:

- Must be in the best interests of the individual.
- Must be undertaken in a manner that is least restrictive to the individual's rights.

The framework used to assess mental capacity in Scotland is the Adults with Incapacity (Scotland) Act 2000. In Northern Ireland, decision making ability is governed by common law.

With regard to medical treatment, clinicians should provide patients with a clear explanation of the nature and likely benefits of a treatment as well as its potential risks and side-effects. An adult who has capacity has the right to refuse treatment, even if this refusal results in death or serious disability. When patients refuse essential treatment, clinicians should ascertain whether they have the capacity to consent to treatment and have made a free decision without coercion.

When making decisions about capacity, you should not hesitate to discuss the case with colleagues, or even a medicolegal defence organization. The process of assessment should be clearly and comprehensively documented in the medical notes.

Advance Decisions

An Advance Decision (or 'living will') is a statement of an individual's wishes regarding the healthcare and medical treatment they would wish to have (or not wish to have), if they were to become incapable of making decisions on these matters in the future. The individual must be over the age of 18, and must have capacity to make the statement. The Advance Decision can become valid when the individual loses capacity to consent to (or refuse) treatment in the future. Advance Decisions are legally enforceable under the MCA in England and Wales.

In Scotland and Northern Ireland, the equivalent of an Advance Decision is called an 'Advance Directive'. These are not considered under mental health legislation, and are not legally enforceable. However, respecting the advance refusal of a competent adult is a requirement of Articles 5 and 8 of the Human Rights Act 1998. The wishes of the individual should be taken into consideration when acting or making a decision on their behalf.

Proxy decision making

A Power of Attorney is a legal document that enables an individual (who has capacity and is over the age of 18) to nominate another person ('Attorney') to make decisions on their behalf in the event that they become incapable of doing so in the future. The decisions allowed to be made may be specified, and may include healthcare, welfare and financial matters. If the individual lacks capacity and has not made a Power of Attorney, it is possible for the courts to appoint these powers to individuals. Laws regarding Power of Attorney vary between England and Wales, Scotland, and Northern Ireland.

COMMUNICATION

- Having a serious mental illness does not preclude a patient from having the capacity to consent to physical treatment, as long as their illness does not interfere with their understanding of relevant information and the decision making process.

- The Mental Health Acts make provision for the compulsory treatment of mental disorders only, not for the compulsory treatment of physical disorders. Therefore, a patient can never be detained under the MHA to treat a physical disorder, and patients are within their rights to refuse physical treatment as long as they are deemed to have capacity. Patients who require urgent physical treatment, but who do not have capacity, may be treated without their consent (but in their best interests) under the Mental Capacity Act 2005.

COMMON LAW

Common law refers to law that is based on previous court decisions (case law), rather than laws made in Parliament (statute law). The Mental Health Act is an example of statutory law, whereas providing immediate life-saving treatment to an unconscious patient (unable to consent) is justified under common law.

Many doctors and nurses who are not familiar with mental health legislation are often concerned about infringing patients' rights, and may not act at all (e.g. a man with a life-threatening alcohol withdrawal delirium is allowed to leave the ward with no one attempting to stop him).

The common law *doctrine of necessity* allows for treatment of physical or mental disorders in adults who are unable to consent in emergency situations. Treatment must be in the best interests of the individual, and must be necessary to sustain life, to prevent serious deterioration or to alleviate severe pain or suffering. The doctrine of necessity is applicable only in emergency situations, and – if necessary – treatment should be continued under statute law (e.g. MHA, MCA) as soon as practically possible.

When considering an action under common law, always ask yourself whether your actions would be defensible in court. Your actions should be consistent with what most individuals with your level of training would do in the same situation. Choosing not to act when you should is indefensible, and would be construed as negligent.

HINTS AND TIPS

It is permissible under common law to restrain and medicate patients who are mentally disordered and who present an imminent danger to themselves or others. However, it is bad practice to repeatedly impose psychiatric medication on informal patients. They should be assessed and treated under the appropriate Section of the Mental Health Act.

HUMAN RIGHTS LEGISLATION

Human rights are commonly understood as 'inalienable fundamental rights to which a person is inherently entitled simply because she or he is a human being'. The Universal Declaration of Human Rights was established in 1948, and subsequently the European Convention on Human Rights (ECHR) in 1953. These are considered to be international law. The UK has introduced its own statute law, the Human Rights Act 1998 (HRA).

There are some fundamental incompatibilities between the Human Rights Act 1998 and mental health legislation. The Mental Health Act 2007 has gone some way to address these; however, it is still important to be aware of some important aspects of human rights legislation.

Article 3 of the ECHR states that 'no one shall be subjected to torture or to inhuman or degrading treatment or punishment'. This is an absolute right, and is always applicable. When a patient is in hospital (whether detained or not), practices that could be considered to be 'inhuman or degrading' may include the use of excessive force during restraint, maintaining high levels of sedation to compensate for staff shortages, a lack of privacy or adequate sanitation, or treatment without consent in cases where it is not medically necessary (under common law or under the MHA). Public authorities have a duty under the HRA to protect the human rights of patients in their care.

Article 8 of the ECHR protects the right to respect for private and family life, home and correspondence. It also sets out, in general terms, circumstances when an interference (also known as a restriction) with this right is acceptable. However, interference must be lawful, necessary and proportionate. Under mental health legislation, seclusion (keeping and supervising a patient alone in a room that may be locked) can occasionally be used; however, if this is not justified as being lawful, necessary and proportionate, it may be a violation of the human rights of the patient.

Article 5 of the ECHR protects the right to liberty; however, it also sets out specific circumstances in which this can be limited. Inappropriate use of the MHA (including undue delays in tribunal or appeal processes) can result in an unlawful restriction of liberty, which may be in violation of Article 5 of the ECHR.

There are also instances when failure to appropriately use mental health legislation may be considered to be in violation of an individual's human rights. Article 2 of the ECHR is an absolute right to life, and professionals or authorities who fail to protect life may be considered to be in violation of the law (e.g. failing to detain a severely depressed and suicidal patient who later completed suicide was considered by the UK Supreme Court to be a violation of Article 2 of the ECHR).

As exemplified, the interface between mental health legislation and human rights legislation is incredibly complex, and beyond the scope of this book to discuss in detail. However, it is important to be mindful of human rights law and these potential difficulties, and to seek advice from an expert if in doubt.

FITNESS TO DRIVE

Both mental illness and psychiatric medication can impair fitness to drive. Clinicians should be aware of the following legal provisions:

- It is the responsibility of the Driver and Vehicle Licensing Authority (DVLA) to make the decision as to whether an individual is fit to continue driving.

- It is the driver's responsibility to inform the DVLA of any condition that may impair his/her driving ability.
- It is the doctor's responsibility to advise patients to inform the DVLA of any condition that may interfere with their driving (e.g. psychotic episode, manic episode, dementia). Doctors may be contacted by the DVLA for further clinical information, or invited to prepare a medical report.
- Doctors may, and indeed have a duty to, breach confidentiality considerations and contact the DVLA medical advisor themselves if patients fail to take this advice and the potential impairment is serious. The same applies to patients who, due to their illness (e.g. dementia, psychosis), are unable, or unlikely, to contact the DVLA.

Mental health service provision 5

Objectives

After this chapter you should have an understanding of:
- The history of mental health services
- The role of:
  - General practitioners
  - Primary care liaison teams
  - Community mental health teams
  - The care programme approach
  - Out-patient clinics
  - Day hospitals
  - Assertive outreach teams
  - Home treatment teams
  - Early intervention in psychosis teams
  - Admission units

HISTORY

Until the 18th century, the mentally ill in the UK received no formal psychiatric care, and those who were not looked after by their families were kept in workhouses and private institutions. In 1845, the Lunatics Act led to the building of an asylum in every county so that those patients with severe mental illness could be cared for in large remote asylum communities. Since the introduction in the 1950s of chlorpromazine, the first effective medication for schizophrenia, there has been a significant decline in the numbers of patients in psychiatric hospitals. The attempts to reduce the cost of in-patient care, and the criticism levelled at asylums regarding the 'institutionalization' of patients and the loss of patient autonomy, led to the closure of the large asylums and the rise of community care. Today, most mentally ill patients are assessed and managed in the community and hospital admission, when indicated, is usually only brief in duration.

PRIMARY CARE

Up to 95% of mental illness is seen and managed exclusively in primary care by general practitioners (GPs), with mild to moderate mood and anxiety disorders and alcohol abuse being the most common conditions. Depression, which is the most common mental illness treated, is frequently associated with symptoms of anxiety as well as physical complaints.

It is important to note that up to half of all mentally ill patients go undetected in primary care. This is because many of these patients present with physical, rather than psychological, symptoms. Also, some patients are reluctant to discuss emotional issues with their doctor, due to feelings of embarrassment or uncertainty about how they will be received.

Some GPs have the option of referring patients with mild symptoms or those going through a life crisis (e.g. bereavement) to a practice counsellor (see p. 25). Practice and district nurses may be helpful in screening for, and educating patients about, mental illness.

Primary care liaison teams exist in many areas. These act as a single point of contact for GPs to refer to. Referrals are allocated to psychiatrists, psychologists, community mental health nurses (CPNs) or occupational therapists as appropriate. This means the GP does not have to work out which professional is best placed to help the patient before referring; the team can discuss this among themselves. Some patients will continue to receive intervention at a primary care level and others will require secondary care. Figure 5.1 lists the common reasons for referral from primary to secondary mental health care.

SECONDARY CARE

Community mental health teams

In the UK, specialist psychiatric care in the community is mostly coordinated by regional community mental health

41

Fig. 5.1 Reasons for referral to secondary mental health services

- Moderate to severe mental illness, e.g. schizophrenia, bipolar affective disorder, severe depressive or anxiety disorders, personality disorder
- Patients who pose a serious risk of harm to self, others or property
- Uncertainty regarding diagnosis
- Poor response to standard treatment, despite adequate dose and compliance
- Specialist treatment required, e.g. psychological therapy, specialist medication regimens

teams (CMHTs), which consist of a multidisciplinary team of psychiatrists, CPNs, social workers, psychologists, occupational therapists and support workers. Team members usually operate from a base which is easily accessible to the community they serve, although local GP surgeries are also used to see patients. Patients who are unable to come to the CMHT member's location are often seen at home.

Care programme approach

The approach taken by the secondary psychiatric services is called the care programme approach (CPA), introduced by the Department of Health in 1991. This approach applies to all patients under specialist psychiatric care and includes community-, hospital- and prison-based patients. The key components of the CPA are:

- The systematic assessment of patients' health and social care needs.
- The formation of an agreed care plan which addresses these identified needs.
- The allocation of a *care coordinator* (previously called 'keyworker') to keep in touch with the patient to monitor and coordinate the care of these needs. This is usually a CPN, social worker or psychiatrist.
- Regular review meetings, which include all relevant professionals, patients and their carers, to adjust the care plan, if necessary.

Patients may be placed on a *standard* or *enhanced* CPA according to the severity of their needs.

HINTS AND TIPS

The diverse and multiple needs of patients with mental health problems make a multidisciplinary approach indispensable in psychiatry. A multidisciplinary team consists of members with medical, psychological, social and occupational therapy expertise.

Out-patient clinics

Psychiatric out-patient clinics take place in CMHT centres, GP surgeries and hospital buildings. Types of clinics include psychiatrist's clinics for new referrals and follow-up patients, and special purpose clinics (e.g. depot injections clinics, clozapine monitoring clinics).

Day hospitals

Day hospitals are non-residential units that patients attend during the day. They are an alternative to in-patient care for patients who, although distressed, are able to go home in the evening and on weekends. Having a supportive family is helpful in this regard. They may also be used for patients who have just been discharged from hospital, but who still need a high level of support, as a form of 'partial hospitalization'. They are now mainly used for older adults.

Assertive outreach teams

These are like CMHTs and involve a multidisciplinary team but provide a more intensive service, providing more flexible and frequent patient contact. They are targeted at challenging patients who have not engaged well with mainstream mental health services in the past. The patients who use this service often have histories of severe and enduring mental illness, significant social problems and complex needs and are at high risk. The nature of their illness requires more focused and intensive input.

Home treatment teams

There is increasing emphasis on treating patients at home, and avoiding expensive and disruptive in-patient admissions. A hospital admission can be very challenging for anyone, particularly someone with an acute mental illness. Treatment at home also allows practical problems with housing and activities of daily living to be better identified and addressed. Most regions now have home treatment teams (also called crisis teams) who can provide short periods of support (a few days to weeks) to people who might otherwise have to be admitted. They can also facilitate earlier discharge than would otherwise be possible. Such teams include similar professionals to a CMHT but generally are available out of hours and can visit patients more often (e.g. multiple times per day, if required). Medication, practical help and psychological therapy can be offered.

Early intervention in psychosis teams

There is some evidence that the longer a psychotic episode goes untreated, the poorer the prognosis, suggesting that early treatment is preferable. However, not all mild or vague symptoms of possible psychosis go on to become a definite psychotic episode, meaning it can be hard to know when to start treatment (e.g. a person who is suspicious of others, but not holding a certain belief of persecution). Specialist teams exist in many regions to manage such cases, offering assessment, medication, psychological strategies and education for patients and families. Teams are open to psychosis secondary to any diagnosis (e.g. schizophrenia, bipolar disorder, substance-induced) and generally accept people aged 14–35 years.

In-patient units

Occasionally, community care is not possible and hospital admission is necessary. Reasons for admission include the following:

- To provide a safe environment when there is: (1) high risk of harm to self or others, or (2) grossly disturbed behaviour.
- A period of in-patient assessment is needed (e.g. of response to treatment or when the diagnosis is uncertain).
- It is necessary to institute treatment in hospital (e.g. electroconvulsive therapy, clozapine therapy – although both of these can be initiated as out-patients if the patient is at low risk of complications).

There are various types of in-patient units. These range from a general adult acute ward for uncomplicated admissions to psychiatric intensive care units (PICUs) for severely disturbed patients who cannot be adequately contained on an open ward. High security units (also called 'special hospitals', e.g. Broadmoor, Rampton) are for mentally ill offenders who pose a grave risk to others.

Rehabilitation units

These units aim to reintegrate patients whose social and living skills have been severely handicapped by the effects of severe mental illness and institutionalization into the community. Admissions are often for months to years. The approach taken is holistic, and uses the 'Recovery Model', i.e. learning to live well with ongoing symptoms, rather than aim for complete remission of symptoms.

Accommodation

Certain patients, who are unable to live independently due to severe and enduring mental illness, may need *supported accommodation*. Types of supported accommodation range from warden-controlled property to homes with trained staff on hand 24 hours a day.

The patient with thoughts of suicide or self-harm

6

● **Objectives**

After this chapter you should have an understanding of:
- The definitions of self-harm, suicide and attempted suicide
- The risk factors that must always be assessed
- The importance of exploring alcohol and substance misuse in the suicidal patient

Case summary

The duty psychiatrist is asked for his opinion on Mr SA, a 28-year-old unemployed, recently divorced man, who was brought in by his landlord. The landlord had called round on the off-chance to discuss payment arrears, only to find the door unlocked and Mr SA asleep on his bed with an empty box of paracetamol tablets and several empty cans of lager littered around the floor. He also found a hastily scribbled suicide note on the bedside table, addressed to Mr SA's children. Mr SA was easily roused but was upset to have been found and initially refused the landlord's persistent pleas that they should go along to the hospital. Only when he was violently sick did he finally agree.

The doctor in the accident and emergency (A&E) department reports that, other than the smell of alcohol on his breath, Mr SA's medical examination was normal. Blood tests revealed raised paracetamol levels, but these were not sufficiently high to require medical admission. The A&E doctor is concerned because Mr SA is ambivalent about further acts of self-harm or suicide, saying that his 'life is a failure' and that 'there is nothing worth living for'. Before coming to see the patient, the duty psychiatrist proceeds to ask the A&E doctor some routine questions.

(For a discussion of the case study see the end of the chapter)

While many psychiatric illnesses can be associated with self-harm or suicidal intent (both as a presenting feature and a chronic symptom), many patients who self-harm or attempt suicide are not previously known to mental health services. Assessments of these patients are often made by non-psychiatric staff and so it is vital that primary care clinicians are, firstly, able to detect and manage any underlying mental illness and, secondly, have a sound approach to assessing and managing risk.

DEFINITIONS AND CLINICAL FEATURES

Self-harm is a blanket term used to describe any intentional act done with the knowledge that it is potentially harmful. It can take the form of self-poisoning (overdosing) or self-injury (cutting, burning, hitting). The motives for self-harm are vast and include emotional relief, self-punishment, attention seeking, and can even be a form of self-help (albeit maladaptive) by way of channelling an intolerable emotional experience into a discrete physical sensation. *Suicide* is the act of intentionally and successfully ending one's own life. *Attempted suicide* refers to an unsuccessful suicide bid.

> **HINTS AND TIPS**
>
> Self-harm is one of the top five reasons for acute medical admissions for both men and women in the UK. In addition, it is estimated that a large number of people do not attend hospital following self-harm.

ASSESSMENT OF PATIENTS WHO HAVE INFLICTED HARM UPON THEMSELVES

Patients who present with self-harm have a 100-fold greater chance of completing suicide in the following year in comparison to the general population, emphasizing the need for comprehensive risk assessment. It is incredibly difficult reliably to predict suicide, but numerous

---

Fig. 6.1   Risk factors for suicide

Epidemiological factors:
Male of any age (although younger females more likely to self-harm)
Being lesbian, gay, bisexual, or transgender (particularly younger people)
Prisoners (especially remand)
Being unmarried (single, widowed, divorced)
Unemployment
Working in certain occupations (farmer, vet, nurse, doctor)
Low socioeconomic status
Living alone, social isolation

Clinical factors:
Psychiatric illness or personality disorder (see Fig. 6.2)
Previous self-harm
Alcohol dependence
Physical illness (especially debilitating, chronically painful, or terminal conditions)
Family history of depression, alcohol dependence or suicide
Recent adverse life-events (especially bereavement)

---

studies have shown that certain epidemiological and clinical variables are more prevalent among those who have completed suicide (Fig. 6.1) and it is important to bear these in mind when assessing risk. No patient questionnaire or suicide risk scoring system has been shown to be better than thorough clinical assessment.

The key areas to assess are:

1. Suicide risk factors.
2. Suicidal intent (including circumstances surrounding the act).
3. Mental state examination.
4. Current social support.

HINTS AND TIPS

Suicide remains the most common cause of death for men and women under the age of 35 years.

COMMUNICATION

Suicidal patients often feel distressed and guilty. One of the most important therapeutic aspects of the assessment is to convey empathy and optimism.

Suicide risk factors

Figure 6.1 summarizes the most important epidemiological and clinical risk factors for suicide.

46

HINTS AND TIPS

One way to remember to ask for suicide risk factors is to learn them as a list, and screen for them fairly early in the assessment.

Psychiatric illness

About 90% of patients who commit suicide have a diagnosed or retrospectively diagnosable mental disorder. However, only around a quarter have contact with mental health services in the year before completing suicide. Patients recently discharged from in-patient psychiatric care are at an elevated risk of suicide, particularly for the first couple of weeks. Figure 6.2 summarizes the most important psychiatric conditions associated with suicide.

COMMUNICATION

Every patient with suicidal ideas, no matter how unlikely it seems, should be asked about alcohol or substance misuse. Taking a non-judgemental stance is likely to enhance the therapeutic relationship, and help the patient feel understood.

Physical illness

Many disabling or unpleasant medical conditions can be associated with self-harm and suicide. Often, a patient may have comorbid depression that will respond to treatment. However, a minority have no mental illness and make a 'rational' decision to die. The most common examples are:

- Chronic and painful illnesses.
- Central nervous system diseases (e.g. epilepsy, multiple sclerosis, Huntington's disease).
- Cancer (especially of the genitals or breast).
- Endocrine and metabolic conditions (e.g. Cushing's disease, porphyria).

Recent adverse life events

Stressful life events are more common in the 6 months prior to a suicide attempt, and include relationship break-ups, health problems, legal/financial difficulties, or problems at home or within the family.

Suicidal intent

Suicidal intent, which is commonly defined as the seriousness or intensity of the wish of a patient to terminate his or her life, is suggested by the following:

Fig. 6.2 Association between psychiatric disorders and suicide

Psychiatric disorder	Comments
Unipolar depression	20-fold increase in risk compared to general population. Risk greatest in patients with anxiety/agitation or severe insomnia, and higher in patients having received in-patient treatment in the past
Bipolar affective disorder	15-fold increase compared to general population. One in three sufferers either attempt or complete suicide. More common in depressive phase, but can also happen in manic or mixed affective episodes
Schizophrenia	8.5-fold increase in risk compared to general population. Highest risk is young, intelligent, unemployed males with good insight and recurrent illness
Alcohol dependence	Lifetime risk 3–4%. Highest amongst elderly males, poor work record, social isolation, previous self-harm
Personality disorders	Highest in borderline personality disorder: 10% will die by suicide. Also strong association with antisocial and narcissistic personality disorders. Often have comorbid depression or substance misuse
Eating disorders	Anorexia nervosa is the mental illness with strongest association with suicide (increases risk over 30-fold compared to general population). Risk increased 7.5-fold in bulimia nervosa

The attempt was planned in advance

A lethal suicide attempt typically involves days or weeks of planning. It is rarely an impulsive, spur-of-the-moment idea (the exception is the psychotic patient who impulsively responds to hallucinations or delusions). Planning is strongly suggested by the evidence of final acts. These include the making of a will or the leaving of a suicide note.

Precautions were taken to avoid discovery or rescue

For example, a patient might check into a hotel room in a distant town or ensure that no friends or family will be visiting over the ensuing hours or days.

A dangerous method was used

Violent methods (hanging, jumping from heights, firearm use) are suggestive of lethal intent. That said, use of an apparently ineffective method (e.g. taking six paracetamol tablets) might reflect lack of knowledge of the lethal dose needed, rather than a lack of intent to die. Therefore, it should be ascertained whether the method used was seen as dangerous from the patient's perspective.

No help was sought after the act

Patients who immediately regret their action and seek help are probably less at risk than those who do not seek help and wait to die.

Mental state examination

This should ideally be conducted in a calm, quiet and confidential setting, preferably when the patient has had a chance to rest and is not under the influence of drugs or alcohol. Check specifically for:

- **Current mood state:** does the patient appear to be suffering from a depressive illness? Assess for features of hopelessness, worthlessness or agitation (all of which are associated with a higher risk of completed suicide).
- **Other psychiatric illness:** does the patient appear preoccupied, delusional or responding to hallucinations? Is there evidence of eating disorder, substance abuse or cognitive impairment?
- **Current suicidality:** is the act now regretted, or is there strong intent to die? What does the patient plan to do if discharged?
- **Protective factors:** what aspects of the patient's life (family, children and dependents) would guard against further acts? Lack of protective factors, or dismissal of their importance, is a worrying sign.

The following questions might be helpful when asking about suicidal ideation:

- Have you been feeling that life isn't worth living?
- Do you sometimes feel like you would like to end it all?
- Have you given some thought as to how you might do it?
- How close are you to going through with your plans?
- Is there anything that might stop you from attempting suicide?

PATIENT MANAGEMENT FOLLOWING SELF-HARM OR ATTEMPTED SUICIDE

Management planning should follow assessment of risk factors and mental state. It is important to remember that self-harm and suicidality are not discrete illnesses, and are instead symptoms reflecting a complex interplay of mental disorders, personality types and social circumstances. Rather than taking the form of a prescribed care pathway, management of the suicidal or self-harming patient requires clinical judgement, taking into consideration the needs of the individual patient and the availability of local resources. This can often be anxiety provoking for healthcare workers.

Formulation of a management plan should be made after a thorough review of any available past history, including care programmes or crisis plans. It is always desirable to obtain a collateral history from a family member or close friend. A good plan should include both short- and long-term management strategies.

Immediate management considerations include the following:

- Is the patient in need of in-patient psychiatric care to preserve their safety? If so, can this be achieved on a voluntary basis, or is the use of mental health legislation required?
- Would the patient benefit from the input of home treatment, outreach, or crisis teams (see Ch. 5)?
- Does the patient have existing social supports that could be called upon?
- Reducing access to means of self-harm: does the patient have a collection of tablets or rope remaining in their home they could dispose of? Should they be placed on weekly dispensing of prescription medication?

Longer term management involves the modification of factors that could increase the risk of further acts of self-harm or suicidality, and may include:

- Treatment of psychiatric illness (medication, self-help, psychological therapies, community mental health team, addiction services, out-patient appointments, GP follow-up).
- Optimizing social functioning (social work, Citizens Advice Bureau, community groups and activities, encouragement of family support, voluntary support agencies).
- Crisis planning (relaxation or distraction techniques, telephone counselling services, information on accessing emergency psychiatric services).

DISCUSSION OF CASE STUDY

Self-harm risk assessment

Mr SA's epidemiological risk factors are that he is a young man, recently divorced, unemployed and apparently lives alone in social isolation. His clinical risk factors are that he may have alcohol problems and has recently experienced adverse life events (divorce, financial difficulties). The evidence of final acts (suicide note) and the failure of Mr SA to seek help after the act suggest strong suicide intent. The fact that he would not have been discovered but for the landlord's timely arrival indicates a degree of forward planning, although his leaving of the door unlocked and his willingness to go to hospital after vomiting suggests some ambivalence. Mr SA had clearly consumed a significant quantity of alcohol at the time of the overdose, which could have clouded his judgement and given him courage which he otherwise might have lacked. On mental state examination, Mr SA has ongoing suicidal ideation and cognitive features of worthlessness and hopelessness, which are known to be associated with suicide.

Further management

The duty psychiatrist should ask about all the epidemiological and clinical risk factors, specifically about: past or current mental illness (is Mr SA known to the mental health services?); previous episodes of self-harm; alcohol or substance dependence; physical illness; family history of depression, alcohol dependence or suicide; and recent adverse life events. The duty psychiatrist will also be interested in Mr SA's current social support in order to try and help him formulate the most appropriate management plan.

As this is a complex risk assessment, the duty psychiatrist will probably have to reassess the patient himself, especially as regards detecting mental illness on mental state examination. The psychiatrist might ask the A&E doctor to keep Mr SA overnight, so that a mental state examination can be performed in the morning when he is refreshed and no longer under the influence of alcohol. A hospital admission or follow-up by a community mental health team seems to be the most likely outcome.

Now go on to Chapter 18 and Chapter 22 to read about affective and personality disorders and their management.

After this chapter you should have an understanding of:
- The definition of a depressive disorder and how this differs from sadness
- The mood symptoms of a depressive disorder
- How depressive disorders can also present with cognitive and psychotic symptoms
- The differential diagnosis of a depressive disorder
- The fact that suicidality always has to be assessed in the depressed patient
- How to assess someone complaining of depression

Case summary

Mrs LM, a 32-year-old married housewife with two children aged 4 and 6 years, presented to her family doctor stating that she was persistently unhappy and had been crying repeatedly over the past few weeks. She had no previous psychiatric history or significant medical history and her only regular medication was oral contraception. She had moved to the area 3 years earlier when her husband was promoted and, at first, appeared to have integrated well into the neighbourhood by involving herself in the organization of a toddlers' group. Unfortunately, the group had dissolved a few months ago when her co-organizer and only close confidante had moved away. Deprived of her most important social outlet, Mrs LM found herself increasingly dominated by her young children. Although usually an outgoing person, she noticed that her motivation to keep in touch with other mothers from the group had started to dwindle. At the same time, she started feeling persistently weary even though her work schedule had not increased, and often awakened 2–3 hours earlier in the morning. Although her appetite had not increased, she had turned to food for 'comfort' and had gained over 14 lb in weight. Mrs LM also candidly admitted that she was drinking more alcohol than usual. She described feeling incompetent because she was always miserable and had become too tired to look after the children. She felt guilty for burdening her husband and started crying when talking about her loss of interest in sex and her feelings of unattractiveness. Mrs LM maintained that no aspect of her life gave her pleasure and when asked specifically by her doctor, admitted that she had started to wonder whether her children and husband would be better off without her.

(For a discussion of the case study see the end of the chapter)

Feeling sad or upset is a normal part of the human condition; thus, a patient presenting with emotional suffering does not necessarily warrant a psychiatric diagnosis or require treatment. However, psychiatrists agree that when patients present with a certain number of key depressive features, they are probably suffering from some form of psychopathology that will require, and usually respond to, specific kinds of treatment.

DEFINITIONS AND CLINICAL FEATURES

Core symptoms

Whereas feelings describe a short-lived emotional experience, mood refers to a patient's sustained, subjectively experienced emotional state over a period of time. Patients may describe a depressed mood in a number of ways, such as feeling sad, dejected, despondent, 'down in the dumps', miserable, 'low in spirits' or 'heavy-hearted'. They are unable to just lift themselves out of this mood and its severity is often out of proportion to the stressors in their surrounding social environment.

The term 'affect' has two uses in psychiatry. It can be used synonymously with mood or emotion, as in the affective (mood) disorders. However, it is most often used to describe the transient natural fluctuations of emotional state that occur from moment to moment. For example, you might notice a patient is tearful when discussing the death of their mother but smiles when discussing their holiday plans. The range and appropriateness of a patient's affect is documented as part of the mental state exam. People with depression may have a reduced range of affect, with a monotonous voice and minimal facial expression (see Ch. 1).

The ICD-10 classification system specifies three core symptoms of depression:

- Depressed mood, which varies little from day to day and is unresponsive to circumstances (although diurnal variation may be present, with mood worse in the mornings).
- Markedly reduced interest in almost all activities, associated with the loss of ability to derive pleasure from activities that were formerly enjoyed (partial or complete anhedonia).
- Lack of energy or increased fatigability on minimal exertion leading to diminished activity (anergia).

It is useful to consider the other symptoms associated with depressed mood under the subheadings biological, cognitive and psychotic symptoms.

Biological (somatic) symptoms

In the past psychiatrists used to distinguish between 'endogenous' or 'reactive' depression. 'Endogenous' depression (also called somatic, melancholic, vital or biological depression) was assumed to occur in the absence of an external environmental cause and have a 'biological' clinical picture. This is opposed to so-called 'reactive' or 'neurotic' depression where it is assumed that the patient is, to some degree, understandably depressed, reacting to adverse psychosocial circumstances. However, most depression is a mixture of the two, and an 'understandable depression' does not require any less treatment than a 'spontaneous depression'. 'Biological' symptoms are still important to enquire about as if present they suggest a more severe depression; however, they are no longer viewed as providing information on aetiology.

Early morning wakening

Although patients may get to off to sleep at their normal time, they wake at least 2 hours earlier than they would usually, and then find it impossible to get back to sleep again. Further disturbances of sleep in depression include: difficulty falling asleep (initial insomnia), frequent awakening during the night and excessive sleeping (hypersomnia). Although all of these contribute to the diagnosis of depression, only early morning wakening is a biological symptom.

Depression worse in the morning

Diurnal variation of mood means that a patient's abnormal mood is more pronounced at a specific time of day. A depressive mood consistently and specifically worse in the morning is an important biological symptom.

Marked loss of appetite with weight loss

Although some depressed patients have an increased appetite and turn to 'comfort eating', only a dramatic reduction in appetite with weight loss (5% of body weight in last month) is regarded as a biological symptom. Note that the reversed biological features of overeating and oversleeping are sometimes referred to as atypical depressive symptoms.

Psychomotor retardation or agitation

The term 'psychomotor' is used to describe a patient's motor activity as a consequence of their concurrent mental processes. Psychomotor changes in depression can include retardation (slow, monotonous speech, long pauses before answering questions, or muteness; leaden body movements and limited facial expression, i.e. blunted affect) or conversely agitation (inability to sit still; fidgeting, pacing or hand-wringing; rubbing or scratching skin or clothes). Note that psychomotor changes must be severe enough to be observable by others, not just the subjective experience of the patient.

Loss of libido

Sensitive questioning will often reveal a reduction in sex drive that may lead to guilt when the sufferer feels unable to satisfy their partner.

Cognitive symptoms

Cognition has two meanings in psychiatry: it refers broadly to brain processing functions (e.g. concentrating, learning, making decisions) and also more specifically to the thoughts patients have about themselves and the world, which are conclusions arrived at by cognition, e.g. I failed my maths exam, therefore I will fail all exams (see p. 28).

Reduced concentration and memory

Depressed patients report difficulty in sustaining attention while doing previously manageable tasks. They often appear easily distracted and may complain of memory difficulties.

> **COMMUNICATION**
>
> Questions about concentration can include asking if they can follow their favourite TV programme or read a novel.

Poor self-esteem

Self-esteem includes the interrelated concepts of personal efficacy and personal worth. Depressed patients may have thoughts that they are no longer competent to meet life's challenges and that they are no longer worthy of happiness and the healthy assertion of their needs.

Guilt

Depressed patients often have guilty preoccupations about minor past failings. This guilt is often inappropriate and out of proportion to the original 'offence'. Patients often have guilty thoughts about the very act of developing the depressed mood itself.

Hopelessness

Depressed patients can have bleak and pessimistic views of the future, believing that there is no way out of their current situation.

Suicide or self-harm

Depressed patients frequently have thoughts of death and harming themselves. In severe cases suicidal ideation may lead to an actual suicide attempt. At these times, patients may believe that they are faced with insurmountable difficulties or are trying to escape a relentlessly painful emotional state. Self-harm and suicide are discussed fully in Chapter 6.

> **COMMUNICATION**
>
> Risk needs to be assessed in every patient. During an assessment, the subject can be broached by saying that it is common for people who are depressed to feel that life is not worth living, and asking the patient if this has occurred to them. Suicidality can then be formally assessed as discussed in Chapter 6.

Psychotic symptoms

In severe depressive episodes, patients may suffer from delusions, hallucinations or a depressive stupor; these are termed psychotic symptoms (see Ch. 9). Delusions and hallucinations can be classified as 'mood congruent' or 'mood incongruent', which describes whether the content of the psychotic symptoms is consistent with the patient's mood. Delusions and hallucinations in depression are generally mood congruent and so may involve an irrational conviction of guilt or sin or the belief that parts of the body are dead or wasting away. Hallucinations may take the form of accusatory or defamatory voices criticizing the patient in the second person (auditory hallucination) or the smell of rotting flesh (olfactory hallucination).

In severe episodes, psychomotor retardation may progress to the point of unresponsiveness, lack of voluntary movement (akinesis) and near or total mutism. Severe motor symptoms are probably more common in schizophrenia and bipolar affective disorder, but they can and do occur in unipolar depression (see page 71).

DIFFERENTIAL DIAGNOSIS

Careful history taking and examination should reveal whether the patient presenting with low mood is suffering from a primary mood disorder, or whether their depression is secondary to a medical condition, psychoactive substance or other psychiatric condition. Figure 7.1 presents the differential diagnosis. An algorithm for the diagnosis of mood disorders is presented on page 62.

Differential diagnosis of low mood
Mood disorders • Depressive episode • Recurrent depressive disorder • Dysthymia • Bipolar affective disorder • Cyclothymia Schizoaffective disorder Secondary to a general medical condition Secondary to psychoactive substance use (including alcohol) Secondary to other psychiatric disorders • Psychotic disorders • Anxiety disorders • Adjustment disorder (including bereavement) • Eating disorders • Personality disorders • Dementia

Fig. 7.1 Differential diagnosis for the patient presenting with low mood

Fig. 7.2 ICD-10 criteria for a depressive episode

Depressive episode
Symptoms should be present for at least 2 weeks *At least two of the following core symptoms*: • Depressed mood • Loss of interest and enjoyment • Reduced energy or increased fatigability
AND ... *At least two of the following*: • Reduced concentration and attention • Reduced self-esteem and self-confidence • Ideas of guilt and unworthiness • Bleak and pessimistic views of the future • Ideas or acts of self-harm or suicide • Disturbed sleep • Diminished appetite
Severity *Mild*: total of four or more symptoms, most normal activities continued
Moderate: total of five or more symptoms, great difficulty in continuing normal activities
Severe: total of seven or more symptoms including all three core symptoms, unable to continue normal activities
Severe with psychotic symptoms: in cases with delusions, hallucinations or profound psychomotor retardation

Mood (affective) disorders

Depressive episode

The ICD-10 has set out certain diagnostic guidelines for diagnosing a depressive episode (Fig. 7.2). The minimum duration of the episode is 2 weeks and at least two of the three symptoms of depressed mood, loss of interest or pleasure and increased fatigability should be present. A depressive episode can be graded mild, moderate or severe depending on the number and severity of symptoms. A depressive episode occurring with hallucinations, delusions or a depressive stupor is always coded as 'severe with psychotic features'.

Recurrent depressive disorder

Around 80% of patients who have an episode of depression will go on to have more episodes (the lifetime average is five). Recurrent depressive disorder is diagnosed when a patient has another depressive episode after their first.

Dysthymia

This is a chronically depressed mood that usually has its onset in early adulthood and may remain throughout the patient's life, with variable periods of wellness in between. The patient's mood is seldom severe enough to satisfy the formal criteria for a depressive episode and does not present with discrete episodes as in recurrent depressive disorder. Sometimes dysthymia has its onset in later adult life, often after a discrete depressive

episode, and is associated with bereavement or some other serious stress. Note that patients may develop a depressive episode on a baseline mood of dysthymia (so called 'double depression').

Bipolar affective disorder/cyclothymia

Unipolar depression means that the patient's mood varies between depressed and normal. When patients suffer from episodes of either depressed or elevated mood (often, but not always, punctuated by periods of normal mood), the disorder is termed bipolar, as the mood is considered to deviate from normal to either a depressed or elated (manic) pole. When this instability of mood involves only mild elation and mild depression it is termed cyclothymia. Bipolar illness and cyclothymia are discussed in Chapter 8.

Schizoaffective disorder

A diagnosis of schizoaffective disorder can be made when patients present with both mood (depression or mania) symptoms and schizophrenic symptoms within the same episode of illness. It is important that these symptoms occur simultaneously, or at least within a few days of each other. As you can imagine, this is a difficult diagnosis to establish, as it is not uncommon to have psychotic symptoms in a severe episode of depression (depressive episode with psychotic features); likewise, depressive symptoms often occur in patients with schizophrenia. Schizoaffective disorder is discussed in more detail in Chapter 9.

Depression secondary to psychiatric or general medical disorders, or to psychoactive substances

The mood disorders described above are considered primary; however, depressive symptoms are non-specific and can occur secondary to a range of other conditions. For example, a patient who has schizophrenia, an anxiety disorder, a personality disorder, an eating disorder or dementia may experience low mood as a consequence. If the depressive symptoms meet criteria for a depressive episode they have 'comorbid depression'.

Many general medical conditions are associated with an increased risk of depression (Fig. 7.3). In some cases this may be due to a direct depressant effect on the brain. However, any condition that causes prolonged suffering is a risk factor for depression, for example, chronic pain.

Both prescribed (Fig. 7.4) and illicit drugs can be aetiologically responsible for symptoms of depression. Remember that alcohol is the psychoactive substance that is probably most associated with substance-induced depression.

Low mood may be one of several symptoms that appear when a patient has had to adapt to a significant change in life (e.g. divorce, retirement, bereavement). If the symptoms are not severe enough to be diagnosed as depression but are clearly related to a stressful life event, an adjustment disorder can be diagnosed (see Ch. 12).

ASSESSMENT

History

The following questions might be helpful in eliciting the key symptoms of depression:

Core symptoms

- Have you been cheerful or quite low in mood or spirits lately?
- Do you find that you no longer enjoy things the way you used to?
- Do you find yourself often feeling very tired or worn out?

Biological symptoms

- Do you find your mood is worse in the mornings or evenings?
- What time did you wake up before your mood became low? What time do you wake up now?

Fig. 7.3 General medical conditions associated with low mood

Neurological	Endocrine	Infections	Others
Multiple sclerosis	Cushing's disease	Hepatitis	Malignancies (especially pancreatic cancer)
Parkinson's disease	Addison's disease	Infectious mononucleosis	Chronic pain states
Huntington's disease	Thyroid disorders (especially hypothyroidism)	Herpes simplex	Systemic lupus erythematosus
Spinal cord injury	Parathyroid disorders	Brucellosis	Rheumatoid arthritis
Stroke (especially left anterior infarcts)	Menstrual cycle-related	Typhoid	Renal failure
Head injury		HIV/AIDS	Porphyria
Cerebral tumours		Syphilis	Vitamin deficiencies (e.g. niacin)
			Ischaemic heart disease

Fig. 7.4 Prescribed drugs causing low mood

Antihypertensives	Steroids	Neurological drugs	Analgesics	Other
Beta-blockers	Corticosteroids	L-dopa	Opiates	Antipsychotics
Methyldopa	Oral contraceptives	Carbamazepine	Indometacin	Interferon (alpha and beta)

- Has anyone mentioned you seem slowed up or restless?
- Sometimes when people are depressed they have a poor sex drive. Has this happened to you?

Cognitive symptoms

- How do you see things turning out in the future?
- Do you ever feel that life's not worth living?
- Are you able to concentrate on your favourite TV programme?

Examination

A basic physical examination, including a thorough neurological and endocrine system examination, should be performed on all patients with depression.

Investigations

Social

- Collateral information from general practitioner (GP), community mental health team, family.
- Consider home visit to assess self-care, ability to care for family, home structure.
- Consider interviewing immediate family to gain objective evidence of disturbed interpersonal family dynamics.

Psychological

- Patient may be asked to keep a mood diary.
- Self-report inventories for quantitative ratings of mood, e.g. Beck Depression Inventory (BDI), Hospital Anxiety and Depression Scale (HADS).

Physical

Physical investigations are performed to: (1) exclude possible medical or substance-related causes of depression; (2) establish baseline values before administering treatment that may alter blood chemistry (e.g. antidepressants may cause hyponatraemia, lithium may cause hypothyroidism); (3) assess renal and liver functioning, which may affect the elimination of medication; and (4) screen for the physical consequences of neglect, such as malnutrition.

- Full blood count: check for anaemia (low haemoglobin), infection (raised white count), and a high mean cell volume (MCV; a marker of high alcohol intake).
- Urea and electrolytes (hyponatraemia, renal function).

- Liver function tests and gamma glutamyl transpeptidase (γGT) (also a marker for high alcohol intake).
- Thyroid function tests (hyper- or hypothyroidism) and calcium (hypercalcaemia).

If indicated:

- C reactive protein (CRP) or erythrocyte sedimentation rate (ESR) (if infection or inflammatory disease suspected).
- Vitamin B_{12} and folate (if deficiencies suspected).
- Urine drug screen (if drug use is suspected).
- ECG should be done in patients with cardiac problems as tricyclic antidepressants and lithium may prolong the QT interval and have the potential to cause lethal ventricular arrhythmia.
- EEG (if epileptic focus or other intracranial pathology is suspected).
- CT brain scan (if evidence of neurological or cognitive deficit).

HINTS AND TIPS

Despite much research on the dexamethasone suppression test (DST), there is no reliable blood test to indicate the presence of depression. However, one biological finding that is strongly associated with depression is a reduction in the latency (time to onset after falling asleep) of rapid eye movement (REM) sleep.

DISCUSSION OF CASE STUDY

Mrs LM meets the criteria for a depressive episode, at least moderate in severity. She has had all three core symptoms of depression for longer than 2 weeks: depressed mood, loss of interest or pleasure and fatigability. She also has biological symptoms of early morning awakening and loss of libido. The GP has also elicited cognitive symptoms of feelings of incompetence (reduced self-esteem) and guilt and possible thoughts of self-harm. As this is a first episode, the diagnosis of recurrent depressive disorder is not appropriate. Dysthymia is not a suitable diagnosis as the period of low mood is far too short, the severity of the present episode too great and the deterioration in functioning too marked. There appear to be no instances of elated mood or increased energy, excluding a diagnosis of bipolar affective disorder or cyclothymia.

In order to grade the severity of the depression it would be useful to enquire about all the biological, cognitive and psychotic components of depression. In all cases of suspected depression it is imperative to enquire about thoughts and/or plans of suicide or self-harm (see Ch. 6 for a full discussion). It is also important to rule out secondary causes of depression; these include general medical conditions (Fig. 7.3), psychoactive substance use (Fig. 7.4) and other psychiatric conditions. Mrs LM admitted to using increased quantities of alcohol. Patients often use alcohol as a form of self-medication to alleviate feelings of dysphoria; however, alcohol can aggravate and in some cases even cause depressive symptoms. Mrs LM's use of oral contraception long before the onset of her depressive symptoms suggests that it is unlikely that this prescribed drug is causing her depression.

Now go on to Chapter 18 to read about the mood disorders and their management.

The patient with elevated or irritable mood

After this chapter you should have an understanding of:
- The definitions of a hypomanic episode, a manic episode, a mixed affective episode and bipolar affective disorder
- The mood and cognitive symptoms of a hypomanic or manic episode
- The characteristic psychotic symptoms of a manic psychosis and how they differ from schizophrenia
- The differential diagnosis of a manic episode
- How to communicate with a socially disinhibited patient
- How to assess someone presenting with elevated mood

Case summary

Feeling that she was no longer able to cope, Mrs EM consulted her general practitioner (GP) about a Mental Health Act assessment for her husband, Mr EM, a 37-year-old freelance writer. He had no psychiatric history other than a period of depression 2 years ago. He had progressively needed less sleep over the past 2 weeks and had not slept at all for 48 hours. Recently, he had started taking on increasing amounts of work and seemed to thrive on this due to an 'inexhaustible source of boundless energy'. He told his wife and all his friends that he had a new lease of life, as he was 'happier than ever'. Mrs EM became concerned when he developed lofty ideas that he was a world expert in his field, remaining convinced of this even when she tried to reason with him, and would talk incessantly for hours about elaborate and complicated writing schemes. Mr EM's behaviour had become markedly uncharacteristic over the past day or two, when he started making sexually inappropriate comments to his neighbour's wife, and presented her with reams of poetry which he had spent the night writing. When Mrs EM suggested that he visit the GP, Mr EM became verbally aggressive saying that she was trying to bring him down because she was threatened by his 'irresistible sex appeal and wit'. Mrs EM was unable to reason with him and noticed that he struggled to keep to the point of the conversation, often bringing up issues that seemed completely irrelevant. The GP

noted that, other than a recent bout of flu, Mr EM had no medical problems and was not using any prescribed medication.

(For a discussion of the case study see the end of the chapter)

Just as spells of feeling sad and miserable are quite normal to the human experience, so too are periods where we feel elated, excited and full of energy. Although an irritable or elevated mood is not in itself pathological, it can be when grossly and persistently so, and when associated with other manic psychopathology.

DEFINITIONS AND CLINICAL FEATURES

In Chapter 7 we observed how a disturbance in mood in addition to various other cognitive, biological and psychotic symptoms all contribute to the recognition of a depressive episode. A similar approach is taken to hypomanic and manic episodes; these occur on the opposite pole of the mood disorder spectrum to depression.

Mood

The hallmark of a hypomanic or manic episode is an elevated or irritable mood. Patients often enjoy the experience of elevated mood and might describe themselves as feeling: 'high', 'on top of the world', 'fantastic' or 'euphoric'. This mood has an infectious quality, although those who know the patient well clearly see it as a deviation from normal. However, some patients tend to become extremely irritable or suspicious when manic and do not enjoy the experience at all. They have a low frustration tolerance and any thwarting of their plans can lead to a rapid escalation in anger or even delusions of persecution. When manic and depressive symptoms rapidly alternate (e.g. within the same day), this is termed a *mixed affective episode*.

> **HINTS AND TIPS**
>
> Patients with mania experience irritability (80%) or labile or fluctuating mood (69%) just as often as euphoria (71%).

Biological symptoms

Decreased need for sleep

This is a very important early warning sign of mania or hypomania. Sleep disturbance can range from only needing a few hours sleep a night to a manic patient going for days on end with no sleep at all. Crucially, it is not associated with fatigue.

Increased energy

This initially results in an increase in goal-directed activity and, when coupled with impaired judgement, can have disastrous consequences, e.g. patients may instigate numerous risky business ventures, go on excessive spending sprees, or engage in reckless promiscuity that is unusual for them. However, in severe episodes actions can become repetitive, stereotyped and apparently purposeless, even progressing to a *manic stupor* in the extremely unwell. If left untreated, excessive overactivity can lead to physical exhaustion, dehydration and sometimes even death. On mental state examination, increased energy can be seen as *psychomotor excitation*: the patient is unable to sit still, frequently standing up, pacing around the room and gesticulating expansively.

> **HINTS AND TIPS**
>
> Irrespective of how obvious the diagnosis might appear, it is always important to routinely examine for affective symptoms such as a decreased need for sleep (81%), grandiosity (78%), racing thoughts (71%), distractibility (68%) and sexual disinhibition (57%).

Cognitive symptoms

Elevated sense of self-esteem or grandiosity

Hypomanic patients may overestimate their abilities and social or financial status. In severe cases, manic patients may have delusions of grandeur (see later).

Poor concentration

Manic patients may find it difficult to maintain their focus on any one thing as they struggle to filter out irrelevant external stimuli (background noise, other objects or people in the room), making them, as a consequence, highly distractible.

Accelerated thinking

A manic patient may subjectively experience their thoughts or ideas racing even faster than they can articulate them. When patients have an irrepressible need to express these thoughts verbally, making them difficult to interrupt, it is termed *pressure of speech*. When thoughts are rapidly associating in this way in a stream of connected (but not always relevant) concepts it is termed *flight of ideas*. Some hypomanic patients express themselves by incessant letter writing, poetry, doodling or artwork.

> **COMMUNICATION**
>
> Assessing manic patients can be made difficult by their distractibility and disinhibition. Adopt a polite but firm approach and redirect the patient back to the questions you need to ask.

Impaired judgement and insight

This is typical of manic illness and sometimes results in costly indiscretions that patients may later regret. Lack of insight into their illness can be a difficult barrier to overcome when trying to engage patients in essential treatment.

Psychotic symptoms

Psychotic symptoms are far more common in manic than in depressive episodes and include disorders of *thought form, thought content and perception*.

Disordered thought form

Disordered thought form (see Ch. 9 and Figure 9.3) commonly occurs in schizophrenia, but is regularly seen in manic episodes with psychotic features and to a lesser degree in psychotic forms of unipolar depression. The most common thought form disorders in mania are circumstantiality, tangentiality and flight of ideas. However, signs of thought disorder most typical for schizophrenia can also be seen in manic episodes, e.g. loosening of association, neologisms and thought blocking.

Circumstantiality and tangentiality

Circumstantial (over-inclusive) speech means speech that is delayed in reaching its final goal because of the over-inclusion of details and unnecessary asides and diversions; however, the speaker, if allowed to finish, does eventually connect the original starting point to the desired destination. Circumstantiality can also be found in normal people – most families have at least one person who takes forever to finish a story! Tangential speech, on the other hand, is more indicative of psychopathology and sees the speaker diverting from the initial train of thought but never returning to the original point, jumping tangentially from one topic to the next.

Flight of ideas

As described above, this occurs when thinking is markedly accelerated resulting in a stream of connected concepts. The link between concepts can be as in normal communication where one idea follows directly on from the next, or can be links that are not relevant to an overall goal. For example, links made through word play such as a pun or clang association; or through some vague idea which is not part of the original goal of speech, e.g. 'I need to go to bed now. Have you ever smelt my bed of roses? Ah, but a rose by any other name would smell just as sweet!' Even though manic patients may appear to be talking gibberish, a written transcript of their speech will usually reveal that their ideas are related in some, albeit obscure, way.

As patients become increasingly manic, their associations tend to loosen as they find it increasingly difficult to link their thoughts. Eventually they approach the incoherent thought disorder sometimes seen in schizophrenia (see Ch. 9).

Abnormal beliefs

Patients with elated mood will typically present with *grandiose delusions* in which they believe they have special importance or unusual powers. *Persecutory delusions* are also common, especially in patients with an irritable mood, and often feature them believing that others are trying to take advantage of their exalted status. When the content of delusions matches the mood of the patient, the delusions are termed *mood-congruent*. Very often, patients with elevated mood may have overvalued ideas as opposed to

true delusions, which are important to distinguish, as the former are not regarded as psychotic in nature (see p. 68).

Perceptual disturbance

Some hypomanic patients may describe subtle distortions of perception. These are not psychotic symptoms and mainly include altered intensity of perception such that sounds seem louder (hyperacusis) or colours seem brighter and more vivid (visual hyperaesthesia). Psychotic perceptual features develop when manic patients experience hallucinations. This is usually in the form of voices encouraging or exciting them.

> **HINTS AND TIPS**
>
> Always screen for psychotic symptoms in patients suffering from a manic episode. The prevalence is very high – two-thirds report experiencing psychotic symptoms during such an episode. Interestingly only one third report psychotic symptoms during a depressive episode.

DIFFERENTIAL DIAGNOSIS

Like depression, an elevated or irritable mood can be secondary to a medical condition, psychoactive substance use or other psychiatric disorder. These will have to be excluded before a primary mood disorder can be diagnosed. Figure 8.1 shows the differential diagnosis for patients presenting with elevated or irritable mood.

Fig. 8.1 Differential diagnosis for patient presenting with elevated or irritable mood

Mood disorders
- Hypomania, mania, mixed affective episode (isolated episode or part of bipolar affective disorder)
- Cyclothymia
- Depression (may present with irritable mood)

Secondary to a general medical condition

Secondary to psychoactive substance use

Psychotic disorders
- Schizoaffective disorder (may be similar to mania with psychotic features)
- Schizophrenia

Personality/neurodevelopmental disorders

Delirium/dementia

Mood (affective) disorders

Hypomanic, manic and mixed affective episodes

The ICD-10 specifies three degrees of severity of a manic episode: *hypomania, mania without psychotic symptoms* and *mania with psychotic symptoms*. All of these share the above-mentioned general characteristics, most notably: an elevated or irritable mood and an increase in the quantity and speed of mental and physical activity. Unlike for depressive episodes, the ICD-10 does not specify a certain number of symptoms to establish the diagnosis. It does, however, require the clinician to determine the degree of psychosocial impairment, as well as to code for the presence of psychotic symptoms (Fig. 8.2 – note that the degree of impairment of social functioning rather than number of symptoms is the crucial distinguishing factor between hypomania and mania). As mentioned previously, episodes where patients present with rapidly alternating manic and depressive symptoms are termed *mixed affective episodes*.

Bipolar affective disorder

Most patients who present with a hypomanic, manic or mixed affective episode will have experienced a previous episode of mood disturbance (depression, hypomania, mania or mixed). In this case they should be diagnosed with bipolar affective disorder. Most patients who experience hypomanic or manic episodes also experience depressive episodes, hence, the commonly used term: 'manic-depression'. However, patients who only suffer from manic or hypomanic episodes with no intervening depressive episodes are also classified as having bipolar affective disorder, even though their mood does not swing to the depressive pole. It is good practice to record the nature of the current episode in a patient with bipolar affective disorder (e.g. *'bipolar affective disorder, current episode manic without psychotic features'*).

Cyclothymia

Cyclothymia is analogous to dysthymia (see p. 52) in that it usually begins in early adulthood and follows a chronic course with intermittent periods of wellness in between. It is characterized by an instability of mood resulting in alternating periods of mild elation and mild depression, none of which are sufficiently severe or long enough to meet the criteria for either a hypomanic or a depressive episode.

Depression

There are three common scenarios where a patient with a primary depressive disorder may present with an

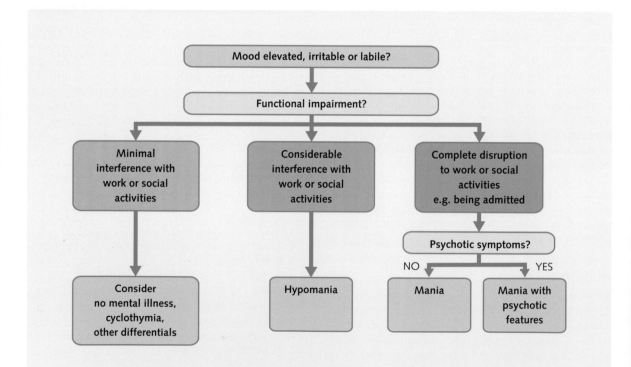

Fig. 8.2 Distinguishing mania from hypomania

elevated or irritable mood. An 'agitated depression' can present with a prominent irritable mood, which, when coupled with psychomotor agitation, can be difficult to distinguish from a manic episode. Secondly, depressed patients who are responding to antidepressants or electroconvulsive therapy (ECT) may experience a transient period of elevated mood. Thirdly, a patient with a recently resolved depressive disorder might misidentify euthymia for hypomania.

Manic episodes secondary to a general medical condition or psychoactive substance use

A medical or psychoactive substance cause of mania should always be sought for and ruled out. Figure 8.3 lists the medical and substance-related causes of mania. The medical condition or substance use should predate the development of the mood disorder and symptoms should resolve with treatment of the condition or abstinence from the offending substance. Absence of previous manic episodes or a family history of bipolar affective disorder also supports this diagnosis.

Schizophreniform disorders

Schizoaffective disorder

See pages 52 and 73. This can be very difficult to distinguish from a manic episode with psychotic features.

Schizophrenia

Patients with schizophrenia can present with an excited, suspicious or agitated mood and therefore can be difficult to distinguish from manic patients with psychotic

Fig. 8.4 Psychopathological distinctions between mania and schizophrenia (these are guidelines only; typically schizophrenic symptoms can occur in mania and vice versa)

Psychopathology	Mania	Schizophrenia
Thought form	Circumstantiality, tangentiality, flight of ideas	Loosening of association, neologisms, thought blocking
Delusions	Most often mood-congruent (grandiose delusions or persecutory delusions)	Delusions unrelated to mood, bizarre delusions, delusions of passivity (e.g. thought insertion, withdrawal, broadcast)
Speech	Pressured speech, difficult to interrupt	Speech is often hesitant or halting
Biological symptoms	Significantly reduced need for sleep, increased physical and mental energy	Sleep less disturbed, less hyperactive
Psychomotor function	Agitation	Agitation, catatonic symptoms or negative symptoms

symptoms. Figure 8.4 compares relevant features that might act as clues to the correct diagnosis.

Personality/neurodevelopmental disorders

Patients with disorders of personality or neurodevelopment often report features similar to hypomania, e.g. impulsivity, displays of temper and lability of mood in borderline personality disorder or attention deficit hyperactivity disorder. However, personality and neurodevelopmental disorders involve stable and enduring behaviour patterns, unlike the more discrete episodes of bipolar affective disorder, which are characterized by a distinct, demarcated deterioration in psychosocial functioning.

Delirium/dementia

See Chapter 14.

Fig. 8.3 Medical and substance causes of mania

Medical conditions	Substances
Cerebral neoplasms, infarcts, trauma, infection (including HIV) Cushing's disease Huntington's disease Hyperthyroidism Multiple sclerosis Renal failure Systemic lupus erythematosus Temporal lobe epilepsy Vitamin B_{12} and niacin (pellagra) deficiency	Amfetamines Cocaine Hallucinogens 'Legal highs' **Prescribed** Anabolic steroids Antidepressants Corticosteroids Dopaminergic agents (e.g. L-dopa, selegiline, bromocriptine)

ASSESSMENT

History

The following questions might be helpful in eliciting the key symptoms of mania/hypomania:

- Have you been feeling particularly happy or on top of the world lately?
- Do you sometimes feel as though you have too much energy compared to people around you?
- Do you find yourself needing less sleep but not getting tired?
- Have you had any new interests or exciting ideas lately?
- Have you noticed your thoughts racing in your head?
- Do you have any special abilities or powers?

Examination

A basic physical examination, including a thorough neurological and endocrine system examination, should be performed on all patients with elevated mood.

Investigations

As for the depressive disorders (page 54), social, psychological and physical investigations are normally performed on manic patients mainly to establish the diagnosis and to rule out an organic or substance-related cause (see Fig. 8.3).

ALGORITHM FOR THE DIAGNOSIS OF MOOD DISORDERS

See Figure 8.5.

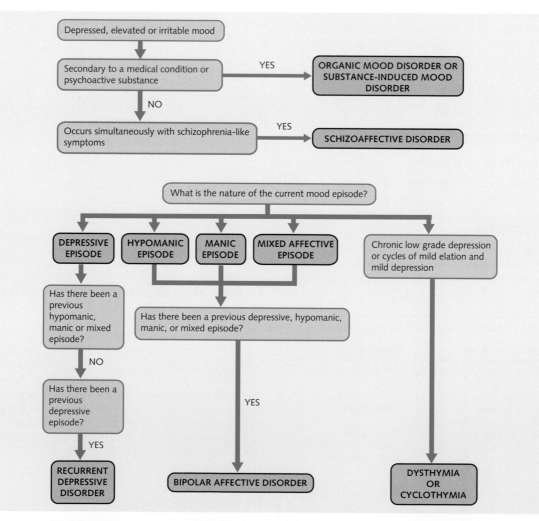

Fig. 8.5 Algorithm for the diagnosis of mood disorders

DISCUSSION OF CASE STUDY

Mr EM appears to be suffering from a *manic episode with psychotic features*. He has an elated mood and has developed the grandiose delusion that he is a world expert (mood-congruent psychotic symptom); note also the rapid switch to irritable mood when confronted. Biological symptoms include the reduced need for sleep and increased mental and physical energy with overactivity. Cognitive symptoms include elevated sense of self-importance, poor concentration, accelerated thinking with pressure of speech and impaired judgement and insight. The episode is classified as manic because of the severe impairment in social and probably work functioning, and because of the psychotic features.

The past psychiatric history is extremely important in this case. A previous mood episode (hypomanic, manic, depressive, mixed) is required in order to make the diagnosis of bipolar affective disorder. Mr EM had a period of depression 2 years prior to developing this manic episode. If this was a genuine depressive episode, corroborated by a collateral history from Mr EM's GP or wife, then the diagnosis would be: *bipolar affective disorder, current episode manic with psychotic features*. Previous psychotic episodes should add schizoaffective disorder and schizophrenia to the differential diagnosis.

Now go on to Chapter 18 to read about the mood disorders and their management.

The psychotic patient ⑨

● Objectives

After this chapter you should have an understanding of:
- The definition of psychosis
- The definitions of: hallucination, pseudohallucination and illusion
- The definitions of: delusion, overvalued idea and obsession
- The phenomenology of psychosis
- The differential diagnosis of psychosis
- How to assess someone presenting with psychotic features

Case summary

Mr PP, aged 23 years, was assessed by his general practitioner (GP) because his family had become concerned about his behaviour. Over the last 6 months his college attendance had been uncharacteristically poor and he had terminated his part-time work. He had also become increasingly reclusive, spending more time alone in his flat, refusing to answer the door or see his friends. After some inappropriate suspiciousness, he allowed the GP into his flat and then disclosed that government scientists had started to perform experiments on him over the last year. These involved the insertion of an electrode into his brain that detected gamma rays transmitted from government headquarters, which issued him with commands and 'planted' strange ideas in his head. When the GP asked how he knew this, he replied that he heard the 'men's voices' as 'clear as day' and that they continually commented on what he was thinking. He explained that his suspicion that 'all was not right' was confirmed when he heard the neighbour's dog barking in the middle of the night – at that point he knew 'for certain' that he was being interfered with. Prompted by the GP, Mr PP also mentioned that a man in his local pub knew of his plight and had sent him a 'covert signal' when he overheard the man conversing about the dangers of nuclear experiments. He also admitted to 'receiving coded information' from the radio whenever it was turned on. The GP found no evidence of abnormal mood, incoherence of speech or disturbed motor function. Mr PP denied use of illicit drugs and appeared physically well. After the GP discussed the case with a psychiatrist, Mr PP was admitted to a psychiatric hospital. He agreed to a voluntary admission, as he was now afraid of staying alone at home.

(For a discussion of the case study see the end of the chapter)

The psychotic patient can present in many varied ways. It is often very difficult to elicit and describe specific symptoms when a patient is speaking or behaving in a grossly disorganized fashion. Therefore, it is important to approach the psychotic patient in a logical and systematic fashion as well as to have a good understanding of the psychopathology involved.

DEFINITIONS AND CLINICAL FEATURES

Psychosis refers to a mental state in which reality is grossly distorted, resulting in symptoms such as delusions, hallucinations and thought disorder. However, patients with schizophrenia and other psychotic disorders often have other symptoms too, e.g. psychomotor abnormalities, mood/affect disturbance, cognitive deficits and disorganized behaviour.

There are many classifications that attempt to describe all the symptoms seen in schizophrenia and psychosis. So, in order to simplify matters it is useful to approach psychotic psychopathology using five somewhat interrelated parameters:

1. Perception.
2. Abnormal beliefs.
3. Thought disorder.
4. Negative symptoms.
5. Psychomotor function.

Perceptual disturbance

Perception is the process of making sense of the physical information we receive from our five sensory modalities.

Hallucinations are perceptions occurring in the absence of an external physical stimulus, which have the following important characteristics:

- To the patient, the nature of a hallucination is exactly the same as a normal sensory experience – i.e. it appears real. Therefore, patients often have little insight into their abnormal experience.
- They are experienced as external sensations from any one of the five sensory modalities (hearing, vision, smell, taste, touch) and should be distinguished from ideas, thoughts, images or fantasies which originate in the patient's own mind.
- They occur without an external stimulus and are not merely distortions of an existing physical stimulus (see illusions).

Illusions are misperceptions of real external stimuli, e.g. in a dark room, a dressing gown hanging on a bedroom wall is perceived as a person. Illusions often occur in healthy people and are usually associated with inattention or strong emotion.

A *pseudohallucination* is a perceptual experience which differs from a hallucination in that it appears to arise in the subjective inner space of the mind, not through one of the external sensory organs. Patients tend to describe these sensations as being perceived with the 'inner eye' or 'mind's eye' (or ear). Although experienced in internal space they are not under conscious control. Examples include: distressing flashbacks in post-traumatic stress disorder or someone hearing a voice inside their own head telling them to harm themselves. These are not viewed as true psychotic experiences. Note that some psychiatrists define pseudohallucinations to mean hallucinations that patients actually recognize as false perceptions, i.e. they have insight into the fact that they are hallucinating. The former definition is probably more widely used.

According to which sense organ they appear to arise from, hallucinations are classified as auditory, visual, olfactory, gustatory or somatic. Special forms of hallucinations will also be discussed. See Figure 9.1 for an outline of the classification of hallucinations.

Auditory hallucinations

These are hallucinations of the hearing modality and are the most common type of hallucinations in clinical psychiatry. Elementary hallucinations are simple, unstructured sounds, e.g. whirring, buzzing, whistling or single words; this type of hallucination commonly occurs in acute organic states. Complex hallucinations occur as spoken phrases, sentences or even dialogue that are classified as:

- *Audible thoughts* (*first person*): patients hear their own thoughts spoken out loud as they think them. When patients experience their thoughts as echoed by a voice after they have thought them, it is termed thought echo.

Fig. 9.1 Outline of classification of hallucinations

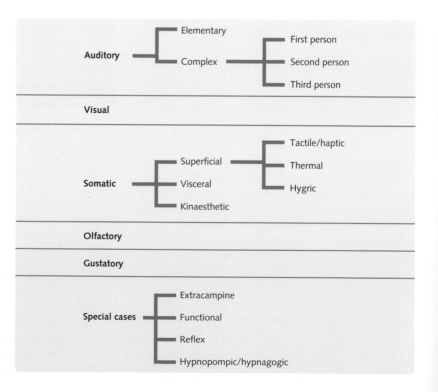

- *Second person auditory hallucinations*: patients hear a voice or voices talking directly to them. Second person hallucinations can be persecutory, highly critical, complimentary or issue commands to the patient (command hallucinations). Second person hallucinations are often associated with mood disorders with psychotic features and so will be critical or persecutory in a depressed patient or complimentary in a manic patient, i.e. mood-congruent hallucinations.
- *Third person auditory hallucinations*: patients hear a voice or voices speaking about them, referring to them in the third person. This may take the form of two or more voices arguing or discussing the patient among themselves; or one or more voices giving a running commentary on the patient's thoughts or actions.

Visual hallucinations

These are hallucinations of the visual modality. They occur most commonly in organic brain disturbances (delirium, occipital lobe tumours, epilepsy, dementia) and in the context of psychoactive substance use (lysergic acid diethylamide (LSD), mescaline, petrol/glue-sniffing, alcoholic hallucinosis). An autoscopic hallucination is the experience of seeing an image of oneself in external space. The Charles Bonnet syndrome describes the condition where patients experience complex visual hallucinations associated with no other psychiatric symptoms or impairment in consciousness; it usually occurs in older adults and is associated with loss of vision. Lilliputian hallucinations are hallucinations of miniature people or animals.

Somatic hallucinations

These are hallucinations of bodily sensation and include superficial, visceral and kinaesthetic hallucinations.

Superficial hallucinations describe sensations on or just below the skin and may be:

- *Tactile* (*haptic*): experience of the skin being touched, pricked or pinched. Formication is the unpleasant sensation of insects crawling on or just below the skin; it is commonly associated with long-term cocaine use (cocaine bugs) and alcohol withdrawal.
- *Thermal*: false perception of heat or cold.
- *Hygric*: false perception of a fluid, e.g. 'I can feel water sloshing in my brain'.
- *Visceral* hallucinations describe false perceptions of the internal organs. Patients may be distressed by deep sensations of their organs throbbing, stretching, distending or vibrating.
- *Kinaesthetic* hallucinations are false perceptions of joint or muscle sense. Patients may describe their limbs vibrating or being twisted. The fleeting but distressing sensation of free falling just as one is about to fall asleep is an example that most people have experienced (see hypnagogic hallucinations below).

Olfactory and gustatory hallucinations

These are the false perceptions of smell and taste. Note that they commonly occur together because the two senses are closely related. Remember that in patients with olfactory or gustatory hallucinations, it is important to rule out epilepsy (especially of the temporal lobe) and other organic brain diseases.

Special forms of hallucination

Hypnagogic hallucinations are false perceptions in any modality (usually auditory or visual) that occur as a person goes to sleep; whereas, hypnopompic hallucinations occur as a person awakens. These occur in normal people and are not indicative of psychopathology.

Extracampine hallucinations are false perceptions that occur outside the limits of a person's normal sensory field, e.g. a patient describes hearing voices from 100 miles away. Patients often give delusional explanations for this phenomenon.

A functional hallucination occurs when a normal sensory stimulus is required to precipitate a hallucination in that same sensory modality, e.g. voices that are only heard when the doorbell rings. A reflex hallucination occurs when a normal sensory stimulus in one modality precipitates a hallucination in another, e.g. voices that are only heard whenever the lights are switched on.

Abnormal beliefs

Abnormal beliefs include primary and secondary delusions and overvalued ideas.

Delusions

A delusion is an unshakeable false belief that is not accepted by other members of the patient's culture. It is important to understand the following characteristics of delusional thinking:

- To the patient, there is no difference between a delusional belief and a true belief – they are the same experience. Therefore, only an external observer can diagnose a delusion. A delusion is to ideation what an hallucination is to perception.
- The delusion is false because of faulty reasoning. A man's delusional belief that his wife is having an affair may actually be true (she may indeed be unfaithful), but it remains a delusion because the reason he gives for this belief is undoubtedly false. For example, she 'must' be having an affair because she is part of a top-secret sexual conspiracy to prove that he is a homosexual.
- It is out of keeping with the patient's social and cultural background. It is crucial to establish that the belief is not one likely to be held by that person's

subcultural group, e.g. a belief in the imminent second coming of Christ may be appropriate for a member of a religious group, but not for a formerly atheist, middle-aged businessman.

It is diagnostically significant to classify delusions as:

- Primary or secondary.
- Mood congruent or mood incongruent.
- Bizarre or non-bizarre.
- According to the content of the delusion.

Primary delusions (autochthonous delusions) do not occur in response to any previous psychopathological state; their genesis is un-understandable. They may be preceded by a delusional atmosphere (mood) where patients have a sense that the world around them has been subtly altered, often in a sinister or threatening way. In this state a fully formed delusion has not yet developed and patients appear perplexed and apprehensive. Note that when a delusion occurs after a delusional atmosphere it is still regarded as primary – the delusional atmosphere is probably a precursor to the fully developed primary delusion. A delusional perception is also a primary delusion and occurs when a delusional meaning is attached to a normal perception; e.g. a patient believed he was a terrorist target because he heard an aeroplane flying in the distance. Primary delusions occur typically in schizophrenia and other primary psychotic disorders. Secondary delusions are the consequences of pre-existing psychopathological states, usually mood disorders (see p. 51 and page 59). Many interrelated delusions that are centred on a common theme are termed systematized delusions.

In mood-congruent delusions, the contents of the delusions are appropriate to the patient's mood and are commonly seen in depression or mania with psychotic features.

Bizarre delusions are those which are completely impossible; e.g. the belief that aliens have planted radioactive detonators in the patient's brain. They are considered to be characteristic of schizophrenia.

Figure 9.2 lists the classification of delusions by their content. It is important that you are able to label a delusion according to its content, so take some time to familiarize yourself with this table.

(see p. 51 and page 59)

HINTS AND TIPS

Note that the term 'paranoid' refers to any delusions or ideas that are unduly self-referent –typically delusions or ideas of persecution, grandeur or reference. It should not be used synonymously with the term persecutory; i.e. when a patient has a false belief that people are trying to harm him, do not say that he is paranoid, rather say that he has persecutory delusions.

Finally, beliefs that were previously held with delusional intensity but then become held with less conviction are termed partial delusions. This occurs when patients start recovering after receiving treatment.

COMMUNICATION

Direct questioning about perceptual experience may alienate a non-psychotic patient and raise undue suspicion in a psychotic patient. To maintain rapport with patients begin these questions with a primer such as: 'I am now going to ask you some questions which may seem a little strange, but are routine questions which I ask all patients'.

Overvalued ideas

An overvalued idea is a plausible belief that a patient becomes preoccupied with to an unreasonable extent. The key feature is that the pursuit of this idea causes considerable distress to the patient or those living around them – it is overvalued. Patients who hold overvalued ideas have usually had them for many years and typically have abnormalities of personality. They are distinguished from delusions by the lack of a gross abnormality in reasoning; these patients can often give fairly logical reasons for their beliefs. They differ from obsessions in that they are not seen as recurrent intrusions. However, one will frequently encounter beliefs that span definitions. Typical disorders that feature overvalued ideas are anorexia nervosa, hypochondriacal disorder, dysmorphophobia, paranoid personality disorder and morbid jealousy (this can also take the form of a delusion).

Thought disorder

Describing the disturbance of a patient's thought form is one of the most challenging tasks facing clinicians. This problem is compounded by two factors. Firstly, it is impossible to know what patients are actually thinking – thought form has to be inferred from their speech and behaviour. Secondly, the unfortunate situation has arisen where various authors in psychiatry have described a different conceptual view of thought disorder, which has resulted in conflicting and confusing classification systems. It is probably not that important that you are able to classify and subgroup thought disorder, but rather that you have a clear understanding of the individual definitions you intend to use and are able to recognize them in the patients that you assess. In this regard, it is particularly helpful if you document and are able to cite examples of the patient's speech in their own words.

Many patients with delusions are able to communicate in a clear and coherent manner; although their beliefs may be false, their speech is organized. However,

Fig. 9.2 Classification of delusions by content

Classification	Content
Persecutory delusions	False belief that one is being harmed, threatened, cheated, harassed or is a victim of a conspiracy
Grandiose delusions	False belief that one is exceptionally powerful (including having 'mystical powers'), talented or important
Delusions of reference	False belief that certain objects, people or events have intense personal significance and refer specifically to oneself, e.g. believing that a television newsreader is talking directly about one
Religious delusions	False belief pertaining to a religious theme, often grandiose in nature, e.g. believing that one is a special messenger from God
Delusions of love (erotomania)	False belief that another person is in love with one (commoner in women). In one form, termed *de Clérambault syndrome*, a woman (usually) believes that a man, frequently older and of higher status, is in love with her
Delusion of infidelity (morbid jealousy, Othello syndrome)	False belief that one's lover has been unfaithful. Note that morbid jealousy may also take the form of an overvalued idea, that is, non-psychotic jealousy
Delusions of misidentification	*Capgras syndrome*: belief that a familiar person has been replaced by an exact double – an impostor *Fregoli syndrome*: belief that a complete stranger is actually a familiar person already known to one
Nihilistic delusions (see Cotard's syndrome, p. 182)	False belief that oneself, others or the world is non-existent or about to end. In severe cases, negation is carried to the extreme with patients claiming that nothing, including themselves, exists
Somatic delusions	False belief concerning one's body and its functioning, e.g. that one's bowels are rotting. Also called *hypochondriacal delusions* (to be distinguished from the overvalued ideas seen in hypochondriacal disorder)
Delusions of infestation (Ekbom's syndrome)	False belief that one is infested with small but visible organisms. May also occur secondary to tactile hallucinations, e.g. formication (see text)
Delusions of control (passivity or 'made' experiences) *Note: these are all first-rank symptoms of schizophrenia*	False belief that one's thoughts, feelings, actions or impulses are controlled or 'made' by an external agency, e.g. believing that one was *made* to break a window by demons Delusions of thought control include: *Thought insertion*: belief that thoughts or ideas are being implanted in one's head by an external agency *Thought withdrawal*: belief that one's thoughts or ideas are being extracted from one's head by an external agency *Thought broadcasting*: belief that one's thoughts are being diffused or broadcast to others such that they know what one is thinking

there is a subgroup of psychotic patients who speak in such a disorganized way that it becomes difficult to understand what they are saying. The coherency of patients with disorganized thinking varies from being mostly understandable in patients exhibiting circumstantial thinking to being completely incomprehensible in patients with a word salad phenomenon (see Fig. 9.3).

The following are important signs of disorganized thinking:

Circumstantial and tangential thinking

See page 59.

Flight of ideas

See page 59.

Loosening of association (derailment/ knight's move thinking)

This is when the patient's train of thought shifts suddenly from one very loosely or unrelated idea to the next. In its worst form, speech becomes a mixture of incoherent words and phrases and is termed 'word salad'. Loosening of association is characteristic of schizophrenia. Note that some psychiatrists, but unfortunately not

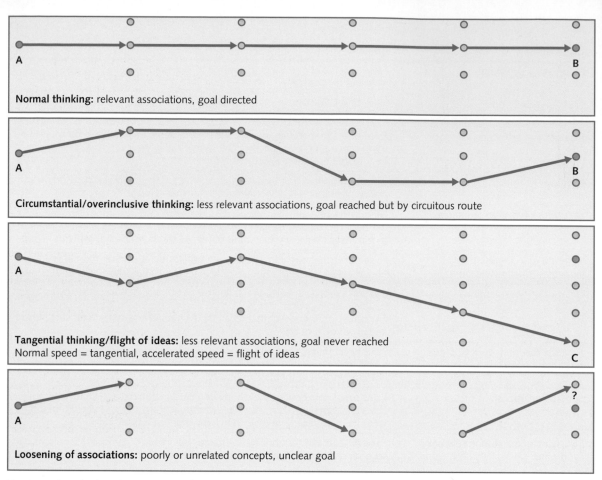

Fig. 9.3 Thought disorder: simplified representation

all, use the term formal thought disorder synonymously with loosening of association.

Thought blocking

This occurs when patients experience a sudden cessation to their flow of thought, often in mid-sentence (observed as sudden breaks in speech). Patients have no recall of what they were saying or thinking and thus continue talking about a different topic.

Neologisms and idiosyncratic word use

Neologisms are new words created by the patient, often combining syllables of other known words. Patients can also use recognized words idiosyncratically by attributing them with a non-recognized meaning (metonyms).

Perseveration

This is when an initially correct response is inappropriately repeated, for example, unnecessarily repeating a previously expressed word or phrase. Palilalia describes the repetition of the last word of a sentence; logoclonia describes the repetition of the last syllable of the last word. Perseveration is highly suggestive of organic brain disease.

Echolalia

This is when patients senselessly repeat words or phrases spoken around them by others – like a parrot.

Irrelevant answers

Patients give answers that are completely unrelated to the original question.

Negative symptoms

Positive symptoms are those that are actively produced and include delusions, hallucinations, loosening of association and bizarre speech or behaviour. This is opposed to negative symptoms that indicate a clinical deficit and include marked apathy, poverty of thought and speech, blunting of affect, social isolation, poor self-care and cognitive deficits. Patients can have positive and negative symptoms simultaneously or, as often happens, develop a negative presentation after initially presenting with predominantly positive symptoms. Remember that patients with a depressed mood or those experiencing significant side-effects from psychotropic medication may also present with negative symptoms.

Psychomotor function

Although a relatively rare phenomenon in industrialized countries, some psychotic patients will present with abnormalities of motor function. Motor system dysfunction in schizophrenia is usually due to the extrapyramidal side-effects of neuroleptic medication (see Ch. 2). However, psychotic patients can occasionally present with impressive motor signs that are not caused by psychiatric medication or a known organic brain disease. Although undoubtedly associated with the patient's abnormal mental state, the cause of this psychomotor dysfunction is far from clarified. The term 'catatonia' literally means extreme muscular tone or rigidity; however, it commonly describes any excessive or decreased motor activity that is apparently purposeless and includes abnormalities of movement, tone or position. Note that catatonic symptoms are not diagnostic of schizophrenia; they may also be caused by brain diseases, metabolic abnormalities or psychoactive substances, and can also occur in mood disorders. Figure 9.4 describes the common motor symptoms seen in schizophrenia.

DIFFERENTIAL DIAGNOSIS

Psychotic symptoms are non-specific and are associated with many primary psychiatric illnesses. They can also present secondary to a general medical condition or psychoactive substance use. See Figure 9.5 for the differential diagnosis for the psychotic patient.

Psychotic disorders

Schizophrenia

There are no pathognomonic or singularly defining symptoms of schizophrenia; it is a syndrome characterized by a heterogeneous cluster of symptoms and signs. The ICD-10 has set out diagnostic guidelines based on the most commonly occurring symptom groups, which have been discussed in the preceding section (Fig. 9.6). It is also important to establish that there has been a clear and marked deterioration in the patient's social and work functioning.

In the past, psychiatrists used Schneider's first-rank symptoms to make the diagnosis of schizophrenia. Kurt Schneider suggested that the presence of one or more first-rank symptoms in the absence of organic disease was of pragmatic value in making the diagnosis of schizophrenia. First-rank symptoms are still referred to so you should familiarize yourself with them; they are presented in Figure 9.7.

Fig. 9.4 Motor symptoms in schizophrenia	
Catatonic rigidity	Maintaining a fixed position and rigidly resisting all attempts to be moved
Catatonic posturing	Adopting an unusual or bizarre position that is then maintained for some time
Catatonic negativism	A seemingly motiveless resistance to all instructions or attempts to be moved; patients may do the opposite of what is asked
Catatonic waxy flexibility (flexibilitas cerea)	Patients can be 'moulded' like wax into a position that is then maintained
Catatonic excitement	Agitated, excited and seemingly purposeless motor activity, not influenced by external stimuli
Catatonic stupor	A presentation of *akinesis* (lack of voluntary movement), *mutism* and *extreme unresponsiveness* in an otherwise alert patient (there may be slight clouding of consciousness)
Echopraxia	Patients senselessly repeat or imitate the actions of those around them. Associated with *echolalia* (see text) – also occurs in patients with frontal lobe damage
Mannerisms	Apparently goal-directed movements (e.g. waving, saluting) that are performed repeatedly or at socially inappropriate times
Stereotypies	A complex movement that does not appear to be goal-directed (e.g. rocking to and fro, gyrating)
Tics	Sudden, involuntary, rapid, recurrent, non-rhythmic motor movements or vocalizations

Fig. 9.5 Differential diagnosis for the psychotic patient

Psychotic disorders
• Schizophrenia
• Schizophrenia-like psychotic disorders
• Schizoaffective disorder
• Delusional disorder
Mood disorders
• Manic episode with psychotic features
• Depressive episode, severe, with psychotic features
Secondary to a general medical condition
Secondary to psychoactive substance use
Dementia/delirium
Personality disorder (schizotypal, borderline, schizoid, paranoid)
Neurodevelopmental disorder (autistic spectrum)

Fig. 9.6 ICD-10 diagnostic guidelines for schizophrenia

One or more of the following symptoms:
a. Thought echo, insertion, withdrawal or broadcast
b. Delusions of control or passivity; delusional perception
c. Hallucinatory voices giving a running commentary; discussing the patient among themselves or 'originating' from some part of the body
d. Bizarre delusions
OR
Two or more of the following symptoms:
e. Other hallucinations that either occur every day for weeks or that are associated with fleeting delusions or sustained overvalued ideas
f. Thought disorganization (loosening of association, incoherence, neologisms)
g. Catatonic symptoms
h. Negative symptoms
i. Change in personal behaviour (loss of interest, aimlessness, social withdrawal)

Symptoms should be present for most of the time during at least 1 month
Schizophrenia should not be diagnosed in the presence of organic brain disease or during drug intoxication or withdrawal

HINTS AND TIPS

Memory aid: if you add 'bizarre delusions' and 'hallucinations coming from a part of the body' to Schneider's first-rank symptoms you will have the (a) to (d) criteria of the ICD-10 diagnostic guidelines for schizophrenia.

Schizophrenia subtypes

Due to the differing presentations of schizophrenia, researchers have tried to identify schizophrenia subtypes. The importance of these subtypes is that they vary in their prognosis and treatment response. The ICD-10 has coded the following subtypes, which are not necessarily exclusive:

• *Paranoid schizophrenia*: dominated by the presence of delusions and hallucinations (positive symptoms). Negative and catatonic symptoms as well as thought disorganization are not prominent. The prognosis is usually better and the onset of illness later than the other subtypes.
• *Hebephrenic (disorganized) schizophrenia*: characterized by thought disorganization, disturbed behaviour and inappropriate or flat affect. Delusions and hallucination are fleeting or not prominent. Onset of illness is earlier (15 to 25 years of age) and the prognosis poorer than paranoid schizophrenia.
• *Catatonic schizophrenia*: a rare form characterized by one or more catatonic symptoms (see Fig. 9.4).
• *Residual schizophrenia*: 1 year of predominantly chronic negative symptoms which must have been preceded by at least one clear cut psychotic episode in the past.

Schizophrenia-like psychotic disorders

Some psychotic episodes with schizophrenia-like symptoms seem to have an abrupt onset (without a prodromal phase), to be precipitated by an acute life stress or to have a duration of symptoms less than that usually observed in schizophrenia. The ICD-10 codes these as acute and transient psychotic disorders. The DSM-IV, on the other hand, suggests diagnoses of schizophreniform disorder and brief psychotic disorder. Often these diagnoses are superseded by a later diagnosis of schizophrenia as the clinical picture evolves.

Fig. 9.7 Schneider's first-rank symptoms of schizophrenia

• Delusional perception
• Delusions of thought control: insertion, withdrawal, broadcast
• Delusions of control: passivity experiences of affect (feelings), impulse, volition and somatic passivity (influence controlling the body)
• Hallucinations: audible thoughts (first person or thought echo), voices arguing or discussing the patient, voices giving a running commentary

Schizoaffective disorder

Schizoaffective disorder describes the presentation of both schizophrenic and mood (depressed or manic) symptoms that present in the same episode of illness, either simultaneously or within a few days of each other. The mood symptoms should meet the criteria for either a depressive or manic episode. Patients should also have at least one, preferably two, of the typical schizophrenic symptoms – symptoms (a) to (d) as specified in the ICD-10 schizophrenia diagnostic guidelines (see Fig. 9.6). Depending on the particular mood symptoms displayed, this disorder can be coded in the ICD-10 as schizoaffective disorder, manic type or schizoaffective disorder, depressed type.

> **HINTS AND TIPS**
>
> When psychiatrists talk about the typical symptoms of schizophrenia, they are generally referring to (a) to (d) of the ICD-10 criteria for schizophrenia (or Schneider's first-rank symptoms), e.g. delusions of control, running commentary hallucinations, etc.

Delusional disorder

In this disorder, the development of a single or set of delusions for the period of at least 3 months is the most prominent or only symptom. It usually has its onset in middle age and expressed delusions may persist throughout the patient's life and include persecutory, grandiose and hypochondriacal delusions. Typically schizophrenic delusions, such as delusions of thought control or passivity, exclude this diagnosis. Hallucinations, if present, tend to be only fleeting and are not typically schizophrenic in nature; brief depressive symptoms may also be evident. Affect, speech and behaviour are all normal and these patients usually have well-preserved personal and social skills. Rarely, patients may present with an induced delusional disorder (*folie à deux*), which occurs when a non-psychotic patient with close emotional ties to another person suffering from delusions (usually a dominant figure) begins to share those delusional ideas themselves. The delusions in the non-psychotic patient tend to resolve when the two are separated.

Mood (affective) disorders

Manic episode with psychotic features

See Chapter 8.

Depressive episode, severe with psychotic features

See Chapter 7.

Psychotic episodes secondary to a general medical condition or psychoactive substance use

A medical or psychoactive substance cause of psychosis should always be sought for and ruled out. Figure 9.8 lists the medical and substance-related causes of psychotic episodes. The medical condition or substance use should predate the development of the psychosis and symptoms should resolve with treatment of the condition or abstinence from the offending substance. Absence of previous psychotic episodes and absence of a family history of schizophrenia also supports this diagnosis.

Delirium and dementia

Visual hallucinations and delusions are common in delirium and may also occur in dementia, particularly diffuse Lewy body dementia (see Ch. 14).

Personality disorder

In general, schizophrenia presents with a clear change in behaviour and functioning, sometimes with a prodrome, whereas patients with a personality or neurodevelopmental disorder have never achieved a normal baseline. Schizotypal (personality) disorder is characterized by eccentric behaviour and peculiarities of thinking and appearance. Although there are no clear psychotic

Fig. 9.8 Medical and substance-related causes of psychotic symptoms

Medical conditions	Substances
Cerebral neoplasm, infarcts, trauma, infection, inflammation (including HIV, CJD, neurosyphilis, herpes encephalitis)	Alcohol
	Cannabis
	'Legal highs'
	Amfetamines
	Cocaine
	Hallucinogens
Endocrinological (thyroid, parathyroid, adrenal disorders)	Inhalants/solvents
Epilepsy (especially temporal lobe epilepsy)	
Huntington's disease	**Prescribed**
Systemic lupus erythematosus	Antiparkinsonian drugs
Vitamin B_{12}, niacin (pellagra) and thiamine deficiency (Wernicke's encephalopathy)	Corticosteroids
	Anticholinergics
Acute intermittent porphyria	

HIV: human immunodeficiency virus
CJD: Creutzfeldt–Jakob disease

symptoms evident and its course resembles that of a personality disorder, the ICD-10 actually describes schizotypal disorder in the chapter on psychotic disorders. This is because it is more prevalent among relatives of patients with schizophrenia and, occasionally, it progresses to overt schizophrenia. Borderline, paranoid and schizoid personality disorders also share similar features to schizophrenia without displaying clear-cut psychotic symptoms. Personality disorders are discussed in greater detail in Chapter 16.

Neurodevelopmental disorder

Social difficulties and rigid thinking are found in both autistic spectrum disorders and schizophrenia. See Chapter 27.

ALGORITHM FOR THE DIAGNOSIS OF PSYCHOTIC DISORDERS

See Figure 9.9.

ASSESSMENT

History

The following questions may be helpful in eliciting psychotic phenomena on mental state examination:

Hallucinations

- Do you ever hear strange noises or voices when there is no one else about?
- Do you ever hear your own thoughts spoken aloud such that someone standing next to you might possibly hear them? (audible thoughts – first person auditory hallucinations)
- Do you ever hear your thoughts echoed just after you have thought them? (thought echo)
- Do these voices talk directly to you or give you commands? (second person auditory hallucinations)
- Do these voices ever talk about you with each other or make comments about what you are doing? (third person auditory hallucinations/running commentary)

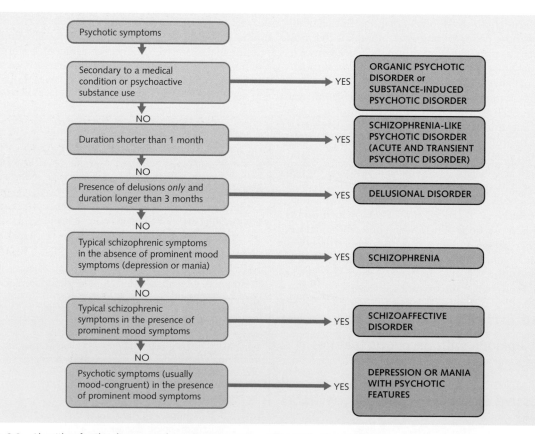

Fig. 9.9 Algorithm for the diagnosis of a patient presenting with psychotic symptoms

Delusions

- Are you afraid that someone is trying to harm or poison you? (persecutory delusions)
- Have you noticed that people are doing or saying things that have a special meaning for you? (delusions of reference)
- Do you have any special abilities or powers? (grandiose delusions)
- Does it seem as though you are being controlled or influenced by some external force? (delusions of control)
- Are thoughts that don't belong to you being put into your head? (thought insertion)

It is important to obtain collateral information from the patient's GP, family and care coordinator (if they have one) to establish premorbid personality and functioning as well as pattern of deterioration.

Examination

A basic physical examination including a thorough neurological and endocrine system examination should be performed on all patients with psychotic symptoms.

Investigations

- Blood investigations are performed to:
  - Exclude possible medical or substance-related causes of psychosis
  - Establish baseline values before administering antipsychotics and other psychotropic drugs that may alter blood composition
  - Assess renal and liver functioning which may affect elimination of drugs that are likely to be taken long-term and possibly in depot form.
- If the patient presents with a first episode of psychosis, a good basic screen comprises full blood count, erythrocyte sedimentation rate, urea and electrolytes, thyroid function, liver function tests, glucose, serum calcium, and a syphilis serology test if syphilis is suspected.
- A urine drug screen should always be done because illicit drugs both cause and exacerbate a psychosis.
- An electrocardiogram (ECG) should be done in patients with cardiac problems as many antipsychotics prolong the QT interval and have the potential to cause lethal ventricular arrhythmia.
- The use of a routine EEG or CT scan to help exclude an organic psychosis (e.g. temporal lobe epilepsy, brain tumour) varies between psychiatric units; they should always be considered in atypical cases, cases with treatment resistance, or if there are cognitive or neurological abnormalities.

DISCUSSION OF CASE STUDY

Mr PP meets the ICD-10 criteria for schizophrenia, paranoid subtype. He has had a marked deterioration in his social and work functioning. He has delusions of persecution (believing he was a victim of government experiments), thought control (believing that ideas were being planted in his head (thought insertion)) and reference (believing that the man in pub was referring specifically to him). His claim that he knew these things after hearing the neighbour's dog bark suggests delusional perception. He also has second person command hallucinations and third person, running commentary hallucinations. 'Receiving coded information' from the radio might be a hallucination or a delusion of reference depending on how Mr PP described this experience subjectively. Mr PP's description that 'all was not right' could indicate the presence of a delusional atmosphere, prior to the development of the full-blown delusions.

It is imperative that a substance-induced psychotic disorder or psychotic disorder secondary to a medical condition is excluded. It would be important to ascertain the duration of Mr PP's psychotic symptoms. It seems as though he has had schizophrenic symptoms for over a month. If the duration of symptoms had been less than a month, it would be advisable to diagnose a schizophrenia-like psychotic disorder, e.g. acute and transient psychotic disorder. It is important to rule out a mood disorder with psychotic features. The presence of a mood episode associated with simultaneous schizophrenic symptoms would suggest a schizoaffective episode. Prominent hallucinations militate against a diagnosis of delusional disorder.

Now go on to Chapter 19 to read more about the psychotic disorders and their management.

The patient with anxiety, fear or avoidance

10

● Objectives

After this chapter you should have an understanding of:
- The definition of anxiety and how it differs from fear
- The clinical features of anxiety
- The different types of anxiety disorders
- The fact that all psychiatric disorders can present with anxiety
- The fact that sufferers of phobias can appear calm if away from the phobic stimulus
- How to assess someone complaining of anxiety

Case summary

Mrs PA, a 32-year-old divorced interior designer, was referred to a consultant psychiatrist by her family doctor because of a 6-month history of sudden, dramatic anxiety attacks accompanied by heart palpitations, profuse sweating, dizziness, a choking sensation and a fear that she was going to die. There appeared to be no logical reason for the attacks and Mrs PA described them as coming on 'out of the blue'. They reached their maximum intensity within 2 minutes and seldom lasted longer than 15 minutes, occurring two to three times a week. Because of these attacks, which occurred in any situation and at any time of day, Mrs PA had stopped going into shops or crowded public places for fear of having an attack and not being able to escape to a safe place and appearing like a 'blubbering fool'. She had started relying on her mother to accompany her on 'absolutely necessary' household excursions 'just in case' she had another attack. Her GP had booked her off work for the past 3 months, as she was too frightened to visit potential clients' houses in the event that she had another attack. Mrs PA told the psychiatrist that she had almost become housebound and felt that she was 'losing her mind'. A full physical examination, routine blood tests including: full blood count, urea and electrolytes, fasting glucose, liver function, thyroid function and calcium concentration as well as an electrocardiogram (ECG) revealed no abnormalities.

(For a discussion of the case study see the end of the chapter)

Feelings of anxiety or fear are both common and essential to the human experience. It is the very uncomfortable nature of this experience that makes anxiety such an effective alerting, and therefore harm-avoiding, device. However, for the same reasons, when anxiety is excessive and unchecked it can create an extremely debilitating condition. To distinguish between normal and psychopathological anxiety it is important to observe the patient's level of functioning. The Yerkes–Dodson law states that the relationship between performance and anxiety has the shape of an inverted U: mild to moderate levels of anxiety improve performance, but high levels impair it. Figure 10.1 demonstrates the Yerkes–Dodson curve.

DEFINITIONS AND CLINICAL FEATURES

Both anxiety and fear are alerting signals that occur in response to a potential threat. Some authors suggest that anxiety occurs in response to threat that is unknown, internal or vague (i.e. objectless); whereas fear occurs in response to a threat from a known, external or definite object.

The experience of anxiety consists of two interrelated components: (1) thoughts of being apprehensive, nervous or frightened and (2) the awareness of a physical reaction to anxiety (autonomic or peripheral anxiety). Figure 10.2 summarizes the physical signs of anxiety. The experience of anxiety may lead to a change in behaviour, particularly an avoidance of the real or imagined threat.

There are two patterns of pathological anxiety:

1. Generalized (free-floating) anxiety does not occur in discrete episodes and tends to last for hours, days or

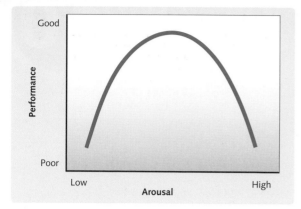

Fig. 10.1 Yerkes–Dodson law (1908)

Fig. 10.2 Physical signs of anxiety
Tachycardia
Palpitations (abnormal awareness of the heart beating)
Hypertension
Shortness of breath/rapid breathing
Chest pain or discomfort
Choking sensation
Tremors, shaking
Muscle tension
Dry mouth
Sweating
Cold skin
Nausea or vomiting
Diarrhoea
Abdominal discomfort ('butterflies')
Dizziness, light-headedness, syncope
Mydriasis (pupil dilatation)
Paraesthesia

even longer and is of mild to moderate severity. It is not associated with a specific external threat or situation (i.e. free-floating) but is rather excessive worry or apprehension about many normal life events (e.g. job security, relationships and responsibilities).

2. Paroxysmal anxiety has an abrupt onset, occurs in discrete episodes and tends to be quite severe. In its severest form, paroxysmal anxiety presents as panic attacks. These are discrete episodes of short-lived (usually less than 1 hour), intense anxiety. They have an abrupt onset and rapidly build up to a peak level of anxiety. They are accompanied by strong autonomic symptoms (see Fig. 10.2), which may lead patients to believe that they are dying, having a heart attack or going mad. This increases their anxiety level and produces further physical symptoms, thereby creating a vicious cycle.

See Figure 10.3 for a comparison of panic attacks and free-floating (generalized) anxiety. Quite often the two co-occur: someone with a background moderately elevated anxiety level can also have superimposed panic attacks.

Paroxysmal anxiety can further be subdivided into episodes of anxiety that occur seemingly spontaneously, without a specific imagined or external threat (see panic disorder, later) and those episodes that occur in response to a specific imagined or external threat. The phobic disorders are the most common cause of paroxysmal anxiety in response to a perceived threat.

A phobia is an intense, irrational fear of an object, activity or situation (e.g. flying, heights, animals, blood, public speaking). Although they may recognize that their fear is irrational, patients characteristically avoid the phobic stimulus or endure it with extreme distress. It is the degree of fear that is irrational in that the feared objects or situations are not inevitably dangerous and do not cause such severe anxiety in most other people. In severe cases, phobic anxiety may progress to frank panic attacks.

DIFFERENTIAL DIAGNOSIS

When considering the differential diagnosis of anxiety you should determine:

- The rate of onset, severity and duration of the anxiety, i.e. is the anxiety generalized or paroxysmal?
- Whether the anxiety is in response to a specific threat or arises spontaneously (unprovoked).
- Whether the anxiety only occurs in the context of a pre-existing psychiatric or medical condition.

Figure 10.4 presents the differential diagnosis for patients presenting with anxiety and Figure 10.5 gives a diagnostic algorithm.

Anxiety disorders

It is useful to consider the primary anxiety disorders under the headings: phobic disorders, non-situational disorders, reaction to stress and obsessive-compulsive disorder.

Phobic disorders

Remember that:

- Phobic disorders are associated with a prominent avoidance of the feared situation.
- The situationally induced anxiety may be so severe as to take the form of a panic attack.

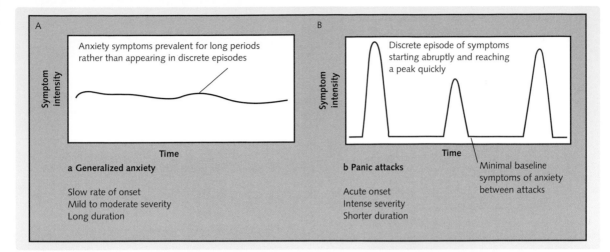

Fig. 10.3 Graphs comparing generalized (free-floating) anxiety (A) and panic attacks (B)

> **Fig. 10.4** Differential diagnosis for patients presenting with anxiety
>
> Anxiety disorders:
> - Phobic disorders
>   - Agoraphobia (with or without panic disorder)
>   - Social phobia
>   - Specific phobia
> - Non-situational disorders
>   - Generalized anxiety disorder
>   - Panic disorder
> - Reaction to stress
>   - Acute stress reaction
>   - Post-traumatic stress disorder
>   - Adjustment disorder
> - Obsessive-compulsive disorder
>   - Secondary to other psychiatric disorders (especially depression and psychosis)
>   - Secondary to a general medical condition
>   - Secondary to psychoactive substance use (especially alcohol use)

Agoraphobia

Agoraphobia literally means 'fear of the marketplace', i.e. fear of public places. In psychiatry today, it has a wider meaning that also includes a fear of entering crowded spaces (shops, trains, buses, elevators) where an immediate escape is difficult or in which help might not be available in the event of having a panic attack. At the worst extreme, patients may become housebound or refuse to leave the house unless accompanied by a close friend or relative.

There is a close relationship between agoraphobia and panic disorder that occurs when patients develop a fear of being in a place from where escape would be difficult in the event of having a panic attack. In fact, studies have shown that in a clinical setting, up to 95% of patients presenting with agoraphobia have a current or past diagnosis of panic disorder. Therefore,

in the ICD-10 you can code agoraphobia as occurring with or without panic disorder.

Social phobia

Patients with social phobia fear social situations where they might be exposed to scrutiny by others that might lead to humiliation or embarrassment. This fear might be limited to an isolated fear (e.g. public speaking, eating in public, fear of vomiting, or interacting with the opposite sex) or may involve almost all social activities outside the home.

Specific phobia

Specific (simple) phobias are restricted to clearly specific and discernible objects or situations (other than those covered in agoraphobia and social phobia). Examples from adult psychiatric samples in order of decreasing prevalence include:

- Situational: specific situations, e.g. public transportation, flying, driving, tunnels, bridges, elevators.
- Natural environment: heights, storms, water, darkness.
- Blood–injection–injury: seeing blood or an injury, fear of needles or an invasive medical procedure.
- Animal: animals or insects, e.g. spiders, dogs, mice.
- Other: fear of choking or vomiting, contracting an illness (e.g. HIV), children's fear of costumed characters.

> **HINTS AND TIPS**
>
> Even if a patient appears calm and denies troublesome anxiety symptoms, always screen for phobias. This is because sufferers of phobic disorders avoid their phobic stimulus. If this is the case, it is also important to establish how severely their lives are curtailed by avoidance.

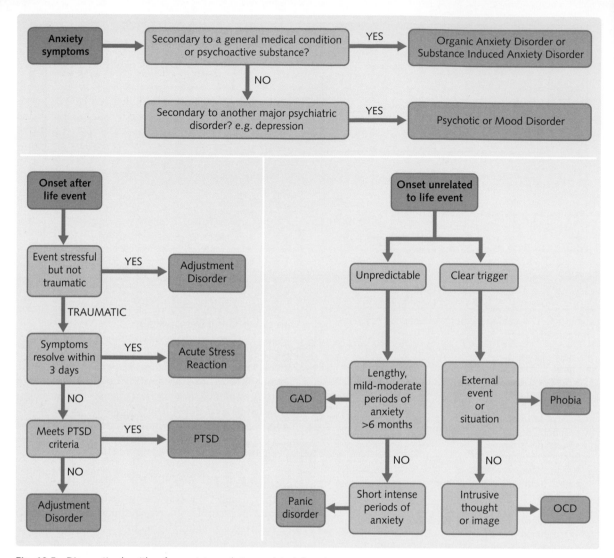

Fig. 10.5 Diagnostic algorithm for anxiety and stress related disorders

Non-situational anxiety disorders

These disorders, unlike the phobic disorders, are characterized by primary anxiety symptoms that are not restricted to any specific situation or circum-stance.

Generalized anxiety disorder

The key element of generalized anxiety disorder is long-standing, free-floating anxiety. Patients describe excessive worry about minor matters and should be apprehensive on most days for about 6 months. The ICD-10 diagnostic guidelines suggest three key elements:

1. Apprehension.
2. Motor tension (restlessness, fidgeting, tension headaches, inability to relax).
3. Autonomic overactivity (see Fig. 10.2).

> **HINTS AND TIPS**
>
> Blood–injection–injury phobias differ from others in that they are characterized by bradycardia and possibly syncope (vasovagal response), rather than tachycardia.

Panic disorder

Panic disorder is characterized by the presence of panic attacks that occur unpredictably and are not restricted to any particular situation (phobic disorders) or objective danger. Panic attacks are so distressing that patients commonly develop a fear of having further attacks; this is known as anticipatory anxiety. Anticipatory anxiety apart, patients are relatively free from anxiety symptoms between attacks.

Remember that many patients with panic disorder will also have concurrent agoraphobia, so in the ICD-10 you can code agoraphobia as occurring with or without panic disorder.

> ### COMMUNICATION
>
> When asking a patient whether they suffer from panic attacks, always define panic attacks for them (i.e. short, discrete episodes of extremely severe anxiety). This is because patients commonly use the term to describe non-specific anxiety.

Reaction to stress and obsessive-compulsive disorder

The disorders associated with a reaction to stress and obsessive-compulsive disorder are discussed in Chapters 12 and 11 respectively.

> ### HINTS AND TIPS
>
> Both agoraphobia and severe social phobia may result in patients becoming housebound and the two disorders can be difficult to distinguish. When in doubt, precedence should be given to agoraphobia.

Other psychiatric conditions

Anxiety is a non-specific symptom and can occur secondary to other psychiatric conditions. See Figure 10.6 for examples of psychiatric problems commonly associated with anxiety.

Note that depression and anxiety are closely intertwined. Not only can anxiety occur secondary to a depressive disorder and vice versa, but some authors have also suggested that the two disorders are aetiologically related. About 65% of patients with anxiety also have depressive symptoms; therefore, when making a diagnosis, it is essential to decide which symptoms came first or were predominant and which were secondary. If symptoms of anxiety occur only in the context of a genuine depressive episode then depression takes precedence and should be diagnosed alone.

Anxiety secondary to a general medical condition or psychoactive substance use

A medical or psychoactive substance cause of anxiety should always be actively sought and ruled out. Figure 10.7 lists the medical and substance-related causes of anxiety. The medical condition or substance use should predate the development of the anxiety and symptoms should resolve with treatment of the condition or abstinence from the offending substance. Absence of previous anxiety or absence of a family history of anxiety disorder also supports this diagnosis. Often symptoms can arise from a combination of a general medical condition and anxiety, as each predispose to the other. For example, if someone is having an acute asthma attack they will naturally feel anxious and breathe even faster. Helping them to calm down may be an important intervention.

Fig. 10.6 Examples of psychiatric problems commonly associated with anxiety

Focus of anxiety	Psychiatric problem
Gaining weight	Eating disorder (see Ch. 17)
Having many physical complaints	Somatization disorder (see Ch. 13)
Having a serious illness	Hypochondriacal disorder (see Ch. 13)
Fear of being poisoned or killed	Delusional beliefs in paranoid schizophrenia (see Ch. 9)
Ruminatory thoughts of guilt or worthlessness	Depression (see Ch. 7)
When having an obsessional thought or resisting a compulsion	Obsessive-compulsive disorder (see Ch. 11)
Separation or abandonment	Personality disorder (emotionally unstable or dependant) (see Ch. 16)
Being rejected or inadequate	Personality disorder (avoidant) (see Ch. 16)

Fig. 10.7 Medical conditions and substances that are associated with anxiety

Medical conditions	Substances		
	Intoxication	Withdrawal	Side-effects of prescribed drugs
Causing dyspnoea	Alcohol	Alcohol	Antidepressants (e.g. SSRIs and
Congestive cardiac failure	Amfetamines	Benzodiazepines	tricyclics in first 2 weeks of use)
Pulmonary embolism	Caffeine	Caffeine	Corticosteroids
Chronic obstructive	Cannabis	Cocaine	Sympathomimetics
airways disease	Cocaine	Nicotine	Thyroid hormones
Asthma	Hallucinogens	Other sedatives and	Compound analgesics containing
Causing increased	Inhalants	hypnotics	caffeine
sympathetic outflow	Phencyclidine	Opiates	Anticholinergics
Hypoglycaemia			Antipsychotics (akathisia)
Phaeochromocytoma			
Causing pain			
Malignancies			
Other			
Cerebral trauma			
Cushing's disease			
Hyperthyroidism			
Temporal lope epilepsy			
Vitamin deficiencies			

ASSESSMENT

History

The following questions may be helpful in eliciting anxiety symptoms:

- Do you sometimes wake up feeling anxious and dreading the day ahead? (any form of anxiety)
- Do you worry excessively about minor matters on most days of the week? (generalized anxiety)
- Have you ever been so frightened that your heart was pounding and you thought you might die? (panic attack)
- Do you avoid leaving the house alone because you are afraid of having a panic attack or being in situations (like being in a crowded shop or on a train) from which escape will be difficult or embarrassing? (agoraphobia)
- Do you get anxious in social situations, like speaking in front of people or making conversation? (social phobia)
- Do some things or situations make you very scared? Do you avoid them? (specific phobia)

Examination

A basic physical examination, including a thorough neurological and endocrine system examination, should be performed on all patients with symptoms of anxiety.

Investigations

The anxiety disorders can only be diagnosed when the symptoms are not due to the direct effect of a substance or medical condition. This stipulation is particularly relevant when considering diagnoses of generalized anxiety disorder and panic disorder. It is impractical to test for each of the large number of drugs and organic conditions capable of producing anxiety symptoms (see Fig. 10.7). It is, however, important to exclude any disease or substance that may be implicated through any clues in the history (e.g. past medical history and drug history) and physical examination. For example, a patient with a rapid pulse and heat intolerance should have thyroid function tests in case thyrotoxicosis is causing the anxiety symptoms. The possibility of withdrawal syndromes (e.g. alcohol, benzodiazepines, opiates) causing anxiety symptoms should also be considered.

DISCUSSION OF CASE STUDY

Repeated, unexpected episodes of short-lived intense anxiety of abrupt onset and rapidly building up to a peak level of anxiety associated with palpitations, sweating, dizziness, a choking sensation and thoughts of being about to die, with no medical cause, suggests a diagnosis of panic disorder.

As is common in many patients with panic disorder, agoraphobia has developed as a super-added problem as evidenced by a fear of going into situations from which escape might be difficult or humiliating. Mrs PA is showing the important sign of avoidance of the feared situation by refusing to go out unless it is essential and then only accompanied by her mother. Note that fear of having another panic attack indicates anticipatory anxiety; fear of having a panic attack in a situation from which escape will be difficult or humiliating, thus resulting in avoidance of those situations indicates agoraphobia – Mrs PA has both.

It is important to rule out depression or other psychiatric conditions as well as medical conditions and psychoactive substance use.

Now go on to Chapter 20 to read about the anxiety disorders and their management.

The patient with obsessions and compulsions

Objectives

After this chapter you should have an understanding of:
- The definitions of an obsession and a compulsion
- The differential diagnosis of a patient presenting with obsessional features
- How to assess someone presenting with obsessionality
- How to determine which disorder the patient is actually suffering from

Case summary

Mr OC is a 22-year-old medical student and has recently moved into his own flat. He describes a 5-month history of recurrent thoughts that he has behaved in a sexually inappropriate way towards his mother. He says that even though on one level he knows that this is impossible, he is unable to push these thoughts away despite trying 'rigorous mental gymnastics'. The only way he is able to relieve the distress he experiences is to actually contact his mother for reassurance that his fears are not true. On most days, he physically has to go and see his mother, and will spend up to 2 hours analysing his behaviour with her until he feels reassured. Whenever he tries to stop himself from seeking reassurance, he feels a rapid escalation in anxiety, thinking that not contacting his mother is evidence that his thoughts 'might be true'. He shudders in horror when asked whether he has ever had any sexual feelings for his mother but admits that these distressing thoughts are 'obviously' his own. He is heterosexual and has recently become engaged. He is extremely embarrassed and was eventually persuaded to see his general practitioner (GP) by his mother and fiancée when he started falling behind with his studies. He says that the whole thing is starting to depress him and that he has lost weight.

*(For a discussion of the case study
see the end of the chapter)*

Obsessions or compulsions are terms that are often used in everyday language, e.g. 'she has an obsession with shoes' or 'he is a compulsive liar'. Psychiatrists, however, use these terms in a very specific way and it is important to elicit, recognize and understand obsessive-compulsive psychopathology.

DEFINITIONS AND CLINICAL FEATURES

Obsessions and compulsions

Obsessions are involuntary thoughts, images or impulses which have the following important characteristics:

- They are recurrent and intrusive, and are experienced as unpleasant or distressing.
- They enter the mind against conscious resistance. Patients try to resist but are unable to do so.
- Patients recognize obsessions as being the product of their own mind (not from without as in thought insertion (see p. 69 and Fig. 11.4)) even though they are involuntary and often repugnant.

Obsessions are not merely excessive concerns about normal life problems, and patients generally retain insight into the fact that their thoughts are irrational. In fact, patients often see their obsessions as foreign to, or against, their 'essence' (ego-dystonic or ego-alien), e.g. a religious man has recurrent thoughts that he has betrayed God (also, see case study).

COMMUNICATION

When asking a patient if they are suffering from obsessional thinking, always define 'obsession'. This is because, like many psychiatric terms, 'obsession' has other, less specific meanings.

Compulsions are repetitive mental operations (counting, praying or repeating a mantra silently) or physical acts (checking, seeking reassurance, handwashing, strict rituals) that have the following unique characteristics:

- Patients feel compelled to perform them in response to their own obsessions (see case study) or irrationally defined 'rules' (e.g. 'I must count to 10 000 four times before falling asleep').
- They are performed to reduce anxiety through the belief that they will prevent a 'dreaded event' from occurring, even though they are not realistically connected to the event (e.g. compulsive counting each night to prevent 'family catastrophe') or are ridiculously excessive (e.g. spending hours handwashing in response to an obsessive fear of contamination).

Compulsions are experienced as unpleasant and serve no realistically useful purpose despite their tension-relieving properties. Similarly to obsessions, patients resist carrying out compulsions. Resisting compulsions, however, causes increased anxiety.

Obsessions and compulsions are often closely linked, as the desire to resist or neutralize an obsession produces a compulsive act (see Fig. 11.1 for examples of the most commonly occurring obsessions and compulsions). It can be difficult enquiring about obsessions and compulsions, especially when patients do not offer them as a presenting complaint. Figure 11.2 suggests some useful questions in eliciting these symptoms.

Fig. 11.1 Examples of the most commonly occurring obsessions and their associated compulsions in descending order

Obsession	Compulsion
Fear of contamination (feared object is usually impossible to avoid, e.g. faeces, urine, germs)	Excessive washing and cleaning. Avoidance of contaminated object
Pathological doubt ('Have I turned the stove off?' 'Did I lock the door?')	Exhaustive checking of the possible omission
Reprehensible violent, blasphemous or sexual thoughts, images or impulses (e.g. impulse to stab husband, having thoughts that one might be a paedophile)*	Act of 'redemption' (e.g. repeating 'Forgive me, I have sinned' 15 times) or seeking reassurance (see case study)
Need for symmetry or precision	Repeatedly arranging objects to obtain perfect symmetry

Patients often have these isolated obsessions without associated compulsions

Fig. 11.2 Questions used to elicit obsessions and compulsions

Do you worry about contamination with dirt even when you have already washed?
Do you have awful thoughts entering your mind despite trying hard to keep them out?
Do you repeatedly have to check things that you have already done (stoves, lights, taps, etc.)?
Do you find that you have to arrange, touch or count things many times over?

DIFFERENTIAL DIAGNOSIS

Obsessions and compulsions may occur as a primary illness as in obsessive-compulsive disorder (OCD) or may be clinical features of other psychiatric conditions. If patients have genuine obsessions or compulsions without other psychiatric symptoms then the diagnosis is simply obsessive-compulsive disorder. For a definite diagnosis the ICD-10 has proposed certain guidelines, as presented in Figure 11.3.

Many other psychiatric conditions may also present with repetitive or intrusive thoughts, impulses, images or behaviours (see Fig. 11.4). However, it is usually possible to differentiate them from OCD by applying the strict definition of obsessions and compulsions. Also, when repetitive thoughts occur in the context of other mental disorders, the contents of these thoughts are limited exclusively to the type of disorder concerned, e.g. morbid fear of fatness in anorexia nervosa, ruminatory thoughts of worthlessness in depression, fear of dreaded objects in phobias. Figure 11.5 lists the differential diagnoses and key distinguishing features of patients presenting with obsessive-compulsive symptomatology. OCD can also be comorbid with other psychiatric conditions, particularly depression and less commonly schizophrenia. Figure 11.6 suggests a diagnosis algorithm that may be useful in differentiating OCD from other psychiatric conditions (see also Fig. 10.5).

Fig. 11.3 ICD-10 diagnostic guidelines for obsessive-compulsive disorder

- Obsessions or compulsions must be present for at least 2 successive weeks and are a source of distress or interfere with the patient's functioning
- They are acknowledged as coming from the patient's own mind
- The obsessions are unpleasantly repetitive
- At least one thought or act is resisted unsuccessfully (note that in chronic cases some symptoms may no longer be resisted)
- A compulsive act is not in itself pleasurable (excluding the relief of anxiety)

Fig. 11.4 Differentiating types of repetitive or intrusive thoughts or images

Term	Description
Obsession	Unpleasant, recurrent, intrusive thought, image or impulse. Patient attributes origin within self. Involuntary and resisted (ego-dystonic)
Hallucination	Involuntary perception occurring in the absence of a stimulus experienced as indistinguishable from a normal perception
Pseudohallucination	Involuntary perception in the absence of stimulus experienced in internal space. Experienced vividly, as opposed to an obsessional image which may lack detail or completeness. Not usually resisted
Rumination	Repeatedly thinking about the causes and experience of previous distress and difficulties. Voluntary, not resisted
Thought insertion	Intrusive thought, image or impulse. Patient attributes origin outside self. May or may not be resisted
Over-valued idea	Plausible belief arrived at logically but held with undue importance. Not resisted or viewed as abnormal
Delusion	Fixed belief arrived at illogically and not amenable to reason. Not culturally normal. May or may not be plausible. Not resisted

Fig. 11.5 Differential diagnosis for patients presenting with obsessions or compulsions

Diagnosis	Diagnostic features
Obsessions and compulsions	
Obsessive-compulsive disorder	At least 2 weeks of genuine obsessions and compulsions (see Fig. 11.3)
Eating disorders (see Ch. 17)	Morbid fear of fatness (over-valued idea) Thoughts and actions are not recognized by patient as excessive or unreasonable and are not resisted (ego-syntonic) Thoughts do not necessarily provoke, or actions reduce, distress *Note: there is a higher incidence of true obsessive-compulsive disorder in patients with anorexia nervosa*
Obsessive-compulsive (anankastic) personality disorder (see Ch. 16)	Enduring behaviour pattern of rigidity, doubt, perfectionism and pedantry Ego-syntonic No true obsessions or compulsions
Mainly obsessions	
Depressive disorder (see Ch. 7)	Obsessive-compulsive symptoms occur simultaneously with, or after the onset of, depression and resolve with treatment Obsessions are mood-congruent, e.g. ruminatory thoughts of worthlessness
Other anxiety disorders (see Ch. 10)	Phobias: provoking stimulus comes from external object or situation rather than patient's own mind Generalized anxiety disorder: excessive concerns about real-life circumstances Absence of genuine obsessions or compulsions
Hypochondriacal disorder (see Ch. 13)	Obsessions only related to the fear of having a serious disease or bodily disfigurement
Schizophrenia (see Ch. 9)	Thought insertion: patients believe that thoughts are not from their own mind Presence of other schizophrenic symptoms Lack of insight
Mainly compulsions	
Habit and impulse-control disorders: pathological gambling, kleptomania, trichotillomania	Repetitious impulses and behaviour (gambling, stealing, pulling out hair) with no other unrelated obsessions/compulsions Concordant with the patient's own wishes (therefore ego-syntonic)
Gilles de la Tourette's syndrome (see Ch. 27)	Motor and vocal tics, echolalia, coprolalia *Note: 35–50% of patients with Gilles de la Tourette's syndrome meet the diagnostic criteria for obsessive-compulsive disorder, whereas only 5–7% of patients with obsessive-compulsive disorder have Tourette's syndrome*

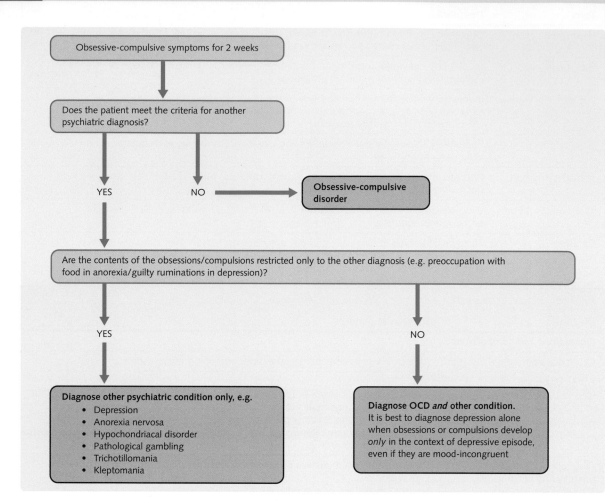

Fig. 11.6 Algorithm for the diagnosis of obsessions and compulsions

You should always consider depression in patients with obsessions or compulsions because:

- Over 20% of depressed patients can have obsessive-compulsive symptoms, which occur simultaneously at or after the onset of depression. They invariably resolve with treatment of the depression.
- Over two-thirds of patients with OCD experience a depressive episode in their lifetime. Obsessions and compulsions are present before and persist after the treatment of depression.
- OCD is a disabling illness and patients often have chronic mild depressive symptoms that do not fully meet the criteria for a depressive episode. These symptoms usually resolve when the OCD is treated and the patient's quality of life improves.

DISCUSSION OF CASE STUDY

Mr OC has genuine obsessions (recurrent, intrusive thoughts that are distressing, resisted and recognized as being from his own mind) and compulsions (repeatedly and excessively seeking reassurance to relieve anxiety caused by obsessions). He also describes symptoms of depression (depressed mood and weight loss).

His most likely diagnosis is obsessive-compulsive disorder (OCD); however, it is important to consider depression. In this case, the depressed mood developed after the obsessive-compulsive symptoms. If Mr OC now met the criteria for a depressive episode then OCD and depression would be diagnosed. He most probably has mild 'reactive' depression, which will resolve when the OCD is treated (see Fig. 11.6).

Now go on to Chapter 20 to read about obsessive-compulsive disorder and its management.

The patient with a reaction to a stressful event or bereavement

Objectives

After this chapter you should have an understanding of:
- The definition of a stressful event
- The different psychiatric disorders that can be induced by stressful or adverse events
- How to distinguish between stress-induced psychiatric disorders
- How to distinguish stress-induced psychiatric disorders from other psychiatric disorders

Case summary

Mrs PT, a 28-year-old divorced woman, was referred to a psychiatrist. She was well and working as a cleaner until 3 months ago when, on her way to work one evening, two men cornered her at a secluded bus shelter. They pushed her to the ground and raped her, threatening to 'slit her throat' if she screamed. The men ran off when they heard someone approaching, leaving Mrs PT shaken but with only superficial cuts and bruises. She felt low in mood for a few days after the assault, but attempted to carry on with her job and forget what had happened. In the month that followed, Mrs PT avoided all attempts by her family and friends to talk about the incident. She became socially withdrawn, only leaving the house to go to work. After a month, she started having nightmares about the incident and would wake up drenched in sweat. Her work colleagues noticed that she had become 'jumpy and quick-tempered' and that sudden movements or noises startled her. She had also started avoiding public transportation and refused to watch television for fear that something might remind her of the rape. Mrs PT finally sought medical help after her work supervisor found her lying on the floor, seemingly in a trance, screaming 'Leave me alone!' repeatedly. She recounted to her psychiatrist how she 're-lived' the rape in her mind and thought she could hear the the men threatening her, just like they did during the incident. The psychiatrist noticed that Mrs PT could not recall certain important aspects of the assault.

(For a discussion of the case study see the end of the chapter)

It is not unusual to have some psychological symptoms after a stressful event or bereavement. However, in some cases, these symptoms may be more severe than expected, and impact upon everyday functioning. It is important to be able to distinguish a normal reaction to a difficult life event from a specific constellation of symptoms that denote psychopathology requiring clinical attention.

DEFINITIONS AND CLINICAL FEATURES

When assessing someone who may have had a pathological response to a stressful event, it is important to explore two variables: (1) the nature and severity of the life event; and (2) the nature and severity of the person's reaction to the life event.

Nature and severity of the life event

Stress

'Psychosocial stressor' is the term used for any life event, condition or circumstance that places a strain on a person's current coping skills. It is important to remember that what constitutes a 'stressor' is subjective, and dependent on the specific person's ability to adapt or respond to a specific life challenge. For example, one student may breeze through an exam without experiencing any stress, while another may feel incredibly strained because of a perceived (or actual) mismatch between their ability and the demands of the situation. Also note that the same person's coping skills vary throughout their developmental life: the death of a distant relative may be far more stressful for a middle-aged man contemplating his own mortality than for an 'invincible' adolescent.

Traumatic stress

A traumatic stressor occurs outside the range of normal human experience, and its magnitude means that it would be experienced as traumatic by most people. This type of stress occurs in situations where a person feels that their own (or a loved one's) physical or psychological integrity is under serious threat. These include natural disasters, physical or sexual assaults, serious road traffic accidents, terrorist attacks, torture and military combat. Bereavement is a special case of traumatic stress that will be discussed later.

Nature and severity of patient's reaction

Some people seem to experience stressful or traumatic life events with minimal symptoms, while others seem more susceptible to developing a diagnosable disorder. Depending on the severity of the stressor and their underlying vulnerability, patients may develop: (1) an adjustment disorder; (2) an acute stress reaction or post-traumatic stress disorder (PTSD); (3) a dissociative disorder; or (4) another major mental illness such as a depressive, anxiety or psychotic disorder.

Adjustment disorder

Feeling unable to cope is common at times of psychosocial stresses to which we need to adapt or adjust (such as moving house, changing job or becoming a parent). However, when symptoms are considered significant enough to be out of proportion to the original stressor, or cause disturbance of social or occupational functioning, this can be described as an adjustment disorder. For this diagnosis to be made, the emotional and/or behavioural symptoms need to occur within 3 months (according to DSM-IV; ICD-10 states 1 month) of the original stressor. Although it is assumed that the disorder would not have arisen without the original stressor, an individual's personality and vulnerability to stress play an important contributing role. Symptoms usually fully resolve within 6 months of onset, and if this is not

the case, consideration should be given to a different diagnosis.

Usually, adjustment disorder is characterized by mood and/or anxiety symptoms, and this can occasionally be of severity sufficient to cause disturbances of conduct (e.g. reckless driving, aggressive behaviour). Many people with adjustment disorder also experience suicidal ideation.

Acute stress reaction

The symptoms of an acute stress reaction (combat fatigue, psychic shock) develop immediately after, or within a few minutes of, a traumatic stressor. Typically, sufferers will experience an initial 'dazed' state followed by possible disorientation and a narrowing of attention with inability to process external stimuli. In some cases, this may be followed either by a period of diminished responsiveness (to the extreme of a dissociative stupor) or psychomotor agitation and overactivity. Patients may also have amnesia for the episode (see Fig. 12.1 for dissociative amnesia and stupor). These symptoms normally begin to diminish after 24–48 hours, and are usually minimal after 3 days.

Post-traumatic stress disorder

The symptoms of post-traumatic stress disorder (PTSD) usually develop after 1 month but within 6 months of a traumatic stressor, and lead to significant distress or functional impairment. Symptoms include all of the following:

- Repetitive re-experiencing of the traumatic event in the form of:
  - Flashbacks (intrusive, unwanted memories; vivid mental images or dreams of the original experience)
  - Distress caused by internal or external cues that resemble the stressor (at times, patients may dissociate and experience the original event as though it were happening at that moment)
  - Patients may also experience hallucinations and illusions.
- Avoidance of stimuli associated with the stressor, amnesia for aspects of the trauma, as well as emotional numbness and social withdrawal.
- Increased arousal (insomnia, angry outbursts, hypervigilance, poor concentration, exaggerated *startle response*).

Fig. 12.1	Dissociative ('conversion') disorders
Dissociative amnesia	Partial or complete memory loss for events of a traumatic or stressful nature not due to normal forgetfulness, organic brain disorders or intoxication
Dissociative fugue	Rare disorder characterized by amnesia for personal identity, including memories and personality. Self-care and social interaction are maintained. Usually short-lived (hours to days), but can last longer. Very often involves seemingly purposeful travel beyond the individual's usual range, and in some cases a new identity may be assumed
Dissociative stupor	Severe psychomotor retardation characterized by extreme unresponsiveness, lack of voluntary movement and mutism, not due to a physical or psychiatric disorder (that is, not due to depressive, manic or catatonic stupor)
Dissociative anaesthesia and sensory loss	Cutaneous or visual sensory loss that does not correspond to anatomic dermatomes or known neurological patterns
Dissociative motor disorders	Partial or complete paralysis of one or more muscle groups not due to any physical cause
Dissociative convulsions (psychogenic non-epileptic seizures)	Used to be known as 'pseudoseizures'; however, the name has been changed because of concerns that the term 'pseudo' implies a degree of voluntary control (which is not the case). May present similarly to epileptic seizures but tongue-biting, serious injury and urinary incontinence are uncommon. There is also absence of epileptic activity on the electroencephalogram (EEG)
Ganser's syndrome	Complex disorder characterized by 'approximate answers', e.g. when asked what colour the grass is, an approximate response will be 'blue'
Multiple personality disorder (dissociative identity disorder)	Apparent existence of two or more personalities within the same individual. This is a rare and highly controversial diagnosis

HINTS AND TIPS

When assessing a patient with suspected PTSD, remember that head injuries and epilepsy are important differential diagnoses that may present with similar symptoms, and may also have been caused by the initial trauma. Patients with PTSD also have a high rate of comorbid substance misuse, and it is important to be vigilant for symptoms of alcohol or drug intoxication/withdrawal.

Dissociation

In clinical psychiatry, 'dissociation' describes a disruption in the usually integrated functions of consciousness and cognition. In this phenomenon, memories of the past, awareness of identity, thoughts, emotions, movement, sensation and/or control of behaviour become separated from the rest of an individual's personality such that they function independently and are not open to voluntary control. Figure 12.1 describes the more common dissociative disorders.

HINTS AND TIPS

Depersonalization is feeling yourself to be strange or unreal. Derealization is feeling that external reality is strange or unreal. These can be considered as types of dissociation, and may be caused by psychiatric illness (e.g. depression, anxiety, schizophrenia), physical illness (e.g. epilepsy), psychosocial stress and substance abuse.

The ICD-10 requires that there be some evidence of a psychological causation (stressful events or disturbed relationships) in association with the onset of the dissociative symptoms. Also note that the diagnosis of dissociative disorder should not be made if there is evidence of a physical or psychiatric disorder that might explain the symptoms.

Historically, dissociative disorders have been termed 'hysteria'; however, this term is seldom used in modern psychiatry. The term 'conversion disorder' is often but not always used synonymously with dissociative disorders, so it is wise to clarify what exact symptoms are being described if this diagnosis is encountered. Also, it is worth noting that DSM-IV categorizes some dissociative disorders as somatoform disorders (see Ch. 13).

HINTS AND TIPS

Before accepting the diagnosis of a dissociative disorder, a neurological affliction or other psychiatric illness should be aggressively sought for and excluded.

Precipitation or exacerbation of an existing mental illness

The influence of a patient's environment on their mental health cannot be overemphasized. Almost all forms of mental illness (e.g. depression, psychotic illness, anxiety) can be precipitated or exacerbated by psychosocial ('life events') or traumatic stressors. However, unlike the above reactions in this group, there need not be a direct aetiological link with the stressor involved.

BEREAVEMENT

Bereavement is a unique kind of stress experienced by most people during their life, and is considered a normal human experience. A bereavement reaction usually occurs after the loss of a loved person but can also result from other losses, like the loss of a national figure, or a beloved pet. The normal course of grief after bereavement occurs in five phases (Fig. 12.2), although these should not be regarded as a rigid sequence that is passed through only once.

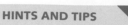

HINTS AND TIPS

The length of a normal bereavement reaction is variable and tends to be longer if the death was sudden and unexpected.

Although most people will meet the criteria for a depressive episode at some stage during the grieving process, bereavement reactions are not pathological and so no psychiatric diagnosis should be made in these cases. However, patients who have been bereaved are at higher risk for developing a depressive illness requiring treatment. The DSM-IV notes the following symptoms are not characteristic of a normal bereavement reaction and suggest the development of a major depressive episode:

1. Guilt (other than events surrounding the death of the loved one).
2. Suicidal ideation (other than feeling better off dead or wanting to be with the deceased).
3. Preoccupation with worthlessness.
4. Marked psychomotor retardation.

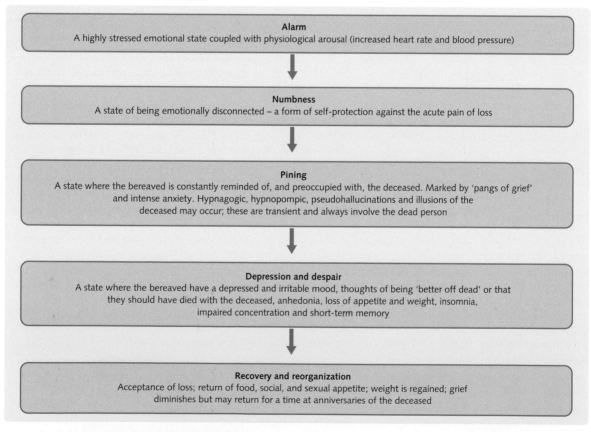

Fig. 12.2 Parkes's stages of normal bereavement

5. Prolonged and marked functional impairment.
6. Hallucinatory experiences (other than transiently seeing or hearing the deceased).

If a bereavement reaction is abnormal, assess for depression. If criteria for a depressive episode are not met, then a diagnosis of adjustment disorder is made.

DIFFERENTIAL DIAGNOSIS

The diagnosis is usually clear following thorough exploration of the nature and severity of both the life event and patient's reaction (see Fig. 12.3 and Fig. 10.5 for a diagnostic algorithm). Even if the onset of symptoms is clearly linked with a stressor, diagnosis of a specific major mental illness (mood disorder, psychotic disorder) should be given if diagnostic criteria are met, as major mental illnesses are often triggered by major stressors.

If a patient presents with psychiatric symptoms after a life-threatening event, always screen for features of depression as well as features of PTSD. This is because the risk of developing depression increases six fold in the 6 months that follow a stressful event.

DISCUSSION OF CASE STUDY

Mrs PT experienced a traumatic stressor in which she believed that her physical integrity was under immediate threat. The event was outside the range of normal human

Fig. 12.3 Differential diagnosis for patients presenting with a reaction to stress or trauma

Adjustment disorder
Acute stress reaction
Post-traumatic stress disorder
Normal bereavement reaction
Dissociative ('conversion') disorder
Exacerbation or precipitation of other psychiatric illness:
• Mood disorders
• Anxiety disorders
• Psychotic disorders (especially acute and transient psychotic disorders)
Malingering (see Ch. 13)

experience and would have been experienced as traumatic by most people. She subsequently developed avoidance of stimuli associated with the trauma (avoided talking or thinking about it, avoided public transportation and television), amnesia for aspects of the trauma and social withdrawal. Later on, she showed signs of increased arousal (startle response, being 'jumpy and quick-tempered'). Finally, Mrs PT repetitively re-experienced the trauma through nightmares, flashbacks and dissociation (re-living and behaving as though the trauma were occurring at that moment through mental imagery and hallucinations). All of the above suggest a diagnosis of post-traumatic stress disorder.

Now go on to Chapter 20 to read about the anxiety disorders and their management.

The patient with medically unexplained physical symptoms

Objectives

After this chapter you should have an understanding of:
- The definitions of somatoform disorder, factitious disorder and malingering
- The different types of somatoform disorders
- The differential diagnosis of a patient presenting with medically unexplained physical symptoms
- The principle that somatoform disorders can only be diagnosed when physical illness has been rigorously excluded
- How to assess someone complaining of medically unexplained physical symptoms

Case summary

Mrs SD, a 32-year-old mother of three, had consulted her GP at least once every 2 weeks for the past year. Her GP had known her for just over a year since she moved to the area after an acrimonious divorce. Her medical history, part of which was obtained from her previous GP, was substantial, and her health difficulties had precluded her from employment. At menarche, she was diagnosed with dysfunctional uterine bleeding and dysmenorrhoea. Later, extensive investigations, including three exploratory laparoscopies, revealed no physical cause for persistent upper abdominal pain with alternating diarrhoea and constipation. Three years ago, Mrs SD presented with urinary frequency and dysuria. Exhaustive investigations including cystoscopy, urodynamic studies and radiography, were all normal. She had also been referred to various specialists including a rheumatologist due to chronic neck pain that she had described as: 'the pain that has ruined mine and my kids' life!' Again, physical examination and investigations revealed no abnormalities. Mrs SD was taking up to 30 codeine tablets daily and could not sleep without two different types of sleeping tablets. Despite a difficult childhood, which featured a violent, alcohol-abusing father, and two abusive marriages that had ended in divorce, Mrs SD refused to contemplate her doctor's suggestion that there might be a psychological explanation for her symptoms. However, she eventually agreed to an appointment with a psychiatrist when she developed hearing loss after her 13-year-old daughter became pregnant.

(For a discussion of the case study see the end of the chapter)

The historical description of the mind–body duality (the relationship between the mind, or *'psyche'*; and the body, or *'soma'*) is well known, and it is clear that the mind and the body are not the separate entities they were once considered. In the same way that physical illness can have an effect on the brain (e.g. delirium), psychological disturbances can manifest as physical symptoms (e.g. dry mouth).

In recent years, medically unexplained physical symptoms have been described as 'functional symptoms' (rather than symptoms as a result of 'structural' or pathological disease). Many specialties have become very adept at identifying and managing symptoms. It is also worth noting that even though no structural disease has been identified, it does not mean that one does not exist – it may remain undiscovered thus far to medical science. For example: epilepsy, migraine, multiple sclerosis and stomach ulcers were historically considered 'functional' illnesses.

However, often the patterns of such symptoms involve multiple systems, or are clearly associated with a great deal of anxiety or obvious psychosocial stressor. If functional symptoms are associated with significant anxiety or stress, or a comorbid psychiatric illness, it can be useful to refer to psychiatry.

Patients with functional symptoms are often stigmatized by healthcare providers, with their genuine difficulties being labelled 'fat folder syndrome', 'all in the mind' and 'the worried well'. Having an understanding of the psychiatric disorders that may mimic physical illness, and the impairment that can result, is invaluable for all junior doctors.

> **COMMUNICATION**
>
> Many of the terms used for medically unexplained symptoms are perceived as stigmatizing but the term 'functional symptoms' is acceptable to most patients and colleagues. Functional symptoms are those without identifiable structural cause. They can be likened to 'software' rather than 'hardware' problems in the body.

DEFINITIONS AND CLINICAL FEATURES

A structural or physical cause should always be considered in response to reported 'physical symptoms'. However, in certain cases, the reported symptoms:

- Do not correspond to, or are clearly not typical of, any known physical condition.
- Are associated with an absence of any physical signs or structural abnormalities.
- Are associated with an absence of any abnormalities in comprehensive laboratory, imaging and invasive investigations.

In these cases, psychiatric illness should be considered, especially when unexplained physical symptoms bear a close relationship with stressful life events or psychological difficulties.

> **COMMUNICATION**
>
> To avoid confusion, you should be able to readily define 'somatoform disorder', 'somatization disorder', 'hypochondriacal disorder', and be able to distinguish them from the 'somatic syndrome of depression', 'factitious disorder' and 'malingering'.

Somatoform disorders

The somatoform disorders are a class of disorders whose symptoms are suggestive of, or take the form of, physical illness. However, there are no detectable structural or neurophysiological abnormalities to explain these symptoms, leading to the presumption that they are caused by psychological factors. Note that these symptoms are not under voluntary control: they occur

unintentionally, as opposed to the intentional feigning or production of symptoms in factitious disorder and malingering.

> **COMMUNICATION**
>
> It is important to acknowledge that even though no physical disease has been found, the functional impairment and distress caused by somatoform disorders is genuine and that the symptoms are neither under conscious control nor are they being feigned. Empathic acknowledgement and explanation can be very therapeutic in itself. Dismissing a patient by telling them that their symptoms are 'all in your mind' is unhelpful and potentially harmful.

Somatization disorder (Briquet's syndrome)

The central features of somatization disorder are multiple, recurrent and frequently changing physical symptoms, with the absence of identifiable physiological explanation. These include:

- Gastrointestinal: nausea, vomiting, diarrhoea, constipation, food intolerance, abdominal pain.
- Sexual or reproductive: loss of libido, ejaculatory or erectile dysfunction, irregular menses, menorrhagia, dysmenorrhoea.
- Urinary: dysuria, frequency, urinary retention, incontinence.
- Neurological: paralysis, paraesthesia, sensory loss, seizures, difficulty swallowing, impaired coordination or balance.

To meet diagnostic criteria, patients should have numerous symptoms from almost all of these systemic groups, not just one or two isolated symptoms.

For the diagnosis of somatization disorder, the ICD-10 suggests that all of the following be present:

- At least 2 years of symptoms with no physical explanation found.
- Persistent refusal by the patient to accept reassurance from several doctors that there is no physical cause for the symptoms.
- Some degree of functional impairment due to the symptoms and resulting behaviour.

Most patients with somatization disorder will have a long history of contact with medical services, during which numerous investigations may have been conducted. This often results in iatrogenic disease with physically explainable symptoms (e.g. abdominal adhesions from frequent exploratory surgery). Due to frequent courses of medication, these patients are often dependent on analgesics and sedatives.

Hypochondriacal disorder

In hypochondriacal disorder, patients misinterpret normal bodily sensations, which lead them to believe that they have a serious and progressive physical disease. These patients tend to ask for investigations to definitively diagnose or confirm their underlying disease. However, despite repeated normal examination and investigations, hypochondriacal patients refuse to accept the reassurance of numerous doctors that they do not suffer from a serious physical illness. This is in contrast to somatization disorder, where patients tend to seek relief from their symptoms.

Body dysmorphic disorder

Body dysmorphic disorder (dysmorphophobia) is a variant of hypochondriacal disorder, in which patients are preoccupied with an imagined or minor defect in their physical appearance. ICD-10 considers this a subtype of hypochondriacal disorder; however, DSM-IV considers it a somatoform disorder in its own right. The symptoms should not be better accounted for by another disorder (e.g. concerns regarding weight and body shape are usually more accurately attributed to an eating disorder). This imagined defect or deformity can concern any part of the body (e.g. a 'crooked nose' or 'ugly hands'). The preoccupation causes significant distress or impairment in functioning.

The psychopathology of both hypochondriacal disorder and body dysmorphic disorder takes the form of an overvalued idea (see p. 68). The belief is not delusional because patients are open to some explanation and their fears can be allayed, at least for a short while. A persistent delusional disorder (somatic delusional disorder) is diagnosed if the belief is held with delusional intensity (see p. 67).

Somatoform autonomic dysfunction

Patients with this disorder have two types of symptoms, both concerning the autonomic nervous system. The first is characterized by objective evidence of autonomic arousal (e.g. sweating, palpitations and tremor). The second is characterized by more subjective symptoms (e.g. pains, burning, heaviness, tightness or feeling bloated). Patients attribute these to a particular organ or system that is largely under autonomic control, e.g. the cardiovascular system (Da Costa's syndrome), the respiratory system (psychogenic hyperventilation), or the gastrointestinal system (irritable bowel syndrome). Although patients with somatization disorder may have autonomic symptoms, they also have numerous other symptoms from multiple systems and the autonomic symptoms are not attributed to only one organ or system as in somatoform autonomic dysfunction.

Persistent somatoform pain disorder

The central feature of this disorder is severe and persistent pain that cannot be fully explained by physical illness. The pain usually occurs in association with emotional difficulties or psychosocial stressors. Although patients with somatization disorder may have symptoms of pain, they also have numerous symptoms from multiple systems and pain is not the overwhelmingly dominant symptom.

Conversion and dissociative disorders

'Conversion' is a psychoanalytical term that describes the hypothetical process whereby psychic conflict or pain undergoes 'conversion' into somatic or physical form to produce physical symptoms. The DSM-IV uses the term to describe the presence of one or more neurological symptoms that are not explained by any known neurological disease. ICD-10 considers these to be dissociative disorders. This book considers these in Chapter 12.

Factitious disorder and malingering

Both factitious disorder and malingering differ from somatoform disorders in that physical or psychological symptoms are produced intentionally or feigned. Patients may give convincing histories that fool even experienced clinicians and often manufacture signs (e.g. warfarin may be ingested to simulate bleeding disorders, insulin may be injected to produce hypoglycaemia, urine may be contaminated with blood or faeces). Certain patients feign psychiatric symptoms such as hallucinations, delusions, depression or dissociation. These patients can go undetected and may receive large doses of psychotropic medication.

Factitious disorder (Münchausen's syndrome)

The central feature of factitious disorder is focus on the primary (internal) gain of assuming the sick role (the aim to be cared for like a patient, usually in hospital). Although symptoms are feigned, it is important to understand that this care-seeking behaviour is usually a manifestation of psychological distress.

Malingering

Malingering patients focus on secondary (external) gain of the secondary consequence of being diagnosed with an illness (avoidance of military service, evading criminal prosecution, obtaining illicit drugs, obtaining benefits or compensation).

Münchausen syndrome by proxy

Also known as 'fabricated or induced illness', this describes a form of abuse where a carer (classically a parent) will seek help for fabricated or induced symptoms in a dependant (classically a child). The psychological aim of the carer is for the dependant to be cared for like a patient. The induction of a factitious disorder can be dangerous (e.g. covert poisoning) and once a diagnosis has been made, the dependent should be removed from the direct influence of the carer, and relevant authorities (most often child/adult protection agencies) alerted. The affected carer should be offered psychiatric help; however, because the disorder is rare, little is known about effective treatment.

DIFFERENTIAL DIAGNOSIS

The differential diagnosis for patients presenting with medically unexplained symptoms is shown in Figure 13.1. The flow chart in Figure 13.2 can help with reaching the correct diagnosis.

An underlying medical condition should be ruled out when patients present with unexplained physical symptoms. Somatization disorder can resemble insidious multi-system diseases such as systemic lupus erythematosus, multiple sclerosis, acquired immune deficiency syndrome (AIDS), hyperparathyroidism, occult malignancy and chronic infections.

Physical complaints often occur in the context of other psychiatric conditions. Patients with schizophrenia may have somatic delusions or visceral somatic hallucinations. However, the explanation of these symptoms is often quite odd and there are usually other psychotic symptoms accompanying the physical complaints. Individuals with depressed mood often present with numerous somatic complaints; these tend to be episodic and

---

Fig. 13.1 Differential diagnosis for patients presenting with medically unexplained symptoms

Somatoform disorders
- Somatization disorder
- Hypochondriacal disorder (including body dysmorphic disorder)
- Somatoform autonomic dysfunction
- Persistent somatoform pain disorder

Factitious disorder
Malingering
Other psychiatric conditions
- Anxiety disorders
- Mood disorders
- Psychotic disorders
- Dissociative disorders

Insidious multi-systemic disease

---

resolve with the treatment of the depression. Patients with panic disorder have multiple somatic symptoms while having panic attacks, but these resolve when the panic subsides. Patients with generalized anxiety disorder may also have multiple somatic preoccupations, but their anxiety is not limited to physical symptoms. Conversion and dissociative disorders (e.g. motor disorders, psychogenic non-epileptic seizures) can present with neurological symptoms without any evidence of an organic cause. However, these symptoms are usually clearly defined and isolated as opposed to the ill-defined, multiple symptoms in somatization disorder. The difficulty in distinguishing other mental disorders from somatization disorder is illustrated by the observation that at least half of patients with somatization disorder have another coexisting mental illness.

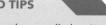

HINTS AND TIPS

Somatization disorder usually has its onset in early adult life. The onset of multiple physical symptoms late in life is more likely to be due to a physical illness.

ASSESSMENT

History

The following questions may be helpful in screening for somatoform disorders on mental state examination:
- Do you often worry about your health?
- Are you bothered by many different symptoms?
- Are you concerned you may have a serious illness?
- Are you concerned about your appearance?
- Do you find it hard to believe doctors when they tell you that there is nothing wrong with you?

Examination

A thorough physical examination with special focus on the presenting problem is imperative when dealing with somatoform complaints.

Investigations

Clinicians dealing with patients with a somatoform disorder need to investigate physical complaints judiciously. It is important to take all symptoms seriously, yet excessive and needless investigations to placate an anxious patient can result in a vicious circle with worsening of symptoms. Invasive investigations can result in

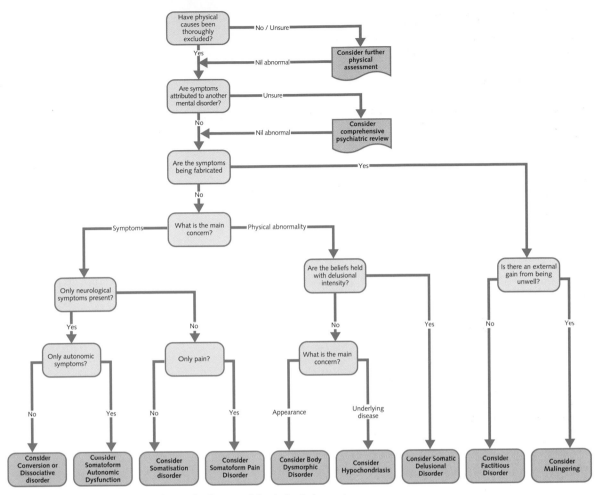

Fig. 13.2   Diagnostic flow chart for medically unexplained physical symptoms

iatrogenic harm. See Figure 20.4 in Chapter 20 for guidance on how to manage these patients.

DISCUSSION OF CASE STUDY

Mrs SD has a long history of multiple, recurrent, frequently changing physical symptoms for which no physical causes have been found despite extensive investigation. She is resistant to the idea that there might be a psychological reason for her symptoms despite the association of her symptoms with psychosocial stress. Her functioning has been impaired, and this has possibly impacted on her children's lives. Because she is focused on symptoms, not the idea that she has a serious and progressive illness, Mrs SD has somatization disorder as opposed to hypochondriacal disorder. As is typical, Mrs SD has a secondary (possibly iatrogenic) substance misuse problem (codeine and sleeping tablets). It would be important to exclude other mental illness, such as depression and anxiety, as causative factors. If there was evidence that Mrs SD intentionally produced or feigned her symptoms then factitious disorder or malingering should be considered.

Now go on to Chapter 20 to read about the somatoform disorders and their management.

After this chapter you should have an understanding of:
- The definitions of cognition and consciousness
- The different classification systems of memory
- The definition of dementia, the subtypes of dementia and how to distinguish them
- The definition and clinical features of delirium
- The definition and clinical features of amnesic syndrome
- The differential diagnosis of cognitive impairment
- How to assess a patient presenting with memory problems or cognitive impairment

Case summary

Mr DD, aged 78 years, lived at home with his wife with carers visiting twice daily. His general practitioner (GP) had referred him to a psychiatrist 6 years earlier, after he started experiencing difficulty remembering things. At first he would forget things like the social arrangements he had made. Later he started forgetting activities he had engaged in only the day before. His wife had noticed a gradual change in his personality in that he became increasingly withdrawn and sullen and, at times, verbally aggressive. His language deteriorated to the point where he would ramble incoherently, even when there was no one else in the room. Despite having smoked for many years, Mr DD seemed unable to recognize his pipe and would stare at it quizzically for hours. He lost the ability to dress himself or complete simple multi-step tasks such as making a cup of coffee.

His wife contacted their GP when one morning Mr DD was too sleepy to get out of bed. The GP arranged hospital admission for further investigation. Nurses were concerned because his consciousness level was fluctuating from hour to hour. He slept through most of the day, but would wander around the ward at night looking very agitated and appeared to have visual hallucinations. The senior nurse pointed out that he had developed a productive cough.

(For a discussion of the case study see the end of the chapter)

Cognitive impairment is common and important, but often under-diagnosed and under-investigated. It is associated with a high morbidity and mortality and you are likely to frequently encounter people with cognitive impairment in most specialities.

DEFINITIONS AND CLINICAL FEATURES

Consciousness

To be conscious is to be aware, both of the environment and of oneself as a subjective being. It is a global cognitive function. It is a poorly understood, complex phenomenon with multiple vaguely defined terms for its abnormalities. It is best to avoid terms such as 'confused', 'obtunded', 'clouding of consciousness', 'stupor' as they are not well defined and mean different things to different specialities. Clinically, the key question is whether someone has a normal or altered consciousness level. This is assessed at a practical level by observing arousal level (hyperaroused or lowered) (Fig. 14.1).

Cognition

This chapter considers 'cognition' in its broadest sense as meaning all the mental activities that allow us to perceive, integrate and conceptualize the world around us. These include the global functions of consciousness, attention and orientation and the specific domains of memory, executive function, language, praxis and perception. The term 'cognition' is used more narrowly in cognitive psychology and cognitive therapy where individual thoughts or ideas are also referred to as 'cognitions'.

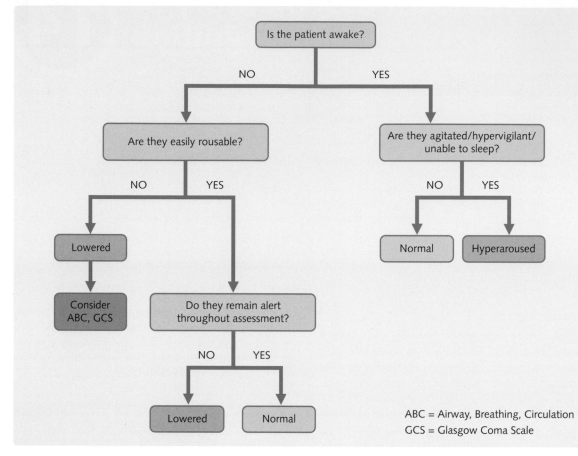

Fig. 14.1 Assessment of consciousness level

Impairments in cognition can be generalized (multiple domains) or specific (one domain only). An altered level of consciousness is generally associated with a generalized impairment in all aspects of cognition, as it is difficult to concentrate on any tasks when feeling very agitated or drowsy.

A very large number of specific cognitive impairments exist (Fig. 14.2). These can be isolated impairments, for example, if they are developmental or secondary to a small cerebrovascular accident, or occur together in disorders of generalized cognitive impairment such as dementia.

Memory

Memory is one of the commonest cognitive domains to be impaired. There are two main ways to categorize memory: the duration of storage (working or long term) or the type of information stored (implicit or explicit). Explicit memory (sometimes called *declarative memory*) includes all stored material of which the individual is consciously aware and can thus 'declare' to others. Implicit memory (sometimes called *procedural memory*) includes all material that is stored without the

individual's conscious awareness, e.g. the ability to speak a language or ride a bicycle.

Explicit memory is the most common type of memory to be disrupted. It can be further subdivided into *semantic* and *episodic* memory. Semantic memory is knowledge of facts, e.g. Edinburgh is the capital of Scotland. Episodic memory is knowledge of autobiographical events, e.g. remembering a trip to Edinburgh when you were 10 years old. See Figure 14.3 for the characteristics of different durations of explicit memory, and how to test them.

COMMUNICATION

There are different ways of classifying memory, and different terms have similar or overlapping meanings. For example, some clinicians use the term 'short-term memory' to mean recent long-term memory whereas others mean working memory. Therefore, when speaking to colleagues it can be useful to define the type of memory referred to by what test was used to measure it.

Fig. 14.2 Specific cognitive impairments

Cognitive domain	Term(s) for Impairment	Description
Language	Dysphasia/aphasia	Loss of language abilities despite intact sensory and motor function, e.g. difficulty in understanding commands or other words (receptive dysphasia) or difficulty using words with correct meaning (expressive dysphasia). Not being able to name items correctly despite knowing what they are (nominal dysphasia) is a subtype of expressive dysphasia
Praxis	Dyspraxia/apraxia	Loss of ability to carry out skilled motor movements despite intact motor function, e.g. inability to put a letter in an envelope, use a tin-opener, button up a shirt
Perception	Dysgnosia/agnosia	Loss of ability to interpret sensory information despite intact sensory organ function, e.g. not able to recognize faces as familiar
Memory	Amnesia	Loss of ability to learn or recall new information, e.g. not able to recall time or recent events, not able to learn new skills
Executive function (umbrella term for many abilities)	Many terms, including: Disinhibition Perseveration Apathy Dysexecutive syndrome	Loss of ability to plan and sequence complex activities, or to manipulate abstract information, e.g. not able to plan the preparation of a meal

Fig. 14.3 Explicit memory types, disorders and tests

Explicit memory type	Capacity Duration	Key brain regions	Tests
Working/ short term	7 ± 2 items 15–30 seconds	Frontal cortex	WORLD backwards Serial 7s
Long term (recent)	Unlimited Minutes to months	Hippocampus Mamillary bodies	Anterograde: delayed recall of an address or objects Retrograde: questions about recent events, e.g. what they had for breakfast
Long term (remote)	Unlimited Lifetime	Frontal and temporal cortex	Questions about past important events. Ask about personal events (episodic), e.g. what school they attended, and general knowledge (semantic), e.g. which USA president was assassinated in the 1960s?

Amnesia refers to the loss of the ability to store new memories or retrieve memories that have previously been stored. Anterograde amnesia occurs after an amnesia-causing event and results in the patient being unable to store new memories from the event onwards (impaired learning of new material), although the ability to retrieve memories stored before the event may remain unimpaired. Anterograde amnesia usually results from damage to the medial temporal lobes, especially the hippocampal formation.

Retrograde amnesia occurs after an amnesia-causing event and results in the patient being unable to retrieve memories stored before the event, although the ability to store new memories from the event onwards may remain unaffected. Retrograde amnesia usually results from damage to the frontal or temporal cortex.

HINTS AND TIPS

Implicit memory (procedural memory) is typically preserved despite severe disruptions to explicit (declarative) memory, probably due to its independent neural location. Implicit memory is associated with basal ganglia circuitry. Explicit memory is associated with the hippocampal and diencephalic structures.

COMMON COGNITIVE DISORDERS

Delirium

If someone has acute or fluctuating cognitive impairment and is drowsy or agitated, they are very likely to have delirium. Psychotic features such as hallucinations or persecutory delusions are often present but are not essential to make the diagnosis. Delirium often fluctuates, so a patient may appear normal on the morning ward round but cognitively impaired and agitated in the evening. Delirium usually resolves when the trigger is treated, but sometimes can be prolonged for weeks or months.

Delirium can be a final common pathway of severe injury to the brain or body, and is a marker of severity of illness (e.g. the 'C' in the CURB65 score for severity of community acquired pneumonia). It has a high mortality, with around a third of sufferers dying during the presentation. It is therefore a medical emergency and the cause should be aggressively investigated and treated (Fig. 14.4). It is particularly common in those with 'at risk' brains, such as those with pre-existing dementia. In individuals with vulnerable brains a relatively minor insult can result in delirium, e.g. dehydration or a new medication. Delirium is also a risk factor for development or worsening of dementia.

The terms 'acute confusional state' and 'encephalopathy' have roughly the same meaning as delirium. Prominent symptoms of delirium are described further below.

HINTS AND TIPS

Risk factors for delirium include an abnormal brain (e.g. dementia or previous serious head injury), age, polypharmacy and sensory impairment.

Impaired consciousness

Patients may have a reduced level of consciousness ranging from drowsiness to coma (hypoactive delirium), or they can be hypervigilant and agitated (hyperactive delirium). Their ability to sustain attention is reduced and they are easily distractible.

Impaired cognitive function

Short-term memory and recent memory are impaired with relative preservation of remote memory. Patients with delirium are almost always disorientated to time and often to place. Orientation to self is seldom lost. Language abnormalities such as rambling, incoherent speech and an impaired ability to understand are common.

Fig. 14.4 Causes of delirium (anything that disrupts homeostasis)

Systemic illness

Infections and sepsis

Anoxia
- Respiratory failure
- Heart failure
- Myocardial infarction

Metabolic and endocrine
- Electrolyte disturbances
- Uraemia
- Hepatic encephalopathy
- Porphyria
- Hypoglycaemia
- Hyper- and hypothyroidism
- Hyper- and hypoparathyroidism
- Hyper- and hypoadrenocorticism (Cushing's syndrome, Addison's disease)
- Hypopituitarism

Nutritional
- Thiamine (Wernicke's encephalopathy), vitamin B_{12}, folic acid or niacin deficiency

Drugs (use or discontinuation)

Prescribed (plus many more)
- Anticholinergics
- Benzodiazepines
- Opiates
- Antiparkinsonian drugs
- Steroids

Recreational
- Alcohol (delirium tremens, see p. 155)
- Opiates
- Cannabis
- Amfetamines

Poisons
- Heavy metals (lead, mercury, manganese)
- Carbon monoxide

Intracranial causes

Space-occupying lesions
- Tumours, cysts, abscesses, haematomas

Head injury (especially concussion)
Infection
- Meningitis
- Encephalitis

Epilepsy
Cerebrovascular disorders
- Transient ischaemic attack
- Cerebral thrombosis or embolism
- Intracerebral or subarachnoid haemorrhage
- Hypertensive encephalopathy
- Vasculitis (e.g. from systemic lupus erythematosus)

Perceptual and thought disturbance

Patients may have perceptual disturbances ranging from misinterpretations (e.g. a door slamming is mistaken for an explosion) to illusions (e.g. a crack in the wall is perceived as a snake) to hallucinations (especially visual and, to a lesser extent, auditory). Transient persecutory delusions and delusions of misidentification may occur.

Sleep–wake cycle disturbance

Sleep is characteristically disturbed and can range from daytime drowsiness and night-time hyperactivity to a complete reversal of the normal cycle. Nightmares experienced by patients with delirium may continue as hallucinations after awakening.

Mood disturbance

Emotional disturbances such as depression, euphoria, anxiety, anger, fear and apathy are common.

> **HINTS AND TIPS**
>
> A physical illness should always be ruled out whenever a patient presents with prominent visual hallucinations because patients with schizophrenia or psychotic mood disorders usually experience auditory hallucinations.

Dementia

Dementia is a syndrome of acquired progressive generalized cognitive impairment associated with functional decline. Consciousness level is normal. Symptoms should be present for 6 months before a diagnosis can be confirmed. The following text describes the general categories of impairment in dementia.

Functional impairment

Functional impairment must be present to make a diagnosis of dementia. Functional impairment means difficulties with basic or instrumental activities of daily living (ADL). Basic ADLs refer to self-care tasks such as eating, dressing, washing, toileting, continence and mobility (being able to make crucial movements such as from bed to chair to toilet). Instrumental ADLs refer to tasks which are not crucial to life but which allow someone to live independently, such as cooking, shopping and housework. As well as being diagnostically important, someone's ability to perform ADLs determines what level of support they need – home carers or 24-hour care.

Memory impairment

Impairment of memory is a common feature of dementia. Recent memory is first affected, e.g. forgetting where objects are placed, conversations and events of the previous day. With disease progression, all aspects of memory are affected, although highly personal information (name, previous occupation, etc.) is usually retained until late in the disease. Note that memory is essential for orientation to person, place and time and this will also be gradually affected, e.g. patients may lose their way in their own house.

Other cognitive symptoms (aphasia, apraxia, agnosia, impaired executive functioning)

See Figure 14.2.

Behavioural and psychological symptoms of dementia

'Behavioural and psychological symptoms of dementia' (BPSD) is an umbrella term for non-cognitive symptoms associated with dementia, including changes in behaviour, mood and psychosis. Behavioural symptoms are very common and include pacing, shouting, sexual disinhibition, aggression and apathy. Depression and anxiety may occur in up to half of all those with dementia. Delusions, especially persecutory, may occur in up to 40% of patients. Hallucinations in all sensory modalities (visual more common) occur in up to 30% of patients. BPSD can be similar to those of delirium, but generally have a more gradual onset and consciousness level is normal. See Figure 14.5 for more ways to differentiate BPSD from delirium.

Neurological symptoms

Between 10% and 20% of patients will experience seizures. Primitive reflexes (e.g. grasp, snout, suck) may also be evident as well as myoclonic jerks.

> **COMMUNICATION**
>
> When seeing a new patient with a likely diagnosis of dementia, always take a collateral history as patients may have poor insight and recall of their difficulties.

Distinguishing the type of dementia

Dementia can result from a primary neurodegenerative process or be secondary to substance use or another medical condition. Early onset dementia begins before

Fig. 14.5 Factors differentiating delirium from dementia		
Feature	Delirium	Dementia
Onset	Acute	Gradual
Duration	Hours to weeks	Months to years
Course	Fluctuating	Progressive deterioration
Consciousness	Altered	Normal
Context	New illness/ medication	Health unchanged
Perceptual disturbance	Common	Occurs in late stages
Sleep–wake cycle	Disrupted	Usually normal
Orientation	Usually impaired for time and unfamiliar people/places	Impaired in late stages
Speech	Incoherent, rapid or slow	Word finding difficulties.
Things you may think	'Why aren't they listening?', 'Why won't they wake up properly?', or 'They need to calm down'	'Why do they keep telling me about the past?', 'Why do they keep asking me the same question?'

Fig. 14.6 Diseases that may cause dementia

Neurodegenerative
- Alzheimer's disease
- Frontotemporal dementia (includes Pick's disease)
- Dementia with Lewy bodies (DLB)
- Parkinson's disease
- Huntington's disease
- Progressive supranuclear palsy

Cerebrovascular disease

Space-occupying lesions
- Tumours, cysts, abscesses, haematomas

Trauma
- Head injury
- Punch-drunk syndrome (dementia pugilistica)

Infection
- Creutzfeldt–Jakob disease (including 'new variant CJD')
- HIV-related dementia
- Neurosyphilis
- Viral encephalitis
- Chronic bacterial and fungal meningitides

Metabolic and endocrine
- Chronic uraemia (also dialysis dementia)
- Liver failure
- Wilson's disease
- Hyper- and hypothyroidism
- Hyper- and hypoparathyroidism
- Cushing's syndrome and Addison's disease

Nutritional
- Thiamine, vitamin B_{12}, folic acid or niacin deficiency (pellagra)

Drugs and toxins
- Alcohol (see p. 119), benzodiazepines, barbiturates, solvents

Chronic hypoxia

Inflammatory disorders
- Multiple sclerosis
- Systemic lupus erythematosus and other collagen vascular diseases

Normal pressure hydrocephalus

age 65 years. A small number of cases are due to treatable, potentially reversible causes (see Fig. 14.6). However, the most common causes of dementia are neurodegeneration and/or vascular disease. Figure 14.7 describes the distinguishing clinical features of the various types of dementias although clinically it is often very difficult to tell exactly what form of dementia is present, and definitive diagnosis can normally only be made by post-mortem. It is important to establish the likely underlying type of dementia because:

- A secondary dementia-causing process (e.g. brain tumour) may be detected and possibly halted.
- The progress of certain types of dementia may be slowed with specific medication (e.g. cholinesterase inhibitors in Alzheimer's disease).
- Certain drugs may be contraindicated in some dementias (e.g. antipsychotics can cause a catastrophic parkinsonian reaction in patients with dementia with Lewy bodies).
- The prognoses of the various dementias differ; this may have practical implications for patients and their families as regards final arrangements, e.g. wills.

- The patient's relatives may enquire about genetic counselling, e.g. Huntington's disease, early-onset Alzheimer's disease.

In a minority of cases the distinction will be obvious, based on other symptoms produced by the disease process, e.g. jerky movements of the face and body (chorea) and a positive family history would be suggestive of Huntington's disease. In the majority of cases, the different dementias may be distinguished to some degree based on a detailed history from the patient and an

Fig. 14.7 Distinguishing clinical features of the commonest types of dementia	
Alzheimer's disease (62%)	Gradual onset with progressive cognitive decline Early memory loss
Vascular dementia (multi-infarct dementia) (17%)	Focal neurological signs and symptoms Evidence of cerebrovascular disease or stroke May be uneven or stepwise deterioration in cognitive function
Mixed (10%)	Features of both Alzheimer's disease and vascular dementia
Lewy body dementia (4%)	Day-to-day (or shorter) fluctuations in cognitive performance Recurrent visual hallucinations Motor signs of parkinsonism (rigidity, bradykinesia, tremor) (not drug-induced) Recurrent falls and syncope Transient disturbances of consciousness Extreme sensitivity to antipsychotics (induces parkinsonism)
Frontotemporal dementia (including Pick's disease) (2%)	Early decline in social and personal conduct (disinhibition, tactlessness) Early emotional blunting Attenuated speech output, echolalia, perseveration, mutism Early loss of insight Relative sparing of other cognitive functions
Parkinson's disease with dementia (2%)	Diagnosis of Parkinson's disease (motor symptoms prior to cognitive symptoms) Dementia features very similar to those of Lewy body dementia
Percentages are prevalence of dementia subtypes in UK population (2007 Dementia UK report).	

informant, physical examination, relevant investigations and follow-up over time. However, the definitive diagnosis of dementia subtype can only be established with absolute certainty on detailed microscopic examination of the brain at autopsy – and not always then.

To aid the clinical distinction of dementia, some authors differentiate cortical, subcortical and mixed dementias based on the predominance of cortical or subcortical dysfunction, or a mixture of the two (see Fig. 14.8 for the features of cortical and subcortical

Fig. 14.8 Features of cortical and subcortical dementias		
Characteristic	**Cortical dementia**	**Subcortical dementia**
Language	Aphasia early	Normal
Speech	Normal until late	Dysarthric
Praxis	Apraxia	Normal
Agnosia	Present	Usually absent
Calculation	Early impairment	Normal until late
Motor system	Usually normal posture/tone	Stooped or extended posture, increased tone
Extra movements	None (may have myoclonus in Alzheimer's disease)	Tremor, chorea, tics
Cortical: Alzheimer's disease and the frontotemporal dementias (including Pick's disease)		
Subcortical: Parkinson's disease, dementia with Lewy bodies, Huntington's disease, progressive supranuclear palsy, Wilson's disease, normal pressure hydrocephalus, multiple sclerosis, HIV-related dementia		
Mixed: vascular dementias, infection-induced dementias (Creutzfeldt–Jakob disease, neurosyphilis and chronic meningitis)		

dementias). Unfortunately, in advanced dementia, of whatever type, there is often a considerable overlap.

HINTS AND TIPS

At this point you might find it helpful to read up on the aetiology and neuropathology of the various neurodegenerative dementias in Chapter 25, pp. 173–176.

DIFFERENTIAL DIAGNOSIS

There are three key questions when a patient presents with possible cognitive impairment:

- Is there objective evidence of cognitive impairment on a standardized test?

- If so, is it acute, chronic, or acute-on-chronic? (this may require a collateral history)
- Is the patient's consciousness level normal or abnormal?

See Figure 14.9 for a diagnostic algorithm and Figure 14.10 for a summary of differential diagnosis.

Acute, acute-on-chronic or fluctuating cognitive impairment: delirium

See Common cognitive disorders section above for clinical features of delirium.

Chronic cognitive impairment

Key questions when a patient presents with chronic cognitive impairment:

- What cognitive domains are impaired? (one or many?)
- Is the impairment stable, fluctuating or progressive?

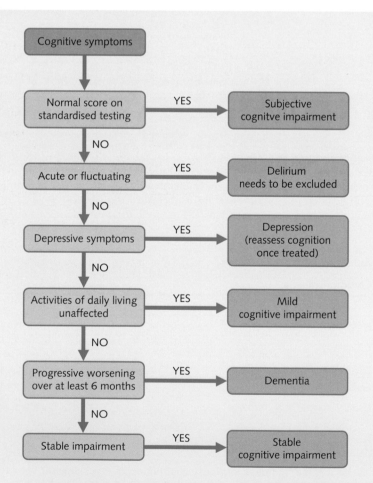

Note: Other differentials of cognitive impairment include intellectual disability, psychotic illness, amnesic syndrome, dissociative disorders, factitious disorder and malingering

Fig. 14.9 Diagnostic algorithm for cognitive symptoms

> **Fig. 14.10** Differential diagnosis of cognitive impairment
>
> Delirium
> Dementia
> Mild cognitive impairment
> Subjective cognitive impairment
> Stable cognitive impairment post insult, e.g. stroke, hypoxic brain injury, traumatic brain injury
> Depression ('pseudodementia')
> Psychotic disorders
> Mood disorders
> Intellectual disability
> Dissociative disorders
> Factitious disorder and malingering
> Amnesic syndrome

- Is the cognitive impairment causing functional impairment?
- Are there any other associated symptoms? (e.g. mood change, personality change, perceptual disturbance).

Chronic impairment in multiple cognitive domains is due most often to dementia, mild cognitive impairment or depression (see Fig. 14.10 for more differentials). Sometimes a patient has an isolated impairment (see Fig. 14.2 for examples), most often due to a head injury or cerebrovascular accident. Causes of isolated amnesia (amnesic syndrome) are considered in more detail at the end of the section (p. 112).

> **HINTS AND TIPS**
>
> When taking the history of a patient with cognitive impairment, always clarify the rate of onset and the course of the symptoms. Delirium is acute in onset, and usually short term, while dementia has a very gradual onset and is a chronic disorder. Lewy body dementia and multi-infarct dementia are the only dementias that feature transient episodes of impaired consciousness as a typical feature. All other dementias do not feature an impairment of consciousness unless complicated by a delirium.

Dementia

See Common cognitive disorders section, above, for clinical features.

Distinguishing between delirium and dementia

Older adults presenting with both physical health problems and generalized cognitive impairment are a very common clinical scenario and it is imperative that you understand how to differentiate between dementia

and delirium. Figure 14.5 summarizes the factors differentiating delirium from dementia – learn it well.

> **HINTS AND TIPS**
>
> Dementia and delirium are by far the most common causes of generalized cognitive impairment. The key question in differentiating them is the duration of impairment: is it acute, chronic or acute-on-chronic? The patient may not be able to tell you, but their notes or a collateral history from a relative or GP can be invaluable.

Mild cognitive impairment

Mild cognitive impairment is objective cognitive impairment (confirmed with a standardized test) that does not interfere notably with activities of daily living. Mild cognitive impairment is a risk state for dementia, with around 10–15% of patients converting to dementia each year. However, in some cases the impairment remains stable or even improves. All the processes that cause dementia can also cause mild cognitive impairment so it is normally investigated in the same way.

Subjective cognitive impairment

Subjective cognitive impairment is when a patient complains of cognitive problems but scores normally on standardized tests. It can reflect anxiety or depression, but can also represent early deterioration in a highly educated individual that is unidentifiable using standard tests. People with subjective memory impairment are at increased risk of later developing mild cognitive impairment or dementia.

Stable cognitive impairment

Some 'one off' insults to the brain can impair one or more aspects of cognition but not cause progressive deterioration. For example, following a cerebrovascular accident, hypoxic brain injury, traumatic brain injury or viral encephalitis. Improvement post insult can occur over several months so it is important not to make a firm diagnosis of stable chronic impairment too soon. Often someone who has had one cerebrovascular accident continues to suffer further episodes, so an initially stable post-stroke cognitive impairment can evolve into vascular dementia.

Depression

Depressive 'pseudodementia' is a term used when patients present with clinical features resembling a dementia that result from an underlying depression. Both depression and dementia can be associated with a gradual onset of low mood, anorexia, sleep disturbance and generalized cognitive and functional impairment, and they can be very difficult to distinguish. If there is uncertainty, treatment for depression is trialled and cognition rechecked after mood has improved. Unfortunately, depression presenting as pseudodementia is a risk factor for later dementia.

Psychosis

Patients with schizophrenia often have multiple cognitive deficits, particularly relating to memory, but unlike dementia, the age of onset is earlier and psychotic symptoms are present from the start. The disturbed behaviour, vivid hallucinations, distractibility and thought disorder of acutely psychotic patients may resemble a delirium. However, careful examination will reveal that the consciousness level is not altered.

Intellectual disability

Patients with intellectual disability have an IQ below 70 with an impaired ability to adapt to their social environment. Unlike dementia, intellectual disability manifests in the developmental period (before age 18) and the level of cognitive functioning tends to be stable over time, not progressively deteriorating. See Chapter 28.

Dissociative disorders

Memory loss and altered consciousness levels can occur in the dissociative disorders (see p. 93), e.g. dissociative amnesia, fugue and stupor. These usually occur in younger adults, there is no evidence of a physical cause and they are usually precipitated by a psychosocial stressor.

Factitious disorder and malingering

See Chapter 13.

Amnesic syndrome

While dementia is the most common cause of chronic memory dysfunction overall, certain brain diseases can cause a severe disruption of memory with minimal or no deterioration in other cognitive functions. This is termed the amnesic syndrome and usually results from damage to the hypothalamic–diencephalic system or the hippocampal region (see Fig. 14.11 for the causes of amnesic syndrome). The amnesic syndrome is characterized by all of the following:

- Anterograde and retrograde amnesia. The impairment of memory for past events is in reverse order of their occurrence, i.e. recent memories are the most affected.
- There is no impairment of attention or consciousness or global intellectual functioning. There is also no defect of short-term (primary or working) memory as tested by digit span.

Fig. 14.11	Causes of amnesic syndrome
Diencephalic damage	**Hippocampal damage**
Vitamin B$_1$ (thiamine) deficiency, i.e. Korsakoff's syndrome: Chronic alcohol abuse Gastric carcinoma Severe malnutrition Hyperemesis gravidarum Bilateral thalamic infarction Multiple sclerosis Post subarachnoid haemorrhage Third ventricle tumours/cysts	Bilateral posterior cerebral artery occlusion Carbon monoxide poisoning Closed head injury Herpes simplex virus encephalitis Transient global amnesia

- There is strong evidence of a brain disease known to cause the amnesic syndrome.

Although there is no impairment of global cognitive functioning, patients with the amnesic syndrome are usually disorientated in time due to their inability to learn new material (anterograde amnesia). Other associated features are confabulation (filling of gaps in memory with details which are fictitious, but often plausible), lack of insight and apathy.

The commonest cause of amnesic syndrome is thiamine deficiency resulting in Wernicke's encephalopathy followed by Korsakoff's syndrome. See pages 119 and 154 for details.

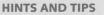

HINTS AND TIPS

Due to their unimpaired intellectual functioning, tendency to confabulate and lack of insight, patients with an amnesic syndrome can appear deceptively 'normal'. Therefore, as in dementia, a collateral history is crucial.

ASSESSMENT

History

The following questions may be helpful in eliciting symptoms of cognitive impairment:
To the patient:

- Do you find yourself forgetting familiar people's names?
- Do you get lost more easily than you used to?
- Are you able to handle money confidently?
- Do you feel being forgetful is stopping you from doing anything?

To the informant:

- Are they repetitive in conversation?

- Has their personality changed?
- Are their memory problems getting in the way of their day to day life?
- Do you have any concerns about their safety?

Examination

Cognitive examination

The key thing when assessing cognition is to use a standardized test and avoid vague descriptions such as 'alert and orientated'. Many patients maintain a good social veneer, making it surprisingly easy to miss cognitive impairment if it is not formally assessed. There is a wide range of tests available of varying comprehensiveness, length and generalizability across cultures. The one you choose depends on the time available and degree of concern about a patient's cognition. In the UK, it is recommended that all hospital in-patients aged > 65 years have their cognition screened whether or not they appear impaired. Figure 14.12 lists the advantages and disadvantages of some widely used screening tests. There are many more cognitive tests which may be useful for specific disorders, e.g. the Wisconsin card test to assess frontal lobe function. Assessment of consciousness level was described in Figure 14.1.

> **HINTS AND TIPS**
>
> Try to ensure the result of a cognitive assessment reflects cognitive abilities rather than other difficulties as far as possible: ensure the patient has their glasses and/or hearing aid, is not hungry, needing the toilet or exhausted.

Physical examination

A physical examination, including a neurological examination, is important in everyone with cognitive impairment as it may provide evidence of:

- Reversible causes of impairment such as hypothyroidism or a space occupying lesion.
- Risk factors for dementia, e.g. hypertension or atrial fibrillation.
- Differential diagnosis of dementia, e.g. a hemiparesis or visual field defect suggestive of a cerebrovascular accident and hence increased risk of vascular dementia.
- Complications of impairment such as self-neglect or injuries from falls.

Investigations

The main aim of investigation in cognitive impairment is to exclude reversible causes (Fig. 14.13). In delirium, additional investigations for acute illness are likely to be appropriate, including an electrocardiogram (ECG) and a septic screen in the presence of infective symptoms or pyrexia.

Although some types of dementia have characteristic radiological findings (Fig. 14.14), these differences are not yet robust enough to be diagnostic. In some rarer forms of dementia, genetic testing may be useful (Huntington's disease and early onset Alzheimer's (see Ch. 25)). If the diagnosis is in doubt or atypical, a more detailed cognitive assessment by a neuropsychologist may be of benefit (usually accessed via a 'memory clinic').

Fig. 14.12 Standardized tests of cognition: advantages and disadvantages

Test	Acronym	Time to perform (min)	Advantages	Disadvantages
Abbreviated Mental Test	AMT	3	Fast	Not sensitive to mild to moderate impairment
Mini-Mental State Exam	MMSE	8	Covers most cognitive domains	Not sensitive to mild impairment Does not test executive function Influenced by premorbid IQ, language and culture
Clock Drawing Test (many varieties available)	CLOX1	2	Tests praxis and executive function Resistant to influence from premorbid IQ, culture and language	Not sensitive to mild impairment Very influenced by poor motor control or visual impairment
Addenbrooke's Cognitive Examination – Revised	ACE-R	20	Tests all cognitive domains Sensitive to mild impairment.	Lengthy Influenced by premorbid IQ, language and culture

Fig. 14.13 Investigations recommended in chronic cognitive impairment

Investigation	Potentially treatable cause
Vitamin B$_{12}$/folate level	Nutrient deficiency/malabsorption
Thyroid function tests, calcium, glucose, urea and electrolytes (U&E)	Hypothyroidism, hypercalcaemia, Cushing's or Addison's disease
CT/MRI head scan	Subdural haematoma, tumour, normal pressure hydrocephalus

The above investigations are recommended by NICE (2010) as a minimum for excluding reversible causes of dementia in the UK. Other investigations may also be appropriate depending on features in the history or examination, e.g. HIV or syphilis serology, heavy metal screen, autoantibodies.

Fig. 14.14 Typical CT appearances for the main forms of dementia

Condition	CT appearance
Normal ageing	Progressive cortical atrophy and increasing ventricular size
Alzheimer's disease	Generalized cerebral atrophy Widened sulci Dilated ventricles Thinning of the width of the medial temporal lobe (in temporal lobe-oriented CT scans)
Vascular dementia	Single/multiple areas of infarction Cerebral atrophy Dilated ventricles
Frontotemporal dementia (including Pick's disease)	Greater relative atrophy of frontal and temporal lobes Knife-blade atrophy (appearance of atrophied gyri)
Huntington's disease	Dilated ventricles Atrophy of caudate nuclei (loss of shouldering)
Creutzfeldt–Jakob disease (CJD)	Usually appears normal
nvCJD (new variant CJD)	nvCJD has a characteristic MRI picture: a bilaterally evident high signal in the pulvinar (post-thalamic) region

DISCUSSION OF CASE STUDY

Mr DD first presented with memory loss for recent events. His personality gradually changed (withdrawn, prone to verbal aggression) and he also developed numerous other cognitive deficits: aphasia (rambling incoherently), agnosia (unable to recognize his pipe), apraxia (unable to dress himself) and impaired executive functioning (unable to make a cup of coffee). This 6-year deterioration in cognitive and functional abilities associated with a normal level of consciousness gives the diagnosis of dementia.

Mr DD then developed a delirium as evidenced by the rapid onset of a fluctuating consciousness level, disturbed sleep–wake cycle, psychomotor agitation and apparent perceptual disturbances (visual hallucinations). It is crucial that the cause of the delirium is diagnosed and treated. In this case, it could be pneumonia as Mr DD had developed a productive cough.

Now go on to Chapter 25 to read about delirium and dementia and their management.

15

After this chapter you should have an understanding of:

- The definitions of a 'substance use disorder' and a 'substance-induced disorder'
- The different types of substance use disorders
- The different types of substance-induced disorders
- The differential diagnosis of substance-induced psychiatric disorders
- How to assess a patient with substance use or substance-induced problems

Case summary

Mr AD, aged 42 years, presented to his general practitioner (GP) smelling of alcohol and complaining of depression, anxiety, marital problems and impotence. He admitted drinking heavily – up to a bottle and a half of whisky per day. He reported drinking increasing amounts over the past year as the same amount no longer gave him the same feeling of well-being. Recently, he noticed that he had to drink in order to avoid shaking, sweating, vomiting and feeling 'on edge'. These symptoms meant having to take two glasses of whisky before breakfast, just to feel better. Mr AD admitted that he had neglected his family and work because of his drinking. Whereas in the past, he would vary what and when he drank, he now tended to drink exactly the same thing at the same time each day, irrespective of his mood or the occasion. He continued to drink although he knew it was harming his liver. He was also concerned about his mental health because, on more than one occasion, he thought he saw an elderly lady, about the same height as the kitchen kettle, walking around the room. Mr AD had no previous psychiatric history or family history of psychiatric illness and was not taking any medication.

(For a discussion of the case study see the end of the chapter)

Psychoactive substances have been used for centuries, and their use is seen in some cultures as entirely acceptable. However, it is important to recognize that psychoactive substances affect specific parts of the brain, which can lead to a range of subjective feelings or behavioural changes. Fortunately, in most cases, these effects are innocuous; however, psychoactive substances may cause symptoms that are difficult to distinguish from psychiatric disorders.

DEFINITIONS AND CLINICAL FEATURES

The term 'psychoactive' refers to any substance that has an effect on the central nervous system. This includes drugs of abuse, alcohol, nicotine, prescribed or over-the-counter medication and poisons or toxins.

This section will introduce five new concepts specifically in relation to psychoactive substance use: hazardous use, harmful use, dependence, intoxication and withdrawal. Figure 15.1 provides an overview of these, and some other substance-related disorders.

Harmful use of substance

Harmful use of a substance is defined as a quantity or pattern of substance use that actually causes adverse consequences, without dependence. It may result in difficulties within interpersonal relationships (e.g. domestic violence, impotence); problems meeting work or educational obligations (e.g. absenteeism); behaviours that have impact on physical health or safety (e.g. drinking in spite of liver disease, drink-driving); or legal difficulties (e.g. arrest for disorderly conduct, stealing to fund habit). This can be remembered using the '4 L's' (love, livelihood, liver, law).

Hazardous use of a substance is defined as a quantity or pattern of substance use that places the user at risk of adverse consequences, without dependence.

Fig. 15.1 Psychoactive substance-related disorders

- Hazardous use of substance
- Harmful use of substance
- Substance dependence (dependence syndrome)
- Substance intoxication (could meet criteria for delirium if severe)
- Substance withdrawal
- Substance withdrawal delirium (including delirium tremens)
- Substance-related cognitive disorders
- Substance-related psychotic disorder
- Substance-related mood disorder
- Substance-related anxiety disorder

COMMUNICATION

Remember the 'four L's' (love, livelihood, liver, law) as a framework for assessing harm arising from substance use.

Substance dependence

HINTS AND TIPS

The confusion regarding use of the term 'addiction' led the World Health Organization (1964) to recommend that the term be abandoned in scientific literature in favour of the term 'dependence'.

Substance dependence describes a syndrome that incorporates physiological, psychological and behavioural elements. If patients exhibit either tolerance or withdrawal, they may be specified as having physiological dependence. However, it is important to note that patients can meet the criteria for the dependence syndrome without having developed tolerance or withdrawal. The dependence syndrome (ICD-10 criteria) is diagnosed if three or more of the following have been present together at some time during the previous year:

1. A strong desire or compulsion to take the substance.
2. Difficulties in controlling substance-taking behaviour (onset, termination, levels of use).
3. Physiological withdrawal state when substance use has reduced or ceased; or continued use of the substance to relieve or avoid withdrawal symptoms.
4. Signs of tolerance: increased quantities of substance are required to produce the same effect originally produced by lower doses.

5. Neglect of other interests and activities due to time spent acquiring and taking substance, or recovering from its effects.
6. Persistence with substance use despite clear awareness of harmful consequences (physical or mental).

HINTS AND TIPS

Patients are physiologically dependent on a psychoactive substance when they exhibit signs of tolerance and/or withdrawal.

Substance intoxication

Substance intoxication describes a transient, substance-specific condition that occurs following the use of a psychoactive substance. Symptoms can include disturbances of consciousness, perception, mood, behaviour and physiological functions. Severity of intoxication is normally proportional to dose or levels.

Substance withdrawal

Substance withdrawal describes a substance-specific syndrome that occurs on reduction or cessation of a psychoactive substance that has usually been used repeatedly, in high doses, for a prolonged period. It is one of the criteria of the dependence syndrome.

ALCOHOL-RELATED DISORDERS

Many people who drink alcohol come to no harm. Indeed, drinking small quantities of alcohol is thought to be linked to many health benefits. Therefore, sensible and modest use of alcohol is not considered to be pathological. Figure 15.2 describes how to calculate the daily intake of alcohol in units and the recommended safe intake limits.

Harmful use of alcohol

Harmful use is defined earlier in the chapter, on page 115. In relation to alcohol, this category is used when drinking causes secondary physical, psychological or social harm to the patient or others around them. People who harmfully drink are not dependent on alcohol: if features of dependence are present, the patient has alcohol dependence syndrome (see below). Figure 15.3 lists the adverse physical, psychological and social consequences of drinking.

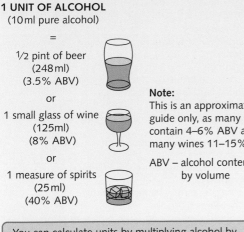

1 UNIT OF ALCOHOL
(10 ml pure alcohol)

=

½ pint of beer
(248 ml)
(3.5% ABV)

or

1 small glass of wine
(125 ml)
(8% ABV)

or

1 measure of spirits
(25 ml)
(40% ABV)

Note:
This is an approximate guide only, as many beers contain 4–6% ABV and many wines 11–15% ABV

ABV – alcohol content by volume

You can calculate units by multiplying alcohol by volume (in %) with volume (in litres),
e.g. ABV x vol = units
For instance, a pint (568 ml) of 5.3% ABV continental lager would contain 5.3 x 0.568 = 3 units

Safe daily alcohol limits
Men: 3–4 units/day (<21 units/week)
Women: 2–3 units/day (<14 units/week)

Note: Alcohol can confer health benefit mainly by giving protection from coronary heart disease, but this only applies to men over 40 and postmenopausal women. The maximum health advantages are obtained by drinking 1–2 units per day.

Fig. 15.2 Safe daily alcohol limits

COMMUNICATION

It is frequently useful to explain that although a patient may not be suffering from alcohol dependence, they could be drinking at harmful levels, and might benefit from an alcohol treatment programme.

Alcohol dependence

After a significant time of heavy, regular drinking, users may develop dependence. In 1976, Edwards and Gross formulated a detailed description of alcohol dependence syndrome: a repeated cluster of symptoms and signs that occur in heavy drinkers (Fig. 15.4). This was a strong influence on the ICD-10 substance dependence syndrome (see earlier in chapter), hence their similarities. It is important to note that alcohol dependence does not just mean physical dependence (although that is an important part of it), but describes a heterogeneous collection of symptoms, signs and behaviours which are determined by biological, psychological and socio-cultural factors. There is a range in the severity of dependence: one dependent drinker may experience a mild tremor while at work while another may shake so much after waking that he is unable to drink a cup of tea in the morning without spilling it.

Acute intoxication

Ingestion of alcohol results in transient psychological, behavioural and neurological changes, the severity of which are roughly correlated to the alcohol concentration in the blood and brain. Initially, this may produce an enhanced sense of well-being, greater confidence and relief of anxiety, which may lead to individuals becoming disinhibited, talkative and flirtatious. As blood levels increase, some drinkers may exhibit inappropriate sexual or aggressive behaviour whereas others might become sullen and withdrawn, with labile mood and possibly self-injurious behaviour. As levels rise further, drinkers can suffer incoordination, slurred speech, ataxia, amnesia (see later) and impaired reaction times, and at very high concentrations, a lowered level of consciousness, respiratory depression, coma and death.

HINTS AND TIPS

Extreme alcohol intoxication states can cause lowered concentration, inability to sustain attention and global cognitive impairment, and can meet diagnostic criteria for delirium (see Ch. 14). However, this should not be confused with delirium tremens, associated with alcohol withdrawal.

Alcohol intoxication can be a potentially life-threatening condition due to the risk of respiratory depression, aspiration of vomit, hypoglycaemia, hypothermia and trauma (e.g. head injury, fractures, or blood loss following accidents or assaults).

Alcohol withdrawal (including delirium)

The development of withdrawal symptoms is part of the dependence syndrome. Figure 15.5 summarizes the continuum of clinical features of alcohol withdrawal, from uncomplicated withdrawal to life-threatening delirium tremens ('the DTs'). However, 'uncomplicated' does not mean not serious. All withdrawal states are potentially life-threatening, as they are associated

Fig. 15.3 Complications of excessive alcohol use

Psychological
- See substance-related disorders – (Fig. 15.1)
- Self-harm or suicidal behaviours

Social
- Absenteeism from, or poor performance at, work or education
- Legal problems (increased risk of violent crime, drink driving, alcohol-related disorderly conduct)
- Interpersonal problems (disharmony with family due to alcohol)
- Financial problems (expense of drinking, unemployment)
- Vagrancy and homelessness

Physical
- *Nervous system*
  Intoxication or withdrawal delirium (delirium tremens)
  Withdrawal seizures
  Cerebellar degeneration
  Haemorrhagic stroke
  Peripheral and optic neuropathy
  Wernicke–Korsakoff syndrome
  Alcohol-related cognitive impairment
- *Gastroenterological system*
  Alcoholic liver disease (fatty liver, alcoholic hepatitis, alcoholic cirrhosis)
  Acute and chronic pancreatitis
  Peptic ulceration and gastritis
  Cancers: oropharynx, larynx, oesophagus, liver

Physical—*cont'd*
- *Cardiovascular system*
  Hypertension
  Arrhythmias
  Ischaemic heart disease (in heavy drinkers)
  Alcoholic cardiomyopathy
- *Immune system*
  Increased risk of infections (especially meningitis and pneumonia)
- *Metabolic and endocrine system*
  Hypoglycaemia
  Hyperlipidaemia/hypertriglyceridaemia
  Hyperuricaemia
  Hypomagnesaemia, hypophosphataemia, hyponatraemia
  Alcohol-induced pseudo-Cushing's syndrome
- *Haematological system*
  Red cell macrocytosis
  Anaemia
  Neutropenia
  Thrombocytopenia
- *Musculoskeletal system*
  Acute and chronic myopathy
  Osteoporosis
- *Reproductive system*
  Intrauterine growth retardation
  Fetal alcohol syndrome
  Impotence, erectile dysfunction
- *Increased incidence of trauma (fractures, head injury, soft tissue injury following accidents or assaults)*

Fig. 15.4 Alcohol dependence syndrome (adapted from Edwards G, Gross MM, 1976. Alcohol dependence: provisional description of a clinical syndrome. British Medical Journal 1:1058–1061)

Alcohol dependence syndrome (adapted from Edwards & Gross 1976)

1. **Narrowing of repertoire**. The range of cues, internal and external, that affect drinking in a normal person influence the pattern of drinking in a dependent person less and less, i.e. drinking becomes increasingly stereotyped. The dependent person will drink the same type of alcohol at the same time each day in the same place.

2. **Increased salience of drinking**. Maintaining the stereotyped pattern of drinking is given priority over other aspects of the patient's life such as home and family life, career and previously enjoyed recreational activities.

3. **Increased tolerance to alcohol**. Increased quantities of alcohol are required to produce the same effect. Patients are able to tolerate blood alcohol levels that would incapacitate non-tolerant drinkers. Note that tolerance to alcohol can sometimes decrease considerably in patients who have been drinking heavily for many years.

4. **Withdrawal symptoms**. A fall in blood alcohol level results in withdrawal symptoms. This will occur when drinkers reduce or stop their alcohol intake. Heavier degrees of dependence may result in early morning withdrawal symptoms after a night's sleep. Withdrawal symptoms include tremors (shakes), nausea and vomiting, sweating and mood disturbances (anxiety, depression, agitation).

5. **Relief or avoidance of withdrawal symptoms by further drinking**. Dependent drinkers may need to nip off to the pub at midday, or worse, have a stiff drink in the morning or, worse still, have a drink in the middle of the night to fend off incipient withdrawal.

6. **Subjective awareness of the compulsion to drink**. Patients sometimes describe this highly subjective symptom as a 'compulsive craving' that is extremely difficult to resist

7. **Rapid reinstatement after abstinence**. Although the dependence syndrome may take many years of heavy drinking to develop, many drinkers may rapidly redevelop dependence when they start drinking again after a significant period of abstinence. For example, within 3 days a drinker might develop severe withdrawal symptoms, and be able to tolerate vast quantities of alcohol despite 2 previous years of abstinence.

Fig. 15.5 Clinical features of alcohol withdrawal
Uncomplicated alcohol withdrawal syndrome • Symptoms develop 4–12 hours after drinking cessation • Tremulousness ('the shakes') • Sweating • Nausea and vomiting • Mood disturbance (anxiety, depression, 'feeling edgy') • Sensitivity to sound (hyperacusis) • Autonomic hyperactivity (tachycardia, hypertension, mydriasis, pyrexia) • Sleep disturbance • Psychomotor agitation
With perceptual disturbances • Illusions or hallucinations (typically visual, auditory, or tactile)
With withdrawal seizures • Develop 6–48 hours after drinking cessation • Occurs in 5–15% of all alcohol-dependant drinkers • Generalized and tonic–clonic • Predisposing factors: previous history of withdrawal fits, concurrent epilepsy, low potassium or magnesium
Withdrawal delirium (delirium tremens) • Develops 1–7 days after drinking cessation, mean 48 hours • Altered consciousness and marked cognitive impairment (i.e. delirium – see Ch. 14 and 25) • Vivid hallucinations and illusions in any sensory modality (patients often interact or are horrified by them; *Lilliputian visual hallucinations*, miniature humans/animals; *formication,* sensation of insects crawling on the skin) • Marked tremor • Autonomic arousal (heavy sweating, raised pulse and blood pressure, fever) • Paranoid delusions (often associated with intense fear) • Mortality: 5–15% from cardiovascular collapse, hypo-/hyperthermia, infection • Predisposing factors: physical illness (hepatitis, pancreatitis, pneumonia)

with autonomic hyperactivity, can include perceptual disturbances and seizures, and might herald the onset of a delirium.

COMMUNICATION

Always check whether previous episodes of alcohol withdrawal have been complicated by medical problems (such as delirium tremens) or psychiatric problems (such as suicidality). These points will be important in determining where detoxification takes place.

Alcohol-related cognitive disorders

Blackouts

Episodes of anterograde amnesia ('blackouts') can occur during acute alcohol intoxication. Memory loss may be patchy, or for a discrete block of time during which nothing can be remembered. Blackouts are common and have been experienced by two-thirds of dependent drinkers and one-third of young men in the general population. Blackouts refer to amnesia, not collapsing or 'passing out' at the end of the night.

Wernicke–Korsakoff syndrome

Both Wernicke's encephalopathy and Korsakoff's psychosis occur because of thiamine (vitamin B_1) deficiency. Although the two disorders were initially described separately it is now clear they represent a continuum, with Wernicke's encephalopathy occurring during acute brain damage due to thiamine deficiency and Korsakoff's being the chronic state that emerges after Wernicke's. Any disorder that is associated with low thiamine can cause Wernicke–Korsakoff's syndrome, but heavy drinkers are at particular risk of this nutritional deficiency because of their poor dietary intake.

Wernicke's encephalopathy is characterized by the classical clinical triad of delirium, ophthalmoplegia (mainly nystagmus, sixth nerve palsy or conjugate gaze palsy), and ataxia (which can be impossible to distinguish from intoxication). Prompt treatment with parenteral thiamine (Pabrinex®) can reduce the likelihood of progression to Korsakoff's psychosis, characterized by extensive anterograde and retrograde amnesia, frontal lobe dysfunction and psychotic symptoms occurring in the absence of delirium. See page 154 for more details of treatment.

Dementia

Long-term alcohol misuse can lead to impairment of memory, learning, visuospatial skills and impulse control associated with cortical atrophy and ventricular enlargement. However, it is difficult to separate the toxic effects of alcohol from the brain damage caused by years of poor nutrition, trauma (e.g. head injury) and comorbid physical illness (e.g. alcoholic liver disease). Subsequent abstinence from alcohol does lead to some improvement in cognitive functioning. See Chapters 14 and 25 for more on dementia.

Alcohol-related psychotic disorder

The interplay between alcohol excess and psychotic symptoms is complex, and is not as simple as 'cause and effect'. While both hallucinations and delusions can occur in the context of heavy alcohol consumption, it is important to remember that alcohol misuse is a common comorbidity in many patients who suffer from disorders associated with psychotic symptoms (e.g. schizophrenia, bipolar affective disorder), and is also strongly associated with overvalued ideas or delusions of infidelity (morbid jealousy, or 'Othello syndrome' – see figure 9.2 on p. 69). However, drinkers may experience psychotic symptoms that resolve completely with abstinence from alcohol. These can range from fleeting perceptual disturbances with retained insight, to more persistent predominantly auditory or visual hallucinations (alcoholic hallucinosis), to persecutory or grandiose delusions. These are distinguished from acute intoxication or alcohol withdrawal delirium by the absence of cognitive impairment and by clarifying when someone last had a drink.

Alcohol-related mood disorder

Again, the relationship between alcohol and depression is complex. Heavy alcohol consumption may cause low mood, and similarly low mood may cause sufferers to drink heavily to 'escape' their difficulties. This problem is often compounded by the social damage that alcohol can have on patients' personal lives (relationships, marriage, employment, finances, physical ill health, criminality, etc.). Differentiating low mood secondary to alcohol and true depressive disorder is very difficult, and usually starts with abstinence (following detoxification if necessary). Because of the potent psychoactive effects of alcohol, pharmacological treatment of depression with antidepressants in a patient who continues to drink heavily is much less likely to be successful than if they remained abstinent.

Problematic drinking is often a consequence of mania (either 'self-medication' or due to disinhibition). However, excessive alcohol can be associated with precipitation or relapse of manic illnesses in sufferers of bipolar affective disorder.

Alcohol-related anxiety disorder

Up to a third of drinkers have significant anxiety symptoms. As in depression, establishing whether alcohol is a cause or a consequence of anxiety disorders is difficult. The anxiolytic properties of alcohol often result in attempts at self-medication in patients with agoraphobia and social phobia, and alcohol withdrawal symptoms can mimic anxiety and panic symptoms. Whatever the direction of the relationship, reducing alcohol consumption is likely to be of benefit.

> **HINTS AND TIPS**
>
> While self-harm and suicide are not discrete mental disorders, they are strongly associated with alcohol misuse. A disproportionately high number of patients who present to hospital after harming themselves are intoxicated, or have a history of heavy drinking. The lifetime risk of suicide in problem drinkers is 3–4%, which is 60–120 times greater than the normal population. This may be due to development of the alcohol-related psychiatric disorders (mainly low mood), the fact that alcohol misuse is often comorbid with many psychiatric illnesses and personality disorders, or through impaired judgement or disinhibition secondary to alcohol.

OTHER SUBSTANCE-RELATED DISORDERS

It is beyond the scope of this book to describe the individual psychiatric consequences of every illicit drug in detail. However, like alcohol, other substance-related disorders are classified as substance use disorders or substance-induced disorders (see Figure 15.1). Common illicit drugs are described in Figure 15.6.

DIFFERENTIAL DIAGNOSIS

Patients using psychoactive substances can present with features similar to primary psychiatric disorder, posing a diagnostic challenge. The relationship between substance use and psychiatric symptoms can be reduced to three diagnostic possibilities:

1. There is a primary psychiatric disorder (e.g. depression or schizophrenia) and the patient is coincidentally using drugs or alcohol (remember that patients suffering from mental illness often use psychoactive substances to obtain relief from their symptoms).

| Fig. 15.6 | Effects of common drugs of abuse | | |
Drug group	Common examples	Psychological effects	Physical effects
Opiates	Heroin dihydrocodeine (DF118), methadone, buprenorphine (Subutex®)	Euphoria, drowsiness, apathy, personality change	Miosis, conjunctival injection, nausea, pruritus, constipation, bradycardia, respiratory depression, coma
Sedatives	Temazepam, diazepam (Valium®), flunitrazepam (Rohypnol) Gamma-hydroxybutyrate (GHB), gamma-butyrolactone (GBL)	Drowsiness, disinhibition, confusion, poor concentration, reduced anxiety, feeling of well-being	Miosis, hypotension, withdrawal seizures, impaired coordination, respiratory depression
Stimulants	Amfetamine, cocaine, crack cocaine, MDMA (Ecstasy), mephedrone, so called 'legal highs' (commonly stimulants)	Alertness, hyperactivity, euphoria, irritability, aggression, paranoid ideas, hallucinations (especially cocaine – formication), psychosis	Mydriasis, tremor, hypertension, tachycardia, arrhythmias, perspiration, fever (especially Ecstasy), convulsions, perforated nasal septum (cocaine)
Hallucinogens	Lysergic acid diethylamine (LSD), magic mushrooms	Marked perceptual disturbances including chronic flashbacks, paranoid ideas, suicidal and homicidal ideas, psychosis	Mydriasis, conjunctival injection, hypertension, tachycardia, perspiration, fever, loss of appetite, weakness, tremors
Cannabinoids	Cannabis, hashish, hash oil	Euphoria, relaxation, altered time perception, psychosis	Impaired coordination and reaction time, conjunctival injection, nystagmus, dry mouth
Dissociative anaesthetics	Ketamine	Hallucinations, paranoid ideas, thought disorganization, aggression	Mydriasis, tachycardia, hypertension
Inhalants	Aerosols, glue, lighter fluid, petrol	Disinhibition, stimulation, euphoria, clouded consciousness, hallucinations, psychosis	Headache, nausea, slurred speech, loss of motor coordination, muscle weakness, damage to brain/bone marrow/liver/kidneys/myocardium, sudden death

2. The symptoms are entirely due to the direct effect of the substance and no primary psychiatric diagnosis exists.
3. Psychiatric symptoms are due to a combination of the above, as occurs when psychoactive substances are used by those with a predisposing vulnerability to the development of mental illness.

The following features suggest a substance-related psychiatric disorder:

- The psychiatric symptoms are known to be associated with the specific drug in question (e.g. psychotic features with amfetamine use).
- There is a temporal relationship (hours or days) between the use of the suspected drug and the development of psychiatric symptoms.
- There is a complete recovery from all psychiatric symptoms after termination of the suspected drug use.

- There is an absence of evidence to suggest an alternative explanation for psychiatric symptoms (e.g. previous history of primary psychiatric illness or family history of psychiatric illness).

COMMUNICATION

You cannot completely exclude the use of substances, or gauge the severity of established misuse, without a collateral history.

ASSESSMENT

History

The CAGE and AUDIT questionnaires (see below) can be helpful in screening for alcohol dependence.

A thorough clinical history should pay particular attention to all substances used, the pattern of use, features of dependence, and consequences of substance use (relationships, employment, physical health, criminality). Past history of psychiatric illness and substance misuse, as well as family history of substance misuse should be explored. Mental state examination is important to establish psychiatric comorbidity or sequelae, current suicidality, and insight into current substance misuse (e.g. whether the patient considers it to be a problem and what they would consider to be helpful).

The CAGE questionnaire is a simple tool to screen for alcohol dependence. If patients answer yes to two or more questions, regard the screen as positive and go on to check if they meet criteria for the alcohol dependence syndrome:

1. Have you ever felt you ought to <u>C</u>ut down on your drinking?
2. Have people ever <u>A</u>nnoyed you by criticizing your drinking?
3. Have you ever felt <u>G</u>uilty about your drinking?
4. Have you ever needed an '<u>E</u>ye-opener' (a drink first thing in the morning to steady your nerves or get rid of a hangover)?

The Alcohol Use Disorders Identification Test (AUDIT) is a 10-item screening questionnaire for problem drinking. It takes 3 minutes to complete and score, and is being used increasingly in many segments of healthcare.

Examination

The physical examination requires an awareness of both the acute and chronic effects of alcohol or substance use and should focus on:

- Evidence of acute use or intoxication (e.g. pupil constriction with opiate use; incoordination and slurred speech with alcohol use).
- Signs of withdrawal (e.g. tremulousness, sweating, nausea and vomiting, tachycardia and pupil dilatation with alcohol withdrawal).
- Immediate and short-term medical complications of substance use (e.g. head injury following alcohol intoxication, infection caused by intravenous drug use).
- Long-term medical complications (e.g. alcohol-related liver disease, hepatitis B or C or HIV infection with intravenous drug use).

Investigations

There is no investigation that is absolutely indicative of substance dependence. A urine or saliva drug-screening test is essential whenever the use of psychoactive substances is suspected, but this is only able to detect a limited number of well-known drugs (not drugs which are new to the market). Breath alcohol level (via a breathalyser) only detects recent alcohol use; however, a high reading in the absence of signs of intoxication suggests some degree of tolerance, which is likely to be indicative of chronic heavy drinking.

Investigations are also useful to identify possible longer term complications of alcohol (see Fig. 15.3) and include a full blood count (mean corpuscular volume, or MCV, may be elevated), urea and electrolytes, liver function tests (gamma glutamyl transpeptidase (γGT) may be raised; elevated aminotransferases (ALT or AST) indicate liver injury), clotting screen (prolonged prothrombin time is a sensitive marker of liver function) and electrocardiogram (ECG).

If the patient has injected drugs consider hepatitis serology and an HIV test; however, ensure that patients are appropriately counselled and provide informed consent. If the patient is suffering from a withdrawal delirium, brain imaging may be necessary to exclude an additional complication (e.g. infection, head injury, brain abscess).

COMMUNICATION

All patients, especially young psychotic patients who are suspected of having a substance-induced psychiatric disorder, should have a urine or saliva drug-screening test. It is important to collect the urine as soon as possible because the half-lives of some drugs are short.

DISCUSSION OF CASE STUDY

Mr AD has an alcohol dependence syndrome as evidenced by his tolerance, withdrawal symptoms, relief of withdrawal by drinking, salience of drinking, narrowing of repertoire and also continued drinking despite awareness of harmful consequences. He has physical (sexual, possibly other systems), social (marital disharmony, neglect of family and work) and psychological (depression, anxiety, hallucinations) complications of his alcohol use. Apart from treating the alcohol dependence, it is important to ensure that his depression, anxiety and hallucinations are not indicative of a primary psychiatric disorder. The visual hallucinations may be suggestive of a withdrawal syndrome or be one of the perceptual disturbances sometimes caused by heavy alcohol use.

Now go on to Chapter 21 to read about the alcohol and substance disorders and their management.

The patient with personality problems 16

Objectives

After this chapter you should have an understanding of:
- The definitions of 'personality trait' and 'personality disorder'
- The different types of personality disorder
- Different approaches to classifying personality problems
- The differential diagnosis of personality disorders
- How to assess a patient presenting with a potential personality disorder

Case summary

The on-call psychiatrist was asked to assess Miss BP, a 27-year-old woman who had been known to mental health services since the age of 17 with symptoms that had been fairly consistent. She lived with her mother, who had contacted services because Miss BP was threatening to jump in front of a bus. Her father had sexually abused her as a child, and she had a long history of self-harm that included self-inflicted cuts and repeated overdoses. Her mother was inclined to challenge her promiscuous behaviour and binge drinking, which led to many heated arguments.
At interview, Miss BP told the psychiatrist that she was feeling 'more depressed than ever' because her mother had suggested that she move into her own house. With gentle questioning, it transpired that she was afraid that her mother would stop caring for her if she moved out. The psychiatrist, who had known Miss BP for years, recognized that this behaviour was not unusual for her and was able to help her to see another perspective to her mother's suggestion. Miss BP's mood quickly lifted and her suicidal ideation resolved.

(For a discussion of the case study see the end of the chapter)

People use the term 'personality' with varying meanings, even within the psychological and psychiatric specialties. Amid the lack of consensus on what defines personality, there is little doubt that some people seem to experience, and interact with, the world in a manner markedly different to other individuals in their culture. The description and management of what has been arbitrarily designated 'personality disorder' is one of the most controversial subjects in psychiatry. Not only are personality disorders associated with significant distress to the sufferer, but they are also associated with great cost to healthcare, social and criminal justice agencies.

DEFINITIONS AND CLINICAL FEATURES

The DSM-IV defines *personality traits* as enduring patterns of perceiving, thinking about, and relating to both self and the environment, exhibited in a wide range of social and personal contexts. It is only when an individual has traits that are persistently inflexible and maladaptive, stable over time, and which cause significant personal distress or functional impairment that a *personality disorder* is said to exist.

Patients with personality disorder tend not to regard their patterns of behaviour as inherently abnormal. Instead, they usually present to healthcare services with a wide range of problems related or consequent to their abnormal personality traits (e.g. self-harm, feelings of depression or anxiety, violence or disorderly conduct, post-traumatic stress disorder, eating disorders, dissociative or somatoform disorders). Having a major psychiatric illness such as schizophrenia does not preclude patients from also having personality disorder.

HINTS AND TIPS

The DSM-IV separates Axis II conditions (e.g. personality disorders) from Axis I conditions (e.g. schizophrenia, affective disorders) so that both are considered when diagnosing a patient.

CLASSIFICATION

The personality disorders can be classified into two groups according to their aetiology. The first group includes 'acquired' personality disorders where the disorder clearly develops after, and is directly related to, a recognizable 'insult'. *Organic personality disorder* results when this 'insult' is some form of brain damage or disease (e.g. a brain tumour or stroke). A common example is seen in patients with frontal lobe lesions, which can be characterized by social disinhibition (e.g. stealing, sexual inappropriateness) and abnormalities of emotional expression (e.g. shallow cheerfulness, aggression, apathy). Patients can also develop enduring personality changes after experiencing a catastrophic event (e.g. concentration camp or hostage situation) or after the development of a severe psychiatric illness.

The second group includes what is referred to in the ICD-10 as the *specific personality disorders* (these are far more prevalent and therefore simply referred to as the 'personality disorders' – as will be done for the rest of this chapter). In this group of personality disorders, it is difficult to find a direct causal relationship between personality traits and any one specific insult, although genetic and environmental factors have been implicated (see Ch. 22). The specific personality disorders usually have their onset in adolescence or early adulthood, and any change in symptoms tends to occur very gradually over long periods of time.

Personality disorders can be further classified according to clinical presentation, specifically which particular maladaptive personality traits are present. In this regard, there are two approaches: the *dimensional* and *categorical* classifications:

The *dimensional approach* hypothesizes that the personality traits of patients with personality disorder differ from the normal population only in terms of degree. Maladaptive personality traits can therefore be seen as existing on a continuum that merges into normality. The dimensional approach is used predominantly in the research of personality disorders and is measured by personality inventories (e.g. Minnesota Multiphasic Personality Inventory – MMPI).

The ICD-10 and DSM-IV use the *categorical approach*, which assumes the existence of distinct types of personality disorder and therefore classifies patients into discrete categories as summarized in Figure 16.1. Despite the widespread use of the categorical approach in clinical practice, it seldom conforms to reality as there is considerable overlap of traits and most individuals do not fit perfectly into these described categories.

In an attempt to further simplify the classification of personality disorders, the DSM-IV has designated three personality clusters based on general similarities. *Cluster A* describes individuals who appear odd or eccentric, and includes paranoid, schizoid and schizotypal personality disorders. *Cluster B* describes individuals who appear dramatic, emotional or erratic, and includes borderline, antisocial (dissocial), histrionic and narcissistic personality disorders. *Cluster C* describes individuals who appear anxious or fearful, and includes avoidant, dependent and obsessive-compulsive (anankastic) personality disorders.

COMMUNICATION

Everybody has a personality that, no matter how 'normal', can have dysfunctional traits (e.g. anger, anxiety, idealization/devaluation, obsessive-compulsive behaviour). These traits often become much more prominent at times of psychological stress, such as mental or physical illness, pain and discomfort, work-related stress, and even tiredness and hunger. It is important to remember that personality *disorders* occur in many settings, remain stable over time, and cause significant personal distress or functional impairment.

HINTS AND TIPS

The term 'borderline personality disorder' is derived from the early 20th century psychoanalysts, who described a group of patients who stood 'on the borderline' between the neuroses and the psychoses.

ASSESSMENT

History

As with other mental illnesses, giving a patient a label of personality disorder gives those involved with their care only a limited amount of information. In fact, the clinical classification of personality disorders is often unreliable and although psychiatrists usually agree that a patient has a personality disorder, there are often differing points of view as regards the subtype of the disorder. Patients with possible personality disorder often present at times of crisis and distress, and therefore diagnosis at first interview can be difficult, because of the quantity of background and collateral information required and because diagnosis requires the features to persist over time.

A practical approach includes making a comprehensive assessment of:

- Sources of distress (thoughts, emotions, behaviour and relationships) to self and others.

Fig. 16.1 Categorical classification of the personality disorders (DSM-IV)	
Cluster A: 'odd or eccentric'	
Paranoid personality disorder	Suspects others are exploiting, harming or deceiving them; doubts about spouse's fidelity; bears grudges; tenacious sense of personal rights; litigious
Schizoid personality disorder	Emotional coldness; neither enjoys nor desires close or sexual relationships; prefers solitary activities; takes pleasure in few activities; indifferent to praise or criticism
Schizotypal personality disorder	Eccentric behaviour; odd beliefs or magical thinking; unusual perceptual experiences (e.g. 'sensing' another's presence); ideas of reference; suspicious or paranoid ideas; vague or circumstantial thinking; social withdrawal
Cluster B: 'dramatic, emotional, erratic'	
Borderline (emotionally unstable) personality disorder	Unstable, intense relationships (fluctuating between extremes of idealization and devaluation); unstable self-image; impulsivity (sex, binge eating, substance abuse, spending money); chronic feelings of emptiness; repetitive suicidal or self-harm behaviour; fluctuations in mood; frantic efforts to avoid (real or imagined) abandonment; transient paranoid ideation; pseudohallucinations; dissociation
Antisocial (dissocial) personality disorder	Repeated unlawful or aggressive behaviour; deceitfulness; lying; reckless irresponsibility; lack of remorse or incapacity to experience guilt; often have *conduct disorder* in childhood – see p. 190 and 197
Histrionic personality disorder	Dramatic, exaggerated expressions of emotion; attention seeking; seductive behaviour; labile shallow emotions
Narcissistic personality disorder	Grandiose sense of self-importance, need for admiration
Cluster C: 'anxious or fearful'	
Dependent personality disorder	Excessive need to be cared for; submissive, clinging behaviour; needs others to assume responsibility for major life areas; fear of separation
Avoidant (anxious) personality disorder	Hypersensitivity to critical remarks or rejection; inhibited in social situations; fears of inadequacy
Obsessive-compulsive (anankastic) personality disorder	Preoccupation with orderliness, perfectionism and control; devoted to work at expense of leisure; pedantic, rigid and stubborn; overly cautious

Note that the ICD-10 includes all the personality disorders described in the DSM-IV clusters above, except for schizotypal and narcissistic personality disorder. However, schizotypal disorder (similar to the DSM-IV's schizotypal personality disorder) is included in the ICD-10's section on psychotic disorders.

- Any comorbid mental illness.
- Specific impairments of functioning at work, home or in social circumstances.

It is usually possible to establish some idea of a patient's personality by taking a detailed history of their life focusing on the areas of education, work, criminality, relationships and sexual behaviour. When patients are not able to describe aspects of their personality, it can be useful to ask how those close to them might describe them. It is also useful – with consent – to obtain collateral information from the patient's family, employer and general practitioner, all of whom might be able to provide information to help distinguish between transient and enduring patterns of behaviour.

It is important to recognize that strong emotional reactions may be elicited by patients with personality disorder (transference and countertransference – see glossary), and that they are often perceived as 'difficult patients' because of this. Being mindful of your own emotions (often strong feelings of anger or anxiety) and taking a non-judgemental and empathic stance during assessment can be greatly beneficial, as well as providing insight into the diagnosis itself.

A number of self-rating questionnaires focused on personality traits are available. These can be helpful in the diagnosis of personality disorder; however, they should not be used as a substitute for a comprehensive clinical history. Structured interviews are also available, although these tend to be used for research purposes and are seldom used clinically.

Examination and investigation

There are no specific physical signs that are diagnostic of personality disorders. However, the consequences of associated behaviours may be seen on examination or investigation, including marks from self-inflicted lacerations or burns, musculoskeletal injuries from assaults or accidents, the sequelae of drug or alcohol misuse, sexually transmitted infections following promiscuity, and so on.

COMMUNICATION

It is difficult to confirm or exclude the diagnosis of personality disorder without taking a reliable collateral history to establish pervasiveness and stability of presentation. It can be difficult for patients to comment on this objectively, especially if they are in a state of distress.

When an individual develops a dramatic personality change after a period of normal personality functioning, consider an *organic personality disorder* or a personality disorder that occurs secondary to experiencing a catastrophic event or developing a severe psychiatric illness.

HINTS AND TIPS

Remember that the cluster A personality disorders may present with features similar to the psychotic disorders (e.g. suspiciousness, social withdrawal and eccentric beliefs) but are differentiated by the absence of true delusions or hallucinations.

DIFFERENTIAL DIAGNOSIS

Almost all the mental illnesses described in this book can feature some of the behaviours that characterize the personality disorders. Examples include social withdrawal, suspiciousness and odd ideas in schizophrenia; self-harm, low mood and poor self-image in depression; aggression, irresponsibility and impulsivity in substance abuse or mania. The diagnostic task is also complicated by the observation that many patients with a major mental illness also have a concurrent personality disorder. Therefore, you should always consider the possibility of major mental illness (DSM-IV: Axis I) before diagnosing a personality disorder (DSM-IV: Axis II), although both can be diagnosed together. *A personality disorder should only be diagnosed when the clinical features begin in adolescence or early adulthood, are relatively stable over time and do not only occur during an episode of a major mental illness (e.g. depressive, manic, psychotic episode).*

DISCUSSION OF CASE STUDY

Miss BP has a chronic condition that first presented in adolescence and has changed little over time. She has a number of maladaptive and inflexible personality traits that manifest as repeated self-mutilation, suicidal behaviour, impulsivity (promiscuity, binge drinking), fluctuations in mood and a desperate fear of abandonment by her mother. These characteristics are consistent with a diagnosis of emotionally unstable personality disorder, borderline type. It would be important to exclude another mental illness that may coexist with the personality disorder, such as depression or harmful use/dependence on alcohol. Note that there is an association between borderline personality disorder and childhood trauma, including physical, emotional and sexual abuse.

Now go on to Chapter 22 to read about the personality disorders and their management.

The patient with eating or weight problems

Objectives

After this chapter you should have an understanding of:
- The definitions of anorexia nervosa and bulimia nervosa
- The psychopathological symptoms of eating disorders
- The physical symptoms and complications of eating disorders
- The differential diagnosis of a patient presenting with low weight

Case summary

Miss ED, a 19-year-old law student, eventually agreed to see a psychiatrist after much persuasion from her mother and general practitioner (GP). Her weight had fallen from 65 kg to 41 kg over the previous 6 months and she appeared emaciated. Her GP had measured her height at 1.65 metres and had calculated her body mass index (BMI) to be 15 kg/m^2. The psychiatrist saw Miss ED alone and spent some time putting her at ease. After an initial reluctance, she admitted that she was repulsed by the thought of being fat and felt that she was still overweight and needed to lose 'just a few more pounds'. She had stopped menstruating 4 months ago and had also noted that she was feeling tired and cold all the time and was finding it difficult to concentrate. The psychiatrist elicited that she only ate one small meal a day and was exercising to the point of almost collapsing. She denied binge eating or self-induced vomiting but did admit to using 20 senna tablets daily. She reported symptoms of depression, but no suicidal ideation. Physical examination revealed a pulse rate of 50 beats per minute and fine downy hair covering her torso.

(For a discussion of the case study see the end of the chapter)

Many people are concerned about what they eat and how this affects their body weight and shape. However, some individuals become morbidly concerned with their body image to the point that their life revolves around the relentless pursuit of thinness. This life-threatening form of psychopathology needs to be distinguished from other physical, psychiatric, or substance-associated causes of weight loss.

DEFINITIONS AND CLINICAL FEATURES

Anorexia nervosa and *bulimia nervosa* are two psychiatric disorders characterized by conscious and deliberate efforts to reduce body weight. There are similarities between the psychopathology of the disorders: a preoccupation with food and being thin, and overvalued ideas involving a dread of fatness and a distorted sense of body shape and weight.

Anorexia nervosa

Anorexia is characterized by overvalued ideas concerning body shape and weight, preoccupation with being thin and intrusive dread of fatness. As a result, a self-imposed low body weight is maintained at least 15% below what is expected for age and height. In adults, the body mass index (BMI: Fig. 17.1) is 17.5 kg/m^2 or less (in children and adolescents, growth charts should be consulted). There is also generalized endocrine disturbance of the hypothalamic–pituitary–gonadal axis, as evidenced by amenorrhoea in post-menarchal women; loss of sexual interest and impotency in men; raised growth hormone and cortisol; and reduced T$_3$. In pre-pubertal sufferers of anorexia, expected weight gain during the growth period is impaired and pubertal events (menarche, breast and genital development) may be delayed or arrested. While not always present, self-induced purging, excessive exercise and use of appetite suppressants or diuretics are often used to enhance weight loss.

Bulimia nervosa

In bulimia nervosa, patients usually have a normal body weight (or weight may even be increased). In addition to sharing similar overvalued ideas with anorexia

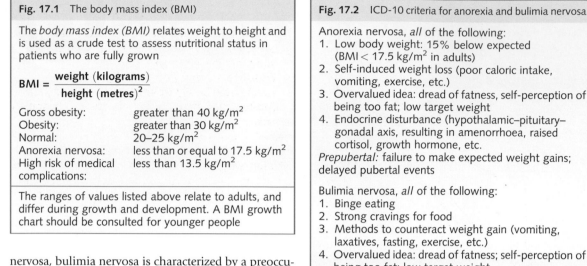

Fig. 17.1 The body mass index (BMI)

The *body mass index (BMI)* relates weight to height and is used as a crude test to assess nutritional status in patients who are fully grown

$$BMI = \frac{weight\ (kilograms)}{height\ (metres)^2}$$

Gross obesity:	greater than 40 kg/m²
Obesity:	greater than 30 kg/m²
Normal:	20–25 kg/m²
Anorexia nervosa:	less than or equal to 17.5 kg/m²
High risk of medical complications:	less than 13.5 kg/m²

The ranges of values listed above relate to adults, and differ during growth and development. A BMI growth chart should be consulted for younger people

Fig. 17.2 ICD-10 criteria for anorexia and bulimia nervosa

Anorexia nervosa, *all* of the following:
1. Low body weight: 15% below expected (BMI < 17.5 kg/m² in adults)
2. Self-induced weight loss (poor caloric intake, vomiting, exercise, etc.)
3. Overvalued idea: dread of fatness, self-perception of being too fat; low target weight
4. Endocrine disturbance (hypothalamic–pituitary–gonadal axis, resulting in amenorrhoea, raised cortisol, growth hormone, etc.
Prepubertal: failure to make expected weight gains; delayed pubertal events

Bulimia nervosa, *all* of the following:
1. Binge eating
2. Strong cravings for food
3. Methods to counteract weight gain (vomiting, laxatives, fasting, exercise, etc.)
4. Overvalued idea: dread of fatness; self-perception of being too fat; low target weight

nervosa, bulimia nervosa is characterized by a preoccupation with eating and an irresistible craving for food that results in binge eating. This is associated with a sense of lack of control, and is invariably followed by feelings of shame and disgust. To counteract this caloric load, patients engage in purging (self-induced vomiting, laxative and diuretic use), fasting or excessive exercise, but can employ any number of ingenious, even dangerous, strategies (e.g. misuse of thyroid drugs, diabetic patients refusing to administer insulin).

Figure 17.2 summarizes the ICD-10 criteria for anorexia and bulimia nervosa.

HINTS AND TIPS

Some patients with anorexia nervosa may also engage in binge eating and purging behaviour, which is characteristic of bulimia nervosa. This does not preclude the diagnosis of anorexia nervosa; the DSM-IV terms this 'anorexia nervosa, binge eating/purging type'. The key diagnostic difference is that patients with anorexia nervosa are significantly underweight and have generalized endocrine abnormalities.

ASSESSMENT

History

It is important to define the extent of the eating disorder, yet at the same time not alienate a patient who might be ambivalent about treatment. Focusing initially on the patient's life history, premorbid personality, social circumstances, family, friendships, relationships and functionality can aid engagement and build rapport. These factors can also be very relevant to the aetiology of the disorder, and useful in determining

appropriate treatment (see Ch. 23). Later in the interview, it is important to focus on weight and eating. Remember that direct questions may lead to confrontation and denial, and a technique that can be helpful to avoid alienating the patient is to 'normalize' symptoms for the purposes of the interview. The following questions may be useful:

Anorexic symptoms

- Body weight and shape can be very important to some people. Do you find that you are quite concerned about your weight?
- A common way of losing weight is to eat less or to exercise a lot. Are these things that you do?
- Sometimes when women lose weight, their periods can become irregular or stop. Has this happened to you?

Bulimic symptoms

- Often when people try to lose weight they have episodes when their eating seems excessive or out of control. Has this ever happened to you?
- After eating a lot, some people can feel guilty and uncomfortable, and can vomit to make themselves feel better. Is this something that you have ever done?
- Sometimes people might use pharmaceutical or street drugs to help control their weight. Have you ever tried this?

Other psychiatric symptoms

Sufferers of eating disorders may report other psychiatric symptoms. Anxiety classically surrounds eating, but may appear more generalized. If symptoms are sufficiently severe to be disorders in their own right, then a comorbid psychiatric illness may be present. Distinguishing depression from anorexia is discussed below (under differential diagnosis).

Physical symptoms

Eating disorders are associated with a number of physical sequelae, and therefore a thorough medical history is required. Physical complications are listed in Figure 17.3. Important factors to ascertain include a menstrual history, episodes of syncope or presyncope, palpitations, tiredness, muscle weakness and sensitivity to cold.

Examination

Both anorexia nervosa and bulimia nervosa cause medical sequelae, and the importance of physical examination cannot be overstated. Patients may be reluctant to be examined; however, this can be facilitated when preceded by a clinical interview in which good rapport is established. Other than measuring height and weight and calculating BMI, important areas to examine are:

- Skin –'lanugo' hair (fine, downy hair on body); loss of head hair; calluses on knuckles (from self-induced vomiting: Russell's sign).
- Dentition – abrasions; tooth decay.
- Cardiovascular – lying and standing blood pressure (postural hypotension may occur if dehydrated); pulse.
- Abdomen – constipation.
- Musculoskeletal – muscle wasting; ability to rise from a squat without using hands; pathological fractures.
- Other – core temperature; mucous membranes (dehydration); facial glands (swollen parotid glands may suggest frequent vomiting).

Investigations

Numerous biochemical and metabolic changes are associated with being underweight and engaging in excessive purging as summarized in Figure 17.3. These complications may be associated with long-term complications or result in sudden death. Investigations should therefore include: electrocardiography (ECG), urea and electrolytes, full blood count, liver function tests, serum glucose and lipids, thyroid function tests and amylase. Changes in hormone levels (cortisol, insulin, luteinizing hormone, follicle stimulating hormone, growth hormone) have been described, but these are of limited diagnostic value and are not routinely measured. Bone density (DXA) scanning may be considered for identification of osteopenia and osteoporosis.

Figure 17.4 shows an algorithm which may help establish diagnosis in patients with a suspected eating disorder.

Fig. 17.3 Medical complications of eating disorders	
Related to starvation	**Related to vomiting**
- Emaciation - Amenorrhoea; infertility; reproductive system atrophy - Cardiomyopathy - Constipation; abdominal pain - Cold intolerance; lethargy - Bradycardia; hypotension; cardiac arrythmias; heart failure - Lanugo: fine, downy hair on trunk; loss of head hair - Peripheral oedema - Proximal myopathy; muscle wasting - Osteoporosis; fractures - Seizures; impaired concentration; depression *Laboratory tests:* - Abnormal liver functions - Raised urea (dehydration) - Raised cortisol - Raised growth hormone - Reduced T_3 - Reduced FSH and LH - Hypercholesterolaemia - Hypoglycaemia - Hypercarotenaemia (yellowing of skin) - Normocytic anaemia - Leucopenia	- Permanent erosion of dental enamel; dental cavities - Enlargement of salivary glands (especially parotid) - Calluses on the back of hands from repeated teeth trauma (Russell's sign) - Oesophageal tears; gastric rupture *Laboratory tests:* - Hypokalaemic, hypochloraemic alkalosis - Hyponatraemia - Hypomagnesaemia - Raised serum amylase

HINTS AND TIPS

Hypokalaemia is a life-threatening complication that can result from repeated vomiting, as well as laxative and diuretic abuse. Gradual correction is safer than rapid correction, so advise patients to eat high potassium foods (e.g. bananas) or use potassium supplements. Severe hypokalaemia is an indication for hospitalization.

DIFFERENTIAL DIAGNOSIS OF PATIENTS WITH LOW WEIGHT

Figure 17.5 lists the other causes of significant weight loss that should be considered, especially when the onset of illness is later than adolescence or early adulthood.

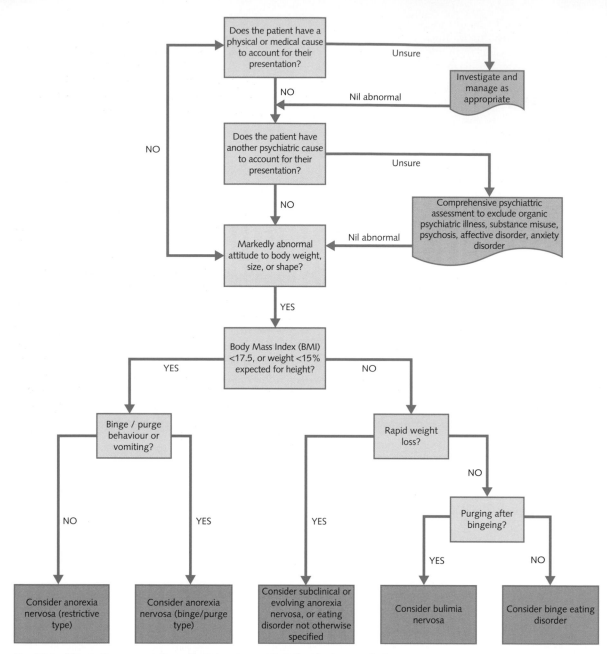

Fig. 17.4 Diagnostic approach for patients in whom eating disorder is suspected

It is very important to exclude physical causes of weight loss, including malignancies, gastrointestinal disease, endocrine diseases (e.g. diabetes mellitus, hyperthyroidism), chronic infections and chronic inflammatory conditions. Note that rare neurological syndromes associated with gross overeating include the Kleine–Levin, Klüver–Bucy and Prader–Willi syndromes.

Severe weight loss may occur in depression, but this is usually associated with a marked loss of appetite and interest in food. Patients with anorexia maintain their appetite until late in the disease and remain interested in food-related subjects (e.g. low-calorie recipes). Note that patients with anorexia and bulimia often have comorbid depression and that depressive symptoms

Fig. 17.5 Differential diagnosis for patient presenting with weight loss

Anorexia nervosa
Bulimia nervosa
Medical causes of low weight
Depression
Obsessive-compulsive disorder
Psychotic disorders
Alcohol or substance abuse
Dementia

HINTS AND TIPS

In the differential diagnosis of weight loss, anorexia and bulimia nervosa are closely associated with the overvalued idea of dread of fatness. Weight loss occurring in depression results from loss of appetite and lack of interest and enjoyment in food.

DISCUSSION OF CASE STUDY

may be secondary to the biological consequences of starvation and thus resolve with subsequent weight gain.

Patients with obsessive-compulsive disorder may lose weight when time-consuming compulsions prevent an adequate diet. Also, obsessions of contamination of food might curtail their caloric intake. As with depression, the issue is clouded by the observation that patients with anorexia nervosa have an increased incidence of obsessive-compulsive disorder, which should only be diagnosed when obsessions or compulsions are unrelated to food or body shape.

Psychotic patients may not eat due to delusions about food or hallucinations commanding them not to. The negative symptoms of schizophrenia (see p. 70) can also result in substantial weight loss.

Poor nutrition often occurs in patients with alcohol or substance abuse and dementia.

Miss ED's body mass index is 15 kg/m^2, which is more than 15% below what would be expected. She admits to a dread of fatness and consequently pursues a target weight significantly below that which is normal or healthy. Her weight loss methods include poor caloric intake, excessive exercise and laxative abuse. Dread of fatness, low body weight and endocrine disturbance (amenorrhoea) are characteristic of anorexia nervosa. The absence of binge eating precludes a diagnosis of bulimia nervosa, but Miss ED does engage in purging (use of laxatives). The depressive symptoms may signify a comorbid disorder or be secondary to the biological effects of malnutrition. Medical complications include amenorrhoea, lethargy, hypothermia, bradycardia and lanugo (fine downy hair on torso).

Now go on to Chapter 23 to read about the eating disorders and their management.

The mood (affective) disorders 18

Objectives

After this chapter you should have an understanding of:
- The epidemiological differences between recurrent depressive disorder and bipolar affective disorder
- The risk factors for depression
- When to consider hospitalization for a depressive or manic episode
- The role of psychological therapies in the treatment of depression
- The strategies to employ when a patient does not respond to 4 weeks of treatment with a SSRI
- Medications used to augment antidepressants in treatment-resistant cases
- The initial treatment of an acutely manic patient
- When to consider the use of electroconvulsive therapy (ECT) in mood disorder
- How to counsel patients regarding prognosis after one manic episode
- The relationship between cyclothymia and bipolar affective disorder

This chapter discusses the disorders associated with the presenting complaints in Chapters 6, 7 and 8, which you might find helpful to read first:

- Suicide and deliberate self-harm (Ch. 6).
- Depressive disorders (Ch. 7).
- Bipolar affective disorder (Ch. 8).
- Cyclothymia and dysthymia (Chs 7 and 8).

DEPRESSIVE DISORDERS

Epidemiology

Figure 18.1 summarizes the epidemiology of the mood disorders.

Aetiology

Depression is a multifactorial disorder, with interacting risk factors from many aspects of a patient's make-up. Genetics, early upbringing and personality can increase vulnerability to depression, with episodes arising depending on the level of acute and chronic stress experienced (see Fig. 18.2).

Genetics

Twin studies show the heritability of depression as 40–50%. The genetic risk is likely to be contributed to by multiple genes of individual small effect. Some genetic influence may only manifest in particular circumstances (gene–environment interactions). For example,

a particular allele of the serotonin transporter gene is associated with an increased risk of depression only in those who experience adverse life events. People who have the allele but do not suffer adverse life events do not experience the increased risk.

Early life experience

Parental separation (e.g. divorce) during childhood increases the risk of depression in adult life. This may partly relate to the loss of a parent, and partly to the disruption of care to the child. Other types of childhood adversity (e.g. neglect, physical and sexual abuse) increase the risk of depression and other psychiatric disorders. Postnatal depression in mothers can be associated with an indifferent early upbringing, leading to poor self-esteem and increased risk of depression in the child.

Personality

Genetics and early upbringing combine to shape personality, so it is unsurprising that some personality features are associated with increased risk of mood disorder. The personality trait 'neuroticism' (anxious, moody, shy, easily stressed) has consistently been found to increase the risk of unipolar depression. Certain personality disorders (e.g. borderline personality disorder, obsessive-compulsive personality disorder) also increase the risk of depression.

Acute stress

Adverse life events are common around the start of a depressive episode, particularly loss or humiliation events such as bereavement, relationship break-up or

Fig. 18.1 Epidemiology of the mood disorders

	Lifetime risk	Average age of onset	Sex ratio (female:male)
Recurrent depressive disorder	10–25% (women) 5–12% (men)	Late 20s	2:1
Bipolar affective disorder	1%	20	Equal incidence
Cyclothymia	0.5–1%	Adolescence, early adulthood	Equal incidence
Dysthymia	3–6%	Childhood, adolescence, early adulthood	2–3:1

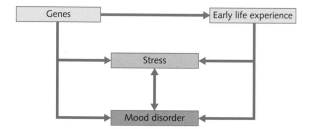

Fig. 18.2 Simplified model of aetiology of mood disorder

redundancy. The life event may not necessarily be causal, as being depressed – or at risk of depression – may also increase the risk of experiencing adverse life events. In recurrent depression, later episodes are less likely to be triggered by life events.

Chronic stress

The psychological and physiological effects of chronic stress may make someone vulnerable to depression and also reduce their ability to cope with more acute stressful life events. Chronic stressors such as poor social support (e.g. lack of someone to confide in), not having employment outside the home and raising young children are associated with depression. Chronic pain and any other chronic illness, particularly heart disease and stroke, are also associated with depression.

Neurobiology

The final common pathway of the multiple aetiological routes to mood disorder is abnormal brain structure and function. It is likely that mood disorders are due to malfunctioning communication between multiple brain regions involved in emotion regulation, rather than just one key abnormal area. Recurrent early-onset depression is associated with reduced volume of the hippocampus, amygdala and some regions of frontal cortex. Depression with onset in later life is associated

with white matter hyperintensities on neuroimaging, thought to represent small silent infarctions.

Neurochemically, multiple interacting neurotransmitter pathways are likely to be important. The two main abnormalities identified in depression are overactivity of the hypothalamic–pituitary–adrenal (HPA) axis and deficiency of monoamines (noradrenaline (norepinephrine), serotonin, dopamine).

Assessment, clinical features, investigations and differential diagnosis

Discussed in Chapters 6, 7 and 8.

Management

A *biopsychosocial* approach is taken to the management of depression, which means that consideration should be given to treating biological, psychological and social aspects of the illness. See Figure 18.3.

Treatment setting

Most patients with depression can be treated successfully in primary care, or in a psychiatric out-patient clinic. Day-hospital attendance may be helpful in patients with chronic or recurrent illness, especially if poor motivation or low self-esteem has led to a reluctance to go outside the home and make contact with others. In-patient admission may be advisable for assessment of patients with:

- Highly distressing hallucinations, delusions or other psychotic phenomena.
- Active suicidal ideation or planning, especially if suicide has previously been attempted or many risk factors for suicide are present (see Ch. 6).
- Lack of motivation leading to extreme self-neglect (e.g. dehydration or starvation).

Detention under mental health legislation may be necessary for patients who need admission but are unwilling to accept in-patient treatment due to reduced

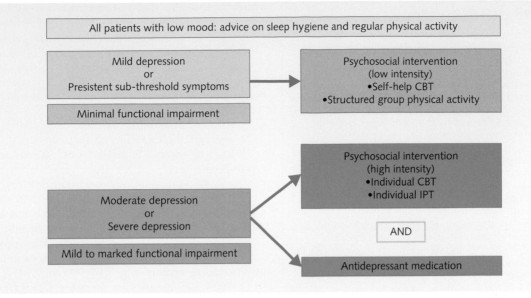

All patients with low mood: advice on sleep hygiene and regular physical activity

Mild depression
or
Presistent sub-threshold symptoms

Minimal functional impairment

Psychosocial intervention
(low intensity)
•Self-help CBT
•Structured group physical activity

Moderate depression
or
Severe depression

Mild to marked functional impairment

Psychosocial intervention
(high intensity)
•Individual CBT
•Individual IPT

AND

Antidepressant medication

Fig. 18.3 Summary of first line treatment for depression (NICE Guidelines 2009)

insight, or lack of capacity to make decisions regarding their treatment (see Ch. 4).

Lifestyle advice

All patients with low mood should be advised to avoid alcohol and substance use, eat a healthy diet, exercise regularly and practice good sleep hygiene (e.g. avoid caffeine and smoking in the evenings, do not sleep during the day, set regular sleep and wake times, do not use the bedroom for studying/watching TV). Patients can be referred to exercise groups; discounts may be available for those suffering from depression.

Psychological treatment

NICE (2009) recommends that psychological treatments are used first line for mild depression, and in combination with drug treatments for moderate–severe depression. The severity of depression is determined in part by the number of symptoms (see Ch. 7) but mainly by the degree of functional impairment (i.e. whether the patient is still able to fulfil their normal social and occupational roles). Chapter 3 covers psychological treatments in detail. Modalities often used in depression are:

- Cognitive-behavioural therapy (CBT).
- Interpersonal therapy (IPT).
- Psychodynamic therapy.
- Family and marital interventions.
- Mindfulness-based cognitive therapy.

HINTS AND TIPS

Patients reluctant to take medication may prefer the idea of 'talking therapies'. It is worth noting that cognitive-behavioural therapy (CBT) can be as effective as antidepressants in treating moderate depressive episodes and that when used after medication it can reduce the rate of relapse up to 4 years later. You may want to discuss both options with the patient, encouraging the use of both but allowing the patient to make the final decision – this often aids concordance.

Pharmacological treatment

NICE (2009) recommends antidepressants only for patients with moderate–severe depression or for patients with persistent subthreshold depressive symptoms or mild to moderate depression who have not benefited from a low-intensity psychosocial intervention. Selective serotonin reuptake inhibitors, or SSRIs (e.g. sertraline, paroxetine, citalopram, fluoxetine), are recommended by NICE (2009) as first line antidepressants because they have fewest side-effects. All antidepressants are similarly effective if prescribed at the correct dose and taken for an adequate length of time. Clinicians therefore tend to choose an antidepressant based not upon efficacy, but upon its side-effect profile (taking into account patient preference and comorbidity), and on which symptoms of depression are most troublesome. Figure 18.4

Fig. 18.4   Choosing an antidepressant

The antidepressants all have a similar efficacy for the treatment of depression. Therefore, the choice of which drug to prescribe depends on:
- Their side-effects: SSRIs have a more favourable side-effect profile over TCAs. Also, side-effects should be matched to a patient's lifestyle, e.g. the weight gain caused by mirtazapine may be preferable to the sexual dysfunction caused by the SSRIs; some patients benefit from the sedation caused by some antidepressants, e.g. amitriptyline, trazodone, mirtazapine (see Ch. 2)
- Previous good response to a specific drug: this is usually re-prescribed
- Safety in overdose: SSRIs are safer in overdose than TCAs and venlafaxine
- For severe depression requiring hospitalization, antidepressants that affect both noradrenaline (norepinephrine) and serotonin may be preferable, i.e. TCAs and high-dose venlafaxine (SSRIs may be slightly less effective in treating depression of severity sufficient to cause hospitalization)
- Atypical depression (i.e. hypersomnia, overeating and anxiety) may respond preferably to MAOIs
- Associated psychiatric symptoms, e.g. patients with obsessions or compulsions, may respond preferably to high dose SSRIs or clomipramine
- Concomitant physical illnesses, e.g. TCAs are contraindicated in patients with a recent myocardial infarction, or arrhythmias

SSRI, selective serotonin reuptake inhibitor; TCA, tricyclic antidepressant; MAOI, monoamine oxidase inhibitor

---

summarizes some of the factors guiding the choice of an antidepressant. See Chapter 2 for more information on antidepressant mechanisms and side-effects.

Antidepressants are most effective in moderate–severe depression, where around 50% of patients will respond (compared with 30% on placebo), when prescribed at an adequate dose for a sufficiently long period (usually 4–6 weeks, longer in older adults), with appropriate patient education and encouragement. When an antidepressant has brought remission of symptoms, it should be continued at full dose (i.e. at the dose that induced the remission) for at least 6 months to reduce the relapse rate. Patients with a history of recurrent depressive disorder may benefit from taking antidepressants for a longer period, perhaps even lifelong in severe cases. The prophylactic effect of antidepressants in reducing relapse has been demonstrated for at least 5 years (with imipramine).

Treatment often fails due to inadequate dose of drug, duration of treatment or poor concordance; therefore, these factors should always be ruled out. However, when a patient has not responded to an antidepressant at the correct dose for the correct length of treatment the following strategies may be employed (often in this order):

- Reassess the diagnosis: is depression the cause of their low mood? Are they using alcohol or substances? Do they have a different psychiatric disorder? Is there an ongoing psychosocial stressor?
- Consider psychological therapy, if this is not already in place.
- Increase the dose of the current antidepressant (e.g. increasing fluoxetine from 20 mg to 40 mg).
- Change to another SSRI (e.g. from fluoxetine to sertraline).
- Change to another antidepressant from a different class (e.g. from sertraline (SSRI) to venlafaxine (SSNRI)).
- Consider augmenting the current antidepressant with lithium or another antidepressant, e.g. mirtazapine (usually done by a psychiatrist). Antipsychotics can also be used as augmenting agents in treatment-resistant depression.
- Consider electroconvulsive therapy (ECT) if criteria met.
- A depressive episode with psychotic features usually requires the adjunctive use of antipsychotic medication.

HINTS AND TIPS

- Patients may tell you that they have already taken antidepressants and that they do not work. People often respond to antidepressants from some classes but not others, so it can still be worth trialling a different antidepressant – you may want to explain this before prescribing.
- Remember that patients are often prescribed inadequate doses for inadequate lengths of time before the medication is changed – this does not represent treatment failure, for which a treatment dose needs to have been prescribed for 6–8 weeks without a response. You may find it useful to document dose and treatment period in your drug history.

Electroconvulsive therapy

See Chapter 2 for information on the administration and side-effects of ECT. Indications for ECT in depression include:

- Poor response to adequate trials of antidepressants.
- Intolerance of antidepressants due to side-effects.
- Depression with severe suicidal ideation.
- Depression with psychotic features, severe psychomotor retardation or stupor.
- Depression with severe self-neglect (poor fluid and food intake).
- Previous good response to ECT.

Course and prognosis

Depression is self-limiting, and without treatment a first depressive episode will generally remit within 6 months to 1 year. However, the course of depression is often chronic and relapsing and around 80% of patients have a further depressive episode, with the risk of future episodes increasing with each relapse.

Depression is one of the most important risk factors for suicide; rates of suicide are over 20 times greater in patients with depression compared with those in the general population.

BIPOLAR AFFECTIVE DISORDER

Epidemiology

Figure 18.1 summarizes the epidemiology of the mood disorders.

Aetiology

Similarly to depression, bipolar disorder is thought to arise from an interaction between genes and environmental stress, with genes being particularly important. Twin studies estimate heritability at 65–80%. First degree relatives of a patient with bipolar disorder have a roughly seven-fold increased risk of bipolar disorder (10%), a two- to three-fold increased risk of unipolar depression (20–30%), and a higher risk of schizophrenia/schizoaffective disorder. Thus genetic susceptibility for severe mental disorder is not disorder-specific: patients with a family history of any of bipolar, schizophrenia or schizoaffective disorder are at increased risk of bipolar disorder. Risk for most patients is likely contributed to by multiple alleles of small individual effect, although some rare high penetrance alleles probably also exist. Many of the mutations identified so far that slightly increase the risk of bipolar disorder also increase the risk of schizophrenia, including genes related to neuronal development, neurotransmitter metabolism (dopamine and serotonin) and ion channels.

The most important environmental risk factor is childbirth. There is a 50% risk of mania post partum in those with untreated bipolar affective disorder.

Neurobiologically, structural and functional abnormalities in brain regions linked to emotion (particularly hippocampus, amygdala, anterior cingulate and corpus callosum) have been identified. Multiple neurotransmitter pathways have been implicated, including an association between increased levels of monoamines and mania.

Assessment, clinical features, investigations and differential diagnosis

Discussed in Chapters 7 and 8.

Management

The main management scenarios are:
- Treatment of acute mania or hypomania.
- Treatment of acute depression.
- Maintenance treatment (prevention of relapse).

Treatment setting

The initial treatment setting depends on the presentation and severity of illness. A manic episode may necessitate a period of hospitalization in cases of:
- Reckless behaviour endangering the patient or others around them.
- Significant psychotic symptoms.
- Impaired judgement (e.g. sexual indiscretion, overspending).
- Excessive psychomotor agitation with risk of self-injury, dehydration and exhaustion.
- Thoughts of harming self or others.

Detention under mental health legislation is often necessary in patients with reduced insight, or in those lacking capacity to make decisions regarding treatment. Patients with bipolar disorder may also require hospital admission for depressive episodes for reasons outlined on p. 134.

Pharmacological treatment

The mainstays of acute and maintenance treatment of bipolar illness are mood stabilizers (lithium and some antiepileptics (sodium valproate/valproic acid, lamotrigine and carbamazepine)) and antipsychotics (which stabilize mood as well as reduce psychotic symptoms).

Treatment of acute mania or hypomania

Antidepressants should be discontinued (this may need to be gradual if half-life is short, to avoid discontinuation symptoms). Short term, benzodiazepines are often helpful in reducing severe behavioural disturbance. An antimanic agent should be started. NICE (2006) recommends an antipsychotic (olanzapine, quetiapine or risperidone), in part because of their benefits in reducing behavioural disturbance. If valproate or lithium have previously been of benefit, they can be restarted, although they take longer to have effect. Because lithium can be harmful if taken for less than 2 years (discontinuation of lithium can precipitate mania), it is not advisable to start lithium in a manic patient who is unlikely to be concordant with long-term treatment. If a patient is already taking an antimanic agent the dose can be increased, or augmentation with a further antimanic agent considered.

Treatment of acute depression in context of bipolar disorder

Antidepressants need to be co-prescribed with an antimanic agent, to avoid precipitating a hypomanic or manic episode. They should not be prescribed for mild depressive symptoms, only moderate–severe. Doses should start low and increase only gradually. SSRIs are first line, or quetiapine can be considered if not already on an antipsychotic (quetiapine also has antidepressant properties). Long-term antidepressants should be avoided, with gradual discontinuation once depression has been in remission for 8 weeks.

Maintenance treatment

Not everyone who has suffered from a manic or hypomanic episode needs long-term prophylactic treatment. NICE (2006) recommends maintenance treatment in those who have had a manic episode associated with serious adverse risk or consequences, a manic episode and another disordered mood episode, or repeated hypomanic or depressive episodes with significant functional impairment or risk. Treatment for at least 2 years is recommended.

If maintenance treatment is indicated, NICE (2006) recommends lithium, valproate or olanzapine. The choice depends on sex, physical comorbidity and patient preference. All mood stabilizers are teratogenic so women of childbearing age should be advised to use reliable contraception, and valproate avoided if at all possible as it is associated with a high risk of neural tube defects. After initiation of valproate, liver and haematological function need to be monitored in the first 6 months. Lithium requires regular blood tests (usually 3-monthly) to monitor plasma level. Discontinuation of lithium can precipitate relapse, meaning net benefit is likely to be gained only after at least 2 years of treatment. Anyone on long-term antipsychotic therapy needs at least annual screening for metabolic syndrome. If one maintenance medication is ineffective, consider switching to an alternative or augmentation with one of the three. If a combination is ineffective, consider carbamazepine. Lamotrigine can be considered for maintenance treatment if the majority of episodes are depressive.

HINTS AND TIPS

Always ask about the number of previous episodes of mania and depression. This will affect the diagnosis and response to treatment. Those that 'rapid cycle' (four or more episodes in 1 year) respond poorly to lithium, and an alternative mood stabilizer may be more appropriate.

HINTS AND TIPS

Do not forget to take a comprehensive family history – including of treatment of psychiatric diagnoses. There is evidence to suggest that the level of response to lithium runs in families.

HINTS AND TIPS

Different preparations of lithium and valproate (which can mean sodium valproate, valproic acid, or semi-sodium valproate) have different bioavailabilities so it is important to specify the preparation when prescribing.

Psychological treatment

Psychotherapy is performed much less commonly in bipolar affective disorder than in unipolar depression; however, it may play a supportive role and help to improve concordance and awareness of early warning signs of relapse.

Electroconvulsive therapy

Although ECT may precipitate a manic episode in bipolar patients, it can be an effective antimanic agent, superior even to lithium, especially in severe mania and mixed states.

Course and prognosis

More than 90% of patients who have a single manic episode go on to have future episodes. The frequency of episodes varies considerably, but on average equates to four mood episodes in 10 years. Between 5% and 15% of patients have four or more mood episodes (depressive, manic or mixed) within 1 year, which is termed *rapid cycling* and is associated with a poor prognosis. Completed suicide occurs in 10–15% of patients.

DYSTHYMIA AND CYCLOTHYMIA

Aetiology

The extent to which the aetiologies of dysthymia and cyclothymia resemble those of depression and bipolar affective disorder is unclear. There are biological similarities between dysthymia and depression; for example, REM (rapid eye movement) latency is decreased in both conditions. Genetic studies link cyclothymia and bipolar affective disorder, as up to a third of patients with the former have a positive family history of the latter.

Epidemiology and course

Figure 18.1 summarizes the epidemiology of the mood disorders. Both dysthymia and cyclothymia have an insidious onset and a chronic course, often beginning in childhood or adolescence. A significant number of patients with cyclothymia will go on to suffer more severe affective disorders, most notably bipolar affective disorder. Dysthymia may coexist with depressive episodes ('double depression'), anxiety disorders and borderline personality disorder.

Assessment, clinical features, investigations and differential diagnosis

Discussed in Chapters 7 and 8.

Management

The two conditions may be treated pharmacologically with the same drugs used in depressive and bipolar affective disorder, but antidepressants should be used with caution in cyclothymia owing to their occasional tendency to turn mild depressive symptoms into hypomania. Psychological therapy may be useful for both conditions.

The psychotic disorders: schizophrenia 19

Objectives

After this chapter you should have an understanding of:
- The prevalence of schizophrenia across socioeconomic classes
- The epidemiological and prognostic differences between men and women with schizophrenia
- How to respond to parents who ask you whether their other child will also develop schizophrenia
- Pharmacological and psychological management of schizophrenia
- A definition of treatment-resistant schizophrenia and its management
- The features of schizophrenia that are associated with a good prognosis
- How to manage acute behavioural disturbance

The main types of psychotic disorder are schizophrenia, schizoaffective disorder, delusional disorder, and acute and transient psychoses. This chapter will concentrate on schizophrenia, the most prevalent and widely researched disorder in this group.

SCHIZOPHRENIA

History

Ideas about the disorder we now term schizophrenia crystallized towards the end of the 19th century. The concept of this disorder has evolved during the 20th century. Important landmarks in the definition of this disorder are:

- 1893: Emil Kraepelin separated affective psychoses (e.g. mania) from non-affective psychoses; he gave the term 'dementia praecox' to clinical conditions resembling the main forms of schizophrenia.
- 1911: Eugen Bleuler coined the term 'schizophrenia' ('splitting of the mind'); his description placed more emphasis on thought disorder and negative symptoms than on positive symptoms.
- 1959: Kurt Schneider defined first rank symptoms, which are now the basis of criteria (a)–(d) of the ICD-10 classification (see Figs 9.6 and 9.7).
- 1970 to the present: the main international classification systems, ICD-10 and DSM-IV, have further clarified the diagnostic criteria. The main distinction between ICD-10 and DSM-IV is that the latter specifies a 6-month duration of symptoms and places a large emphasis on social or occupational dysfunction.

Epidemiology

- The incidence is approximately 15/100 000 individuals per year.
- The prevalence varies geographically but is approximately 1% in most settings.
- The lifetime risk is approximately 1% (see also Fig. 19.1).
- The age of onset is typically between late teens and mid-30s. Women have a later age of onset. Men: 18–25 years; women: 25–35 years.
- Men have a higher incidence than women (ratio of 1.4:1) but equal prevalence (possibly due to a higher rate of mortality among male sufferers).
- There is an increased prevalence in lower socioeconomic classes (classes IV and V). This is more likely to be due to social drift (impairment of functioning caused by schizophrenia results in a 'drift' down the social scale) rather than social causation (poor socioeconomic conditions contribute to the development of schizophrenia).
- There is an increased incidence in urban (inner city) compared to rural areas.
- The incidence and prevalence is higher in migrants, with a relative risk of 4.6.

Aetiology

The aetiology of schizophrenia involves a complex interaction of biological and environmental factors.

Genetic

There is a strong tendency for schizophrenia to run in families. Figure 19.1 shows the lifetime risk of developing schizophrenia if relatives have schizophrenia.

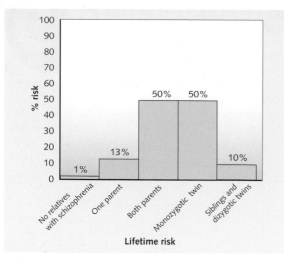

Fig. 19.1 Lifetime risk of developing schizophrenia if relatives have schizophrenia

Twin studies show a higher concordance rate for monozygotic twins (50%) than for dizygotic twins (10%), although this also shows that environmental factors are important, as monozygotic concordance is not 100%. Adoption studies provide further evidence for a genetic factor: babies adopted away from parents with schizophrenia to parents without retain their increased risk, whereas the risk is not increased when babies are adopted to parents with schizophrenia from biological parents without. A number of genetic variations associated with a small to moderate increase in risk have been identified, mainly in genes implicated in neurodevelopment and glutamate and dopamine metabolism. Rare high penetrance genetic variations also exist, for example, deletion of a region of chromosome 22 is associated with a 30% risk of schizophrenia. The overall risk is likely to result from a complex interaction of a large number of genes, and their interaction with environmental factors.

> ### COMMUNICATION
>
> Schizophrenia is not purely genetic in aetiology – environment is also important. You may want to bear this in mind when discussing the diagnosis with patients and their families: parents may find a genetic description accusational while for the patient it will have ramifications about having children themselves.

Developmental factors

Schizophrenia is associated with complications during pregnancy and birth. In addition, the observation that more people with schizophrenia are born in late winter or spring has led to the theory that schizophrenia is linked to second trimester influenza infection.

Brain abnormalities

Structural and functional brain abnormalities are associated with schizophrenia, even in those with first episode psychosis who have never received treatment. Structural imaging is not yet diagnostic, but frequently identified abnormalities include:

- Ventricular enlargement (appears to be associated with negative symptoms).
- Reduced brain size (frontal and temporal lobes, hippocampus, amygdala, parahippocampal gyrus).
- Reduced connectivity between brain regions (particularly frontal and temporal lobes).

Furthermore, people with schizophrenia demonstrate a wide range of cognitive abnormalities, particularly on tasks testing social cognition and memory. They also experience abnormalities of sensory integration leading to 'soft' neurological signs, e.g. abnormalities of stereognosis or proprioception.

Neurotransmitter abnormalities

Based largely on the effects of the conventional antipsychotics (which block dopamine D_2 receptors), the dopamine hypothesis suggests that schizophrenia is secondary to overactivity of the mesolimbic dopamine pathway in the brain. Furthermore, drugs that potentiate this pathway (e.g. amfetamines, antiparkinsonian drugs) are known to cause psychotic symptoms. However, excess dopamine may be a consequence rather than the cause of schizophrenia. Other neurotransmitters, such as serotonin and glutamate, have also been implicated.

Life events

Stressful life events occur more frequently in the month before a first psychotic episode or relapse, and may, therefore, precipitate the illness. However, it may be that the early stages of the illness itself cause the stressful events.

Expressed emotion

When family or carers become over-involved, over-critical or hostile towards a patient with schizophrenia, he or she is more likely to relapse. This interaction has been termed 'high expressed emotion' and exerts an influence if contact is greater than 35 hours a week.

Assessment, clinical features, investigations and differential diagnosis

Discussed in Chapter 9.

Management

There is no known cure for schizophrenia. Management is aimed at improving symptoms and preventing relapse. Long-term medication is the mainstay of treatment, although psychosocial treatment is also very important.

Treatment setting

The initial treatment setting depends on the presentation and severity of illness. Home treatment is preferable but hospitalization is often necessary in cases of first episode psychosis and when there is a significant risk that psychotic symptoms may lead to harm to self or others, or self-neglect. Detention under mental health legislation may be necessary in patients with reduced insight and impaired judgement.

Long-term community management is provided by community mental health teams or assertive outreach teams with the help of a care coordinator and regular follow-up in a psychiatric out-patient clinic. Patients with schizophrenia who have symptoms that are stable and well controlled can be managed in primary care.

Pharmacological treatment

Antipsychotics are of benefit in reducing positive symptoms (e.g. delusions and hallucinations). However, they have little or no benefit on negative symptoms (e.g. apathy and social withdrawal). Differences in efficacy between antipsychotics are small, with the exception of clozapine, which is the most effective antipsychotic known, but is not used first line because of its side-effects. Therefore the main factor influencing choice of antipsychotic is tolerability. Antipsychotics

commonly cause side-effects, and as they are generally long-term medications, it is important to find one whose side-effects the patient feels they can tolerate for the foreseeable future. See Figure 19.2 for a comparison of some common antipsychotic side-effects and see Chapter 2 for more information on antipsychotic side-effects and classification.

Treatment-resistant schizophrenia is defined as a lack of satisfactory clinical improvement despite the sequential use of at least two antipsychotics for 6–8 weeks, one of which should be a second generation antipsychotic. If a patient appears treatment resistant, reassess the diagnosis, check concordance, check psychological therapies have been offered and assess for comorbid substance use. If treatment resistance is confirmed, offer clozapine at the earliest opportunity, assuming there are no contraindications and the patient is in agreement with taking oral medication and attending for regular blood tests. Clozapine is not used as a first line medication due to its significant side-effects including life-threatening agranulocytosis in just less than 1% of patients. Thus, regular haematological monitoring is obligatory (initially weekly, then monthly) and patients are required to be registered with a monitoring service. Clozapine will benefit over 60% of treatment-resistant patients.

Concordance with medication is poor in schizophrenia, with around 75% of patients stopping antipsychotics within 2 years. This frequently leads to relapse. Concordance can be increased by the use of depot intramuscular medication (administered 1–4 weekly), increased social support and patient education.

The length of treatment requires careful consideration as single episodes cannot be predicted and most patients with schizophrenia relapse. After a first episode, prophylactic treatment is recommended for 1–2 years but relapse rates are high (80–98%). Relapse is less likely if withdrawal is gradual, over a few weeks. For most patients, antipsychotics are a long-term, lifelong, treatment.

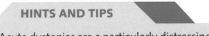
Other pharmacological treatments

Benzodiazepines can be of enormous benefit in short-term relief of behavioural disturbance, insomnia,

Fig. 19.2 Side-effects of commonly used antipsychotics

Antipsychotic	Somnolence	Extrapyramidal side-effects	Weight gain	Drug-specific important side-effects
First generation				
Chlorpromazine	**Very common**	Common	Common	Photosensitivity
Haloperidol*	Common	**Very common**	Common	QTc prolongation on average > 20 ms (baseline ECG recommended)
Flupentixol (Depixol®)*	Common	Common	Common	
Zuclopenthixol (Clopixol®)*	Common	Common	Common	
Second generation				
Olanzapine	**Very common**	Common	**Very common**	
Quetiapine	**Very common**	Common	**Very common**	
Risperidone*	Common	**Very common**	Common	
Aripiprazole	Common	Common	Rare	
Clozapine	**Very common**	Common (tardive dyskinesia very rare)	**Very common**	Agranulocytosis Hypersalivation

*Can be given in long-acting intramuscular injection (depot) form.
ECG, electrocardiogram.

aggression and agitation, but they do not have any specific antipsychotic effect.

Antidepressants and lithium are sometimes used to augment antipsychotics in treatment-resistant cases, especially when there are significant affective symptoms, as is the case in schizoaffective disorders, or in post-schizophrenia depression.

Electroconvulsive therapy (ECT) is now rarely used in schizophrenia. The usual indication is the rare case with severe catatonic symptoms.

HINTS AND TIPS

Early institution of medication may improve prognosis. Early detection is therefore critical. If uncertain, take a collateral history – a family member may well have noticed changes earlier and this may prove invaluable. You will particularly want to bear this in mind with young male patients who often have an earlier onset, a worse outcome and prominent negative symptoms that may have been mistaken for depressive symptoms.

Physical health monitoring

Patients with schizophrenia are at increased risk of cardiovascular disease. This risk is increased further by the use of antipsychotics. Therefore NICE (2009) recommends a health screen should be carried out at least annually, focusing on cardiovascular risk factors. An electrocardiogram (ECG) is needed prior to commencing an antipsychotic if the patient is in hospital, has a history of cardiovascular disease, a family history of sudden cardiac death, or has evidence of cardiovascular disease on examination (e.g. hypertension). Pre-treatment ECGs are also recommended for some antipsychotics at high risk of prolonging the QTc interval (e.g. haloperidol).

Psychological treatments

Historically psychotic disorders were thought to be unresponsive to psychological interventions, but increasing evidence points towards their value in augmenting drug treatments:

- Schizophrenia can be a devastating condition and is associated with significant social morbidity.

Therefore, the importance of support, advice, reassurance and education to both patients and carers cannot be overemphasized.

- Cognitive-behavioural therapy has been shown to be effective in reducing some symptoms in schizophrenia. It is also useful for helping patients with poor insight come to terms with their illness, thereby increasing concordance with medication. It can also help the patient become aware of early warning signs of relapse. It is recommended by NICE (2009) for all patients with schizophrenia.
- Family psychological interventions focus on alliance building, reduction of expressions of hostility and criticism (expressed emotion), setting of appropriate expectations and limits, and effecting change in relatives' behaviour and belief systems. Family intervention has been shown to reduce relapse and admission rates. It is recommended by NICE (2009) for all patients with schizophrenia who live with or are in close contact with their family.

Social inputs

Issues beyond drug and psychological treatment should be addressed to optimize community functioning; these include financial benefits, occupation, accommodation, daytime activities, social supports and support for carers. A variety of agencies can provide these services, notably, health services, social services, local authorities, local support groups and national support groups (SANE, MIND).

All patients with schizophrenia should be assessed for the care programme approach (CPA) to achieve optimum coordination in the delivery of services. Community psychiatric nurses (CPNs), consultant psychiatrists, occupational therapists, psychologists or social workers are appointed as care coordinators. Their primary role is to coordinate the multifaceted aspects of patients' care and to monitor mental state and concordance with medication.

Acute behavioural disturbance

Severe psychomotor agitation or aggressive behaviours frequently occur in acutely ill psychotic patients. Note that in patients who are not well known, it is vital that the correct diagnosis is established. Many other conditions, for example mania, delirium, alcohol and substance withdrawal and dementia, can present with acute aggression and agitation, all of which require special consideration. The algorithm in Figure 19.3 describes the principles of acute management. Many regions also have local protocols.

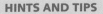

HINTS AND TIPS

Lorazepam is the only benzodiazepine that has a reliable rate of absorption from muscle tissue and therefore should always be used, if at all possible, when benzodiazepines are given intramuscularly. Other advantages include its relatively short half-life (10–20 hours) and its lack of active metabolites during elimination (no accumulation).

Course and prognosis

The course of schizophrenia is highly variable and difficult to predict for individual patients. In general, the disorder is chronic, showing a relapsing and remitting pattern. About 20% have a single lifetime episode with no further relapses. However, more than 50% of patients have a poor outcome characterized by repeated psychotic episodes with hospitalizations, depression and suicide attempts.

About 10% of patients with schizophrenia will die by suicide. Those most at risk are young men who have attained a high level of education and who have some insight into their illness. The periods soon after the onset of illness and in the months following discharge from hospital are particularly high risk, although all patients with schizophrenia are at lifelong increased risk of suicide.

The lifespan for patients with schizophrenia is on average 15 years shorter than for the general population. Causal factors include suicide, increased smoking, socioeconomic deprivation, cardiovascular disease, respiratory disease and accidents.

The overall prognosis for schizophrenia appears to be better in low income as opposed to middle and high income countries; the reasons are unclear but may reflect better extended-family social support or greater social acceptance once recovered. The factors associated with a good prognosis are:

- Female sex.
- Married.
- Older age of onset.
- Abrupt onset of illness (as opposed to insidious onset).
- Onset precipitated by life stress.
- Short duration of illness prior to treatment.
- Good response to medication.
- Paranoid subtype, as opposed to hebephrenic subtype (see p. 72).
- Absence of negative symptoms.
- Illness characterized by prominent mood symptoms or family history of mood disorders.
- Good premorbid functioning.

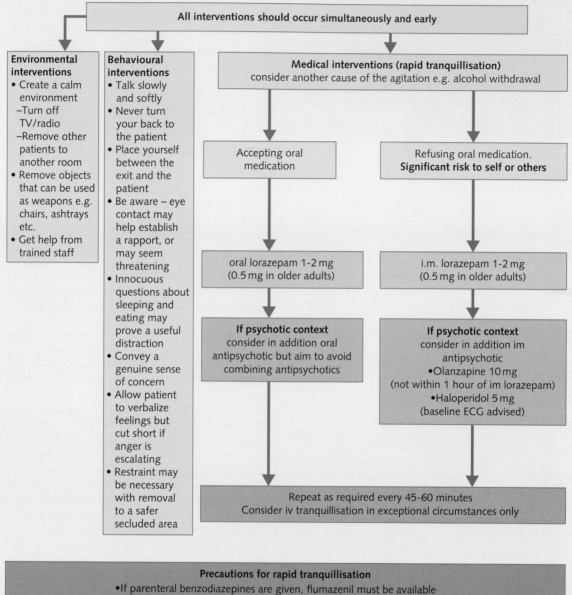

Fig. 19.3 Acute management of the agitated or aggressive patient

The anxiety and somatoform disorders **20**

● **Objectives**

After this chapter you should have an understanding of:
- The key epidemiological differences between anxiety disorders
- The cognitive model for panic attacks
- Indications for benzodiazepines in the treatment of anxiety
- Which anxiety disorders are treated with SSRIs as a first-line pharmacological option
- Why clomipramine is effective in treating obsessive-compulsive disorder (OCD)
- The treatment options for patients with a specific phobia
- The role of medication in treating somatoform disorders

This chapter discusses the most important disorders associated with the presenting complaints in Chapters 10, 11, 12 and 13, which you might find helpful to read first.

ANXIETY DISORDERS

Epidemiology

The anxiety disorders are the most common of all the psychiatric disorders with a combined 1-year prevalence rate of 12–17%. Epidemiological data collected from different countries have shown varying prevalence rates for the individual anxiety disorders, likely reflecting varying thresholds for diagnosis (see Fig. 20.1 for the epidemiology of the anxiety disorders). It is important to remember that anxiety disorders are usually underdiagnosed in primary care settings, or only recognized years after onset. A large UK survey found that only a third of people with clinically significant anxiety disorders were receiving treatment of any kind (psychological or pharmacological).

> **COMMUNICATION**
>
> The anxiety disorders are frequent and closely related in aetiology, symptoms and management. For this reason they are often grouped together along with depression under the heading 'common mental disorders'.

> **HINTS AND TIPS**
>
> In clinical settings, over 95% of patients who present with agoraphobia also have a current diagnosis or a past history of panic disorder. You may want to bear this in mind while screening for symptoms.

> **HINTS AND TIPS**
>
> Anxiety disorders tend to be more common in women than men, apart from social phobia and obsessive-compulsive disorder where the prevalence is about equal.

Aetiology

Genetic and biological factors

Genetic factors contribute moderately to risk for development of most anxiety disorders. There is likely to be considerable genetic overlap with depression. It is possible that different environmental experiences in people with similar genetic vulnerabilities lead to either depression or anxiety, or both.

Panic disorder and obsessive-compulsive disorder (OCD) appear to be the most heritable anxiety disorders, with more than a third of those affected having a first-degree relative with the same diagnosis. OCD shares genetic risk with Gilles de la Tourette's syndrome (see p. 191).

The three main neurotransmitter systems implicated in anxiety disorders are GABA, serotonin and noradrenaline (norepinephrine). Evidence for their role is that these are the neurotransmitters predominantly affected by benzodiazepines, selective serotonin reuptake inhibitors (SSRIs) and tricyclic antidepressants (TCAs). Furthermore, some polymorphisms in genes related to these systems have been found to increase the risk of anxiety disorders.

Obsessive-compulsive symptoms are often reported following damage to the caudate nucleus (e.g. Sydenham's chorea). Amygdala hyperactivation is found in a number

147

Fig. 20.1 Epidemiology of the anxiety disorders

Epidemiology of the anxiety disorders			
Anxiety disorder	One-year prevalence*	Usual age of onset	Sex ratio (female: male)
Generalized anxiety disorder	2.8%	Variable: childhood to late adulthood	2–3:1
Panic disorder (with or without agoraphobia)	3.9%	Late adolescence to mid-30s	2–3:1
Social phobia	3.7%	Mid-teens	About equal
Specific phobia	4.4%	Childhood to adolescence	2:1
Post-traumatic stress disorder	3.6%	Any age – after trauma	2:1
Obsessive-compulsive disorder	2.1%	Adolescence to early adulthood	Equal

*(One year prevalence rates from Narrow et al 2002. Revised prevalence estimates of mental disorders in the United States. Archives of General Psychiatry 59:115–123.)

of anxiety disorders, including post-traumatic stress disorder (PTSD) and social phobia, in response to the relevant anxiety-inducing stimuli. However, anxiety disorders likely reflect abnormalities in networks of brain regions, rather than individual regions alone.

Social and psychological factors

Anxiety disorders have been linked to stressful life events. In PTSD a significant traumatic event is essential to the diagnosis, although only around 10–30% of people who experience such an event go on to develop PTSD. Psychosocial stressors may also precede the onset of symptoms in other anxiety disorders.

Cognitive-behavioural theories suggest that symptoms are a consequence of inappropriate thought processes and over-estimation of dangers, as in the case of panic attacks:

- A cognitive model of the panic attack suggests that an attack may be initiated when a susceptible individual misinterprets a normal body stimulus. For example, a patient may become aware of their heart beating. Instead of dismissing this as normal, they may assume that it is under excessive pressure and that something could be physically wrong. This fear activates the sympathetic nervous system (the 'fight or flight' response), producing a real increase in the rate and strength of the heart beat. A vicious cycle ensues in which the perception of increasing cardiac effort convinces the sufferer that they are on the point of collapse or a myocardial infarction. The resulting crescendo of symptoms may proceed to a full-blown panic attack involving several of the panic symptoms listed in Figure 10.2 (p. 78).

Cognitive-behavioural models for phobias suggest a two-step process:

- A neutral stimulus is paired with an aversive stimulus (classical conditioning, e.g. driving and an accident) or anxiety is felt about an intrinsically aversive stimulus (e.g. a snake).
- The neutral stimulus is then associated with anxiety, and avoiding it reduces anxiety (e.g. not driving after an accident, not going into the reptile house in the zoo). The association thus becomes self-reinforcing (operant conditioning) and it becomes increasingly difficult to be exposed to the neutral stimulus (e.g. not getting into a car at all, not going to the zoo at all).

These theories explain why techniques such as exposure response prevention (see p. 28) are effective.

Assessment, clinical features, investigations and differential diagnosis

Discussed in Chapters 10, 11, 12 and 13.

Management

> **HINTS AND TIPS**
>
> Although patients may have genes and life experiences that predispose them to anxiety disorders, often maladaptive patterns of thinking and behaviour exacerbate and maintain symptoms. This means that psychoeducation and psychological therapies can be very effective.

Psychological therapies are recommended as first-line treatment for anxiety disorders, particularly milder forms. Pharmacological treatments are also of benefit, but longer term treatment is generally required so the risk of side-effects and complications is high. Pharmacological treatment can be offered first line for moderate–severe anxiety disorders if a patient wishes this, or if psychological treatment has been insufficient. In severe cases, combining the two is required. Figure 20.2 summarizes the most important concepts in treating anxiety disorders, based on NICE guidelines for common mental health disorders (2011), generalized anxiety disorder

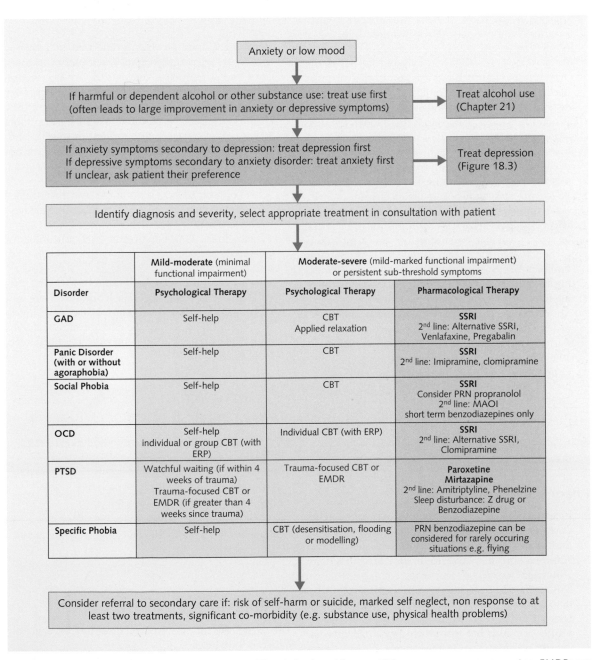

Fig. 20.2 Management of anxiety disorders. CBT: cognitive behavioural therapy, ERP: exposure response preventon; EMDR: eye movement desensitisation and reprocessing therapy; SSRI: selective serotonin reuptake inhibitor; MAOI: monoamine oxidase inhibitor

and panic disorder (2011), PTSD (2005) and OCD (2005). It is important that you familiarize yourself with this diagram, as anxiety disorders are common in primary care settings and 90% are managed there.

Psychological treatment

- There is strong evidence for the use of cognitive-behavioural therapy (CBT) in most anxiety disorders.
- CBT is the first-line treatment for specific phobias, mainly in the form of behaviour therapy, which may involve systematic desensitization, flooding or modelling (see Ch. 28).
- In panic disorder, CBT may help the sufferer to understand that panic attacks can start from a misinterpretation of a normal stimulus, leading to a 'vicious cycle' of spiralling fear and sympathetic activation. When the patient understands this model, the therapist may encourage the patient to break the cycle by promoting rejection of the assumption that the original stimulus (e.g. palpitations) is indicative of impending physical dysfunction (e.g. heart attack).
- Effective treatments in post-traumatic stress disorder include trauma-focused CBT (CBT addressing thoughts and behaviours related to memories of the trauma) or eye movement desensitization and reprocessing therapy (where the patient is asked to think about the trauma while concentrating on a therapist's finger moving from side to side) (see p. 31). Psychological debriefing immediately after trauma is not advised.
- Applied relaxation is used in generalized anxiety disorder. This focuses on being able to relax muscularly during situations in which the patient is or may be anxious.
- Other therapies commonly used in anxiety disorders include supportive, psychodynamic and family therapies although there is less evidence for their efficacy (see p. 26 and p. 29).
- Counselling may be helpful for patients who are experiencing stressful life events, illnesses or bereavements (see p. 25).

Pharmacological treatment

- In general, drugs need to be titrated up to higher doses and take longer to work in anxiety disorders than in depression (e.g. up to 12 weeks at the British National Formulary maximum dose for a trial of an SSRI in OCD).
- SSRIs are first-line treatments for most anxiety disorders due to their proven efficacy and tolerable side-effect profile. Venlafaxine has a similar side-effect profile and also has proven efficacy in generalized anxiety disorder.
- TCAs are generally considered second-line treatments owing to their increased frequency of adverse effects

(e.g. dry mouth, sedation, postural hypotension, tachycardia). Clomipramine, the most serotonergic of the TCAs, has proven efficacy in OCD.
- Restlessness, jitteriness and an initial increase in anxiety symptoms may occur in the first few days of treatment with either the SSRIs or the TCAs, which may reduce concordance in already anxious patients. This can be managed by titrating the dose up slowly or by using benzodiazepines in combination with antidepressants during the first few days of treatment.
- Benzodiazepines are highly effective in reducing anxiety. However, the rapid development of tolerance and dependence means they are not recommended for the majority of anxiety disorders. They can be prescribed as a short-term hypnotic in PTSD, or for infrequent 'as required' use in social phobia (e.g. to allow a speech to be given) or specific phobias (e.g. to allow blood to be taken). They are not recommended for generalized anxiety disorder, panic disorder or OCD.
- A beta blocker such as propranolol can also be used as required to reduce autonomic arousal to anxiety-inducing stimuli.
- Pregabalin is a GABA analogue which is licensed for treatment of generalized anxiety disorder, epilepsy and neuropathic pain.
- The monoamine oxidase inhibitors (MAOIs), despite being effective in some conditions, are not considered first-line treatment for anxiety owing to the possibility of severe side-effects and interactions with other drugs or food components (cheese reaction, see p. 16).

HINTS AND TIPS

Inhibition of serotonin uptake seems to be the essential component of effective drug therapy for obsessive-compulsive disorder as evidenced by the efficacy of the SSRIs and clomipramine. Clomipramine, which predominantly inhibits serotonin reuptake, is more effective than the other tricyclic antidepressants with predominant noradrenaline (norepinephrine) reuptake inhibition (e.g. desipramine, nortriptyline).

Course and prognosis

The prognoses of the anxiety disorders vary greatly between individuals:

- *Generalized anxiety*: is likely to be chronic, but fluctuating, often worsening during times of stress.

- *Panic disorder*: depending on treatment, up to one-half of patients with panic disorder may be symptom-free after 3 years, but one-third of the remainder have chronic symptoms that are sufficiently distressing to significantly reduce quality of life. Panic attacks are central to the development of agoraphobia, which usually develops within 1 year after the onset of recurrent panic attacks.
- *Social phobia*: usually has a chronic course, although adults may have long periods of remission. Life stressors (e.g. a new job), may exacerbate symptoms.
- *Specific phobias*: have an uncertain long-term prognosis, but it is thought that simple phobias that persist from childhood are less likely to remit than those that begin in response to distress in adulthood.
- *Post-traumatic stress disorder*: approximately half of patients will recover fully within 3 months. However, a third of patients are left with moderate to severe symptoms in the long term. The severity, duration and proximity of a patient's exposure to the original trauma are the most important prognostic indicators.
- *Obsessive-compulsive disorder*: the majority have a chronic fluctuating course, with worsening of symptoms during times of stress. About 15% of patients show a progressive deterioration in functioning.

SOMATOFORM DISORDERS

The somatoform disorders: somatization disorder, hypochondriacal disorder (including body dysmorphic disorder), somatoform autonomic dysfunction, persistent somatoform pain disorder, and factitious disorder and malingering were discussed in Chapter 13. This section will focus on the most common of these: somatization disorder and hypochondriacal disorder.

Epidemiology

Figure 20.3 presents the epidemiological data for somatization disorder and hypochondriacal disorder.

Aetiology

The aetiology of somatoform disorders is poorly understood, although episodes often follow the appearance of a stressor.

Somatization disorder may be due in part to genetic factors, with associations identified between somatic symptoms and mutations in genes related to serotonin metabolism and the hypothalamic–pituitary–adrenal (HPA) axis. Childhood sexual abuse increases the risk of the disorder, although not all patients with the disorder have been abused. Growing up in environments where physical distress is more readily acknowledged than psychological distress may have a role. Symptoms often have onset or worsen after a stressor and this may be because emotional states influence the way pain and other bodily sensations are perceived.

Patients with hypochondriacal disorder may have a lower threshold for suspecting illness or may subconsciously covet the gains to be had from adopting the sick role.

Assessment, clinical features, investigations and differential diagnosis

Discussed in Chapter 13.

Course and prognosis

Both somatization disorder and hypochondriacal disorder tend to have a chronic episodic course, with waxing and waning symptoms often exacerbated by stress. Good prognostic features in hypochondriacal disorder include acute onset, brief duration, mild hypochondriacal symptoms, the presence of genuine physical co-morbidity and the absence of a comorbid psychiatric disorder.

Management

Pharmacotherapy will only alleviate symptoms when the patient has a comorbid drug-responsive condition such as an anxiety disorder or depression. Both individual

Fig. 20.3	Epidemiology of somatization disorder and hypochondriacal disorder		
Anxiety disorder	Lifetime prevalence	Usual age of onset	Sex ratio
Somatization disorder	0.2–2%	Before age 25, often in adolescence	Far more common in women (about 10:1)
Hypochondriacal disorder	1–5%	Early adulthood	Occurs in both men and women

---

Fig. 20.4 Role of the general practitioner in managing patients with somatoform disorders

- Arrange to see patients at regular fixed intervals, rather than reacting to the patient's frequent requests to be seen
- Increase support during times of stress for the patient
- Take symptoms seriously, but also encourage patients to talk about emotional problems, rather than just focusing on physical complaints
- Limit the use of unnecessary medication, especially those that may be abused (e.g. benzodiazepines, opiates)
- Treat coexisting mental disorders (e.g. anxiety, depression)
- Limit investigations to those absolutely necessary
- Have a high threshold for referral to specialists
- If possible, arrange that patients are only seen by one or two doctors in the practice to help with containment and to limit iatrogenic harm
- Help patients to think in terms of coping with their problem, rather than curing it
- Involve other family members and carers in the management plan
- Consider referral to a psychiatrist or psychotherapist

---

and group psychotherapy (mainly CBT) may be useful in reducing symptoms by helping patients to cope with their symptoms and develop alternative strategies for expressing their emotions. Figure 20.4 summarizes the role of the general practitioner (GP) in managing patients with somatoform disorders. A supportive relationship with an empathic doctor able to work with the patient to guide understanding of their condition is likely to be the most important intervention.

Alcohol and substance-related disorders

21

Objectives

After this chapter you should have an understanding of:
- The safe levels of alcohol consumption and how many people in the UK exceed those limits
- Psychological theories of alcohol and substance dependence
- What detoxification aims to treat and how it differs from the treatment of dependence
- The differences in the principles of management of community detoxification and delirium tremens
- The most commonly encountered drug problems in patients presenting for treatment
- Non-drug management strategies in the treatment of opiate dependence
- The role of methadone in treating opiate dependence
- The similarities between benzodiazepine and alcohol withdrawal

This chapter discusses the disorders associated with the presenting complaints in Chapter 15, which you might find helpful to read first. Alcohol-related disorders will be presented first, followed by other psychoactive substances.

ALCOHOL DISORDERS

Epidemiology

Prevalence rates vary considerably depending on the geographical location, the age group surveyed and how drinking problems are defined:

- Hazardous drinking was found in 24% of adults in England (33% of men and 16% of women) in 2007. Alcohol dependence was found in 9% of men and 4% of women aged 16–75.
- There were 1 057 000 alcohol-related admissions to English hospitals in 2009/2010. This is nearly twice as many as in 2002/2003 (510 800).
- The annual cost to the National Health Service (NHS) of alcohol-related harm in England was estimated to be £2.7 billion in 2006/2007 prices.
- Just over 12 000 people were estimated to be injured or killed as a result of drink-driving accidents on UK roads in 2010.

Remember that the safe daily alcohol limits are not more than 3–4 units/day for men and 2–3 units/day for women (see Fig. 15.2, p. 117), with at least two alcohol-free days per week. It is thought that 37% of men and 29% of women in Great Britain frequently exceed these limits.

Aetiology

The causes of alcohol dependence are multifactorial and are determined by biological, psychological and socio-cultural factors.

Genetic and biochemical factors

Strong evidence shows a genetic component to alcohol dependence. Family studies show an increased risk of dependence among relatives of dependent individuals. Twin studies indicate that monozygotic twins have a higher concordance rate than dizygotic twins, and adoption studies also indicate a heritable component. The nature of this influence is unclear. It may operate at the level of heritable personality characteristics or it might relate to the body's inherited biochemical susceptibility to alcohol and its consequences. For example, 50% of East-Asians have a deficiency in mitochondrial aldehyde dehydrogenase, leading to flushing and palpitations after small quantities of alcohol; this may explain reduced rates of consumption and dependence in these cultures.

From a biochemical perspective, chronic alcohol consumption produces decreasing activity ('down-regulation') of γ-aminobutyric acid (GABA) systems and increasing activity ('up-regulation') of glutamate (mainly N-methyl-D-aspartate, or NMDA) systems. Both of these changes increase the likelihood of neuroexcitability and withdrawal seizures on cessation of drinking.

Psychological factors

Behavioural models explain dependence in terms of operant conditioning where:

- Positive reinforcement occurs when the pleasant effects of alcohol consumption reinforce drinking behaviour (despite adverse social and medical consequences).
- Negative reinforcement occurs when continued drinking behaviour is reinforced by the desire to avoid the negative effects of alcohol withdrawal symptoms.

An alternative behavioural explanation is the observational learning theory (modelling), which suggests that patterns of drinking are modelled on the drinking behaviour of relatives or peers. Family studies support the idea that drinking habits follow those of older relatives.

The presence of psychiatric (anxiety, bipolar affective disorder, depression, schizophrenia) or physical illness appears to increase the risk of alcohol abuse and dependence, although differentiating cause and effect can be difficult (see Ch. 15, p. 120). There is also evidence linking alcohol dependence with antisocial and borderline personality traits. Possible explanations for this could include any of the following: attempts to self-medicate to relieve symptoms, the use of alcohol as a (maladaptive) coping mechanism, the lack of a supportive environment, impulsivity, or the lack of insight into the risks associated with excessive alcohol.

Social and environmental factors

The cultural attitude towards alcohol affects the prevalence of alcohol-related problems (e.g. lower rates in Jewish societies as opposed to Mediterranean countries). Enormous cross-cultural variation in the way that people behave when drinking alcohol has been noted (e.g. alcohol consumption in the UK, US and Australia is associated with antisocial behaviour and violence, while in Mediterranean countries it is generally more peaceful), suggesting that the effect that alcohol has on behaviour is linked to social and cultural factors rather than solely to the chemical effects of ethanol. Alcohol consumption is greatly affected by price; some evidence exists to suggest that less alcohol is consumed and there are fewer alcohol-related illnesses in countries where it is expensive.

There is an association between certain occupations and deaths from alcoholic liver disease. The highest risk professions are members of leisure and catering trades (publicans especially), doctors, journalists, and those involved with shipping and travel. Furthermore, higher rates of dependence are noted in unskilled workers and the unemployed compared to the higher social classes (this may be partly explained by the 'social drift' caused by alcohol dependence (see p. 118).

The frequency of significant life events increases the risk of harmful drinking. Although the anxiolytic properties of alcohol are often used as a means of coping with stress, the social and physical complications of heavy drinking often lead to even further stress.

Assessment, clinical features, investigations and differential diagnosis

Discussed in Chapter 15.

Management

The management of alcohol-related problems can vary markedly depending on the pattern of use. Advice about reducing intake may be sufficient for hazardous drinkers, and can be delivered by general practitioners (GPs). Dependent drinkers may require a more intensive intervention, delivered by a specialist alcohol advisory service. Management of the latter group can be considered as having two overlapping objectives: the treatment of alcohol withdrawal and the longer term maintenance of abstinence.

Treatment of alcohol withdrawal

All clinicians need to be able to recognize alcohol withdrawal because of its high mortality and morbidity. The treatment of the alcohol withdrawal syndrome is commonly termed 'detoxification'. The following points are important:

- For the majority of patients, an out-patient or community-based detoxification will be safe and effective.
- Contraindications to detoxification in the community include severe dependence, a history of withdrawal seizures or delirium tremens, an unsupportive home environment, or a previous failed community detoxification. In these cases, in-patient detoxification is advised.
- Unplanned, short notice detoxification should only be undertaken if absolutely necessary, e.g. if a patient has to be an in-patient for another reason. In general, detoxification works best when it is planned in advance, to allow the perpetuating factors for dependence to be addressed alongside detoxification.
- In order to relieve severe symptoms and reduce the risk of developing seizures or delirium tremens, a drug with similar neurochemical effects to alcohol is prescribed, usually a benzodiazepine (such as chlordiazepoxide, diazepam or lorazepam). Initially, high doses are given, which are gradually reduced over 5–7 days.
- In order to prevent development of Wernicke–Korsakoff syndrome, thiamine is given. Oral supplements may occasionally be adequate, however in hospital this is often given parenterally in the form of Pabrinex®.

Figure 21.1 summarizes the management of delirium tremens (and Wernicke's encephalopathy).

Fig. 21.1 Management of delirium tremens

Emergency hospitalization essential
Vigorous search for a medical complication, e.g.:
- Infection
- Head injury
- Liver failure
- Gastrointestinal haemorrhage
- Wernicke's encephalopathy

Medication:
- Large doses of a drug with similar neurochemical actions to alcohol, e.g. benzodiazepines. Intravenous therapy seldom needed. Also treats seizures
- Only use antipsychotics (e.g. haloperidol) for severe psychotic symptoms (risk of lowering seizure threshold)
- Large doses of parenteral (intramuscular or slow intravenous) thiamine – two Pabrinex® ampoules twice daily for 5 days. Oral thiamine is not adequate in delirium tremens

Monitoring of temperature, fluid, electrolytes and glucose:
- Risk of hyperthermia, dehydration, hypoglycaemia, hypokalaemia, hypomagnesaemia

General principles for managing delirium (see p. 178)

COMMUNICATION

Some patients think that 'detoxification' refers to the treatment of alcohol dependence; however, it only refers to the management of physical and psychiatric symptoms of withdrawal. Treating alcohol dependence involves addressing biological, psychological and social factors that may have precipitated and perpetuated its development.

HINTS AND TIPS

Delirium tremens is a medical emergency that is common on medical and surgical wards. Despite appropriate care and treatment, it is associated with a mortality rate of 5–15% (estimated to be as high as 35% if untreated), emphasizing the need for prompt recognition and appropriate treatment. Make sure that you know the symptoms (Ch. 15) and management well.

Maintenance after detoxification

Pharmacological therapy
Various pharmacological strategies have been shown to be useful in the maintenance of abstinence from

alcohol. They work best when offered as an adjunct to appropriate psychosocial measures:
- Disulfiram (Antabuse®): blocks the aldehyde dehydrogenase enzyme, causing an accumulation of acetaldehyde if alcohol is consumed. This causes unpleasant symptoms of anxiety, flushing, palpitations, headache and nausea very soon after alcohol consumption. It is contraindicated in patients with compromised cardiorespiratory function.
- Acamprosate (Campral®): enhances GABA transmission and appears to reduce the likelihood of relapse after detoxification by reducing craving. It is safe to use while drinking.
- Naltrexone (Nalorex®): blocks opioid receptors, and appears to both reduce cravings for alcohol, and – when taken in conjunction with normal drinking – reduces the pleasant effect of alcohol, therefore decreasing the desire to drink (the 'Sinclair method').
- The use of antidepressants and benzodiazepines is not recommended as pharmacological means for the maintenance treatment of abstinence from alcohol; however, they can be useful for the treatment of comorbid psychiatric illness.

Psychosocial interventions
Not all interventions are suited to all patients and the care package needs to be tailored accordingly. The various forms of psychosocial intervention that have been shown to be effective in managing alcohol problems include:
- Motivational interviewing: the application of Prochaska and DiClemente's stages of change model (Fig. 21.2).
- Cognitive-behavioural therapy: focusing on cue exposure, relapse prevention work, behavioural contracting.
- Group therapy: psychoeducational, supportive, interpersonal process, skill development, cognitive-behavioural therapy.
- Alcoholics Anonymous: based around a 12-step programme of spiritual and character development.
- Social support: social workers, probation officers and citizens advice agencies may be able to help with homelessness, criminal charges and debt.
- Primary prevention: increasing the cost of alcohol through taxation appears to be the most effective strategy in reducing overall consumption. Limiting availability, curtailing advertising and health education seem less effective measures.

Course and prognosis

Alcohol dependence has a variable course and is often associated with numerous relapses. However, the prognosis is not as poor as is often thought, as some studies show a higher than 65% 1-year abstinence rate

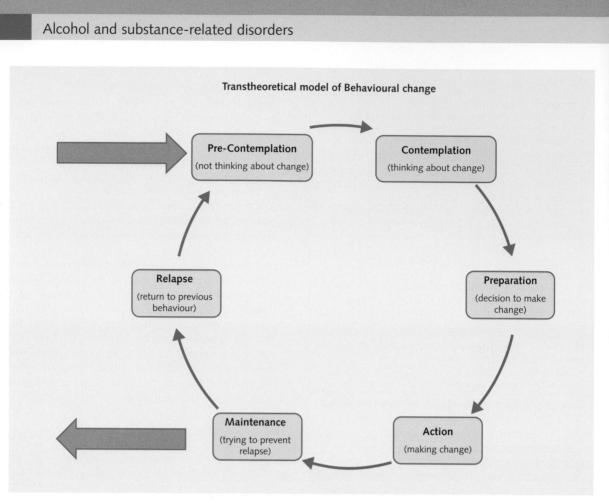

Fig. 21.2 Prochaska and DiClemente stages of change (adapted from Prochaska JO, DiClemente CC, Norcross JC 1992 In search of how people change; applications to addictive behaviours. American Psychologist 47: 1102–1114)

following treatment. Good prognostic indicators include being in a stable relationship, employment, having stable living conditions with good social supports, and having good insight and motivation. In general, alcohol-dependent individuals have a 3.6-fold excess mortality compared with age-matched controls. The lifetime risk of suicide is 3–4%, which is 60–120 times greater than that of the general population.

OTHER PSYCHOACTIVE SUBSTANCES

Epidemiology

- The lifetime prevalence of illicit drug use among adults of all ages was 36.3% in England and Wales in 2010–11 (i.e. over a third of the population have used illicit drugs at least once in their lifetime).
- Although heroin is the most frequently encountered 'problem drug', cannabis was the most commonly consumed used illegal drug in 2010, used by 6.8% of the population. This was followed by powder cocaine (2.1%), and mephedrone (1.4%).
- The prevalence of drug dependence in the general population of England and Wales in 2010–11 was 3.4%. This varies according to age: 10.2% of 16–24-year-olds are dependent compared with 0.3% of 65–74 year olds. This also varies according to sex: 4.5% of all males are dependent compared to 2.3% of females.
- There were 204 473 adults in contact with structured drug treatment services in England in 2010–11 to address their use of heroin (49%), crack cocaine (3%), or both (32%). Most individuals in treatment were male (73.2%).
- Among 11–15-year-olds in England in 2010, 8.2% reported using cannabis in the last year. This has decreased from 13.4% in 2001.

Figure 21.3 summarizes the penalties for possession and dealing the different classes of drugs under the Misuse of Drugs Act 1971.

Fig. 21.3 Misuse of Drugs Act 1971			
The penalties applicable to offences involving drugs are graded broadly according to the harmfulness considered to be attributable to a drug when it is misused. Under the Misuse of Drugs Act 1971, drugs are divided into three groups according to their perceived dangerousness:			
		Penalty for possession	Penalty for dealing
Class A	Ecstasy (MDMA), lysergic acid diethylamide (LSD), diamorphine (heroin), methadone, cocaine (including crack), psilocybin (magic mushrooms) (methamphetamine (crystal meth), any Class B drug prepared for injection	Up to 7 years in prison or an unlimited fine or both	Up to life in prison or an unlimited fine or both
Class B	Amphetamines (not methamphetamine), mephedrone (MCAT), barbiturates, cannabis, methylphenidate (Ritalin®), codeine	Up to 5 years in prison or an unlimited fine or both	Up to 14 years in prison or an unlimited fine or both
Class C	Tranquillizers (diazepam, chlordiazepoxide, lorazepam), γ-hydroxybutyrate (GHB), ketamine, anabolic steroids	Up to 2 years in prison or an unlimited fine or both	Up to 14 years in prison or an unlimited fine or both

Aetiology

Occasional or experimental use of illicit substances is not the same as drug dependence. However, ongoing use of illicit substances over a period of time can lead to development of a dependence syndrome, particularly drugs with a strong potential for the development of dependence (namely opiates and cocaine). Dependence of any drug is associated with stimulation of the brain's 'reward system' (by increasing dopamine release in the mesolimbic pathway). Aetiological factors for illicit drug dependence are not well understood, although they appear to be related to a mixture of biopsychosocial factors. The operant conditioning model described in the alcohol section also applies to other psychoactive substances. Similarly, price, availability and cultural attitudes appear to be key factors influencing the use of illicit substances. In addition, social deprivation, a family environment of substance abuse, conduct disorder in childhood, antisocial personality disorder and severe mental illness all increase the likelihood of substance misuse problems.

Assessment, clinical features, drug classification and differential diagnosis

Discussed in Chapter 15.

Management

Management of illicit drug dependence involves addressing both the physical detoxification process and the maintenance of abstinence by addressing predisposing, precipitating and perpetuating factors within the biological, psychological and sociocultural domains. A detailed description of management strategies regarding the use of all illicit substances is beyond the scope of this book. However, key points on the treatment of opiates and benzodiazepines are below.

Opiates

- Patients should be given education about harm minimization, including the risks of using contaminated injecting equipment (HIV, viral hepatitis, infective endocarditis, etc.) and unsafe sexual behaviour. Clean needles, injecting equipment and condoms can be offered.
- Opiate withdrawal is uncomfortable and distressing, although it is not life-threatening and may be attempted rapidly in mild to moderate dependence. If required, symptoms can be ameliorated by lofexidine, a centrally acting α-adrenoceptor agonist that reduces sympathetic outflow. Other drug treatments, such as antiemetics, antidiarrhoea medication and simple analgesia, can also be beneficial.
- Substitution therapy, where another substance is prescribed as an alternative to illicit opiate use, helps to stabilize the user's life, and to prevent the complications of injecting. One such example is methadone, a long-acting oral opiate. Before prescribing, opiate use must be confirmed by a urine drug screen as serious respiratory depression may result if the patient is not already tolerant to opiates, or if an excessive dose of methadone is given. Methadone may be prescribed indefinitely, but the aim is normally for gradual reduction with long-term abstinence.
- Buprenorphine (Subutex®), a partial opiate agonist, is also used as substitution therapy. Note that because it is only a partial agonist, it may precipitate withdrawal in patients who are dependent on high doses of opiates (equivalent to more than 30 mg methadone daily).

- Once the patient has been detoxified, naltrexone (an opiate antagonist) can be used to block the euphoriant effects of future opiate use. It induces withdrawal if the patient is still dependent.
- Psychological interventions are integral to good therapeutic outcomes and include motivational interviewing, cognitive-behavioural therapy (including relapse prevention), and group therapy.
- Perpetuating sociocultural factors should be addressed as part of the maintenance of abstinence. These can include issues with family and peers, housing and homelessness, prostitution, engagement with healthcare and social services, and criminality.

HINTS AND TIPS

When a patient is admitted to hospital, always confirm methadone and benzodiazepine doses with the main prescriber as soon as possible. Patients can sometimes provide inaccurate information.

Benzodiazepines

Caution must be exercised when attempting withdrawal from benzodiazepines as it can be fatal. The benzodiazepine withdrawal syndrome may include hallucinations, convulsions and delirium. Symptoms can emerge within hours to days, depending on the half-life of the benzodiazepine. Management of benzodiazepine withdrawal involves initially converting drugs with a shorter half-life (e.g. lorazepam) to drugs with a longer half-life (usually diazepam). Doses are then reduced very slowly by a small amount every few weeks, depending on patient response.

HINTS AND TIPS

Sudden discontinuation of a patient's long-term sleeping tablet when they are admitted to hospital can lead to a withdrawal syndrome: only consider this if the patient's condition means benzodiazepines must be avoided, and ideally reduce the dose gradually.

The personality disorders (22)

Objectives

After this chapter you should have an understanding of:
- The differences and similarities in epidemiology between personality disorders
- The psychosocial interventions that may be beneficial in the management of personality disorder
- The role of psychotropic medication in the management of personality disorder
- Strategies for the short- and long-term management of patients with personality disorder
- How personality disorders and other mental illnesses are related in terms of prognosis

This chapter discusses the disorders associated with the presenting complaints in Chapter 16, which you might find helpful to read first.

THE PERSONALITY DISORDERS

Epidemiology

There is a lack of consensus about the definition of personality disorders. Although DSM-IV and ICD-10 classification systems have produced definitions, it is rare for a patient with a personality disorder to neatly match with only one discrete category. It is also unclear whether there is any correlation between diagnostic criteria and the subjective experiences of people identified as having disordered personality. While a number of structured interview schedules and diagnostic instruments have been validated, the level of correlation between these is generally poor. Mental health professionals also remain divided as to how personality disorders should be conceptualized, with some clinicians questioning whether the diagnosis is of any clinical benefit.

Patients with personality disorders have a significantly increased mortality, as well as physical and psychiatric morbidity. Relationships with relatives and friends are adversely affected, and there is a strong association between some types of personality disorder and involvement with healthcare and criminal justice services.

Community studies have shown the prevalence of any personality disorder to be 4–13%, with an increased prevalence in younger age groups (particularly 25–44 years), and an equal distribution between the sexes. This varies according to the population group sampled. It is higher in patients frequently consulting general practitioners (GPs) (10–30%), even higher in psychiatric

out-patient clinics (30–40%), and higher still in psychiatric inpatients (40–50%), self-harming patients (40–80%) and prisons (50–80%).

Figure 22.1 describes the prevalence of the individual disorders and their relevant epidemiology. Note the broad ranges of prevalence from different studies, highlighting the lack of correlation in the current literature.

Aetiology

Different environmental and biological/genetic factors are implicated in the aetiology of different personality disorders, supporting their heterogenicity:

- Monozygotic twins show a higher concordance for personality disorders than dizygotic twins.
- Cluster A personality disorders (see Fig. 16.1) (especially schizotypal) are more common in the relatives of patients with schizophrenia.
- Some authors have suggested that schizoid and schizotypal personality disorders may be neurodevelopmental disorder, possibly within the autistic spectrum.
- Depressive disorders are more common in the relatives of patients with borderline personality disorder.
- Early adverse social circumstances (such as parental alcoholism, physical or emotional neglect, violence, sexual abuse) are associated with the development of cluster B personality disorders (see Fig. 16.1).
- There is a strong association between borderline personality disorder and childhood sexual abuse, although this is not universal.
- Various psychoanalytical theories suggest that disordered attachment between infants and their caregivers lead to difficulties in relationships throughout the rest of life, which may manifest as personality disorders.

Fig. 22.1 Epidemiology of personality disorders

Personality disorder	Prevalence in general population	Comments
Paranoid	0.7–4.4%	More common in males and lower socioeconomic classes More common in relatives of patients with schizophrenia
Schizoid	0.7–4.9%	More common in males and offender populations May be more common in relatives of patients with schizophrenia
Schizotypal	1.6–3.9%	More common in relatives of patients with schizophrenia May be slightly more common in males
Borderline (emotionally unstable)	1.2–5.9%	More prevalent in younger age groups and females Aetiological link with childhood sexual abuse Most contact with services in mid-20s 9% suicide rate Associated with poor work history and single marital status Often comorbid with depression, substance abuse, bulimia and anxiety
Antisocial (dissocial)	0.6–4.5%	Much more common in men Highest prevalence in 25–44-year-olds Associated with school drop-out, conduct disorder and urban settings Very high prevalence in prisons and forensic settings Highly comorbidity with substance abuse
Histrionic	0.4–2.9%	Recent research shows equal gender ratio (previously thought to be more common in women)
Narcissistic	0.1–6.2%	More common in males and forensic settings
Dependent	0.3–0.6%	Comorbid with borderline personality disorder
Avoidant (anxious)	1–5.2%	Equal gender ratio Comorbid with social phobia
Obsessive-compulsive (anankastic)	1.2–7.9%	More common in white, male, highly educated, married and employed individuals

Assessment, clinical features, classification and differential diagnosis

Discussed in Chapter 16.

Management

In the past, there has been considerable debate concerning how (and by whom) patients with personality disorders should be managed. Previously, personality disorders were generally considered to be untreatable. However, advances in diagnosis, psychotherapy and psychopharmacology have equipped clinicians with a variety of treatment options that can be useful in maximizing engagement with services, reducing distress, managing comorbid mental illness and substance misuse, improving relationships and optimizing quality of life.

Patients with borderline personality disorder are frequently encountered in clinical practice, and thus will be the focus of this section.

Principles of managing patients with borderline personality disorder

Patients with borderline personality disorder should not be excluded from health or social care services because of their diagnosis or because they have self-harmed. A consistent and tolerant approach should be taken. Autonomy and choice should be encouraged, with the patient being actively involved in deciding treatment options and in finding solutions to their problems. An optimistic, trusting and non-judgemental relationship should be developed. Endings and transitions may evoke strong emotions and reactions in patients with borderline personality disorder, and as such should be carefully planned and structured to minimize distress. A multidisciplinary approach to care should be considered, as psychological, social and biological treatment modalities all have an important role. A comprehensive assessment should be made of sources of distress to self and others (thoughts, emotions, behaviour and relationships), other comorbid mental illness and specific impairments of functioning at work or home.

Crisis management

It can be useful to develop a crisis management plan in conjunction with the patient, detailing self-management strategies, sources of support (family, friends, telephone-based services), and details on how to access emergency care. This should be shared with the patient and other relevant professionals (GPs, assessment and crisis teams).

Short-term drug treatments can be useful to alleviate distress during a crisis. If possible, this should be agreed in advance with the care team and the patient. Drugs with acceptable side-effects and low dependence profiles are preferable, and should be dispensed in small quantities if there is a risk of overdose. Drugs should not be used in place of other more appropriate interventions.

Before admission to acute in-patient psychiatric care, crisis resolution or home treatment teams should be considered. Admission may be necessary if the management of the crisis involves significant risk to self or others that cannot be managed within other services. If possible, actively involve the patient in the decision, and ensure that it is based on an explicit, joint understanding of the potential benefits (and likely harm) that may result from admission. Agree the length and purpose of the admission in advance. If the patient is detained under mental health legislation, ensure that this is regularly reviewed and that management on a voluntary basis is resumed at the earliest opportunity.

After a crisis has resolved, ensure that the care plan is updated. If drug treatment was started, review this and discontinue if possible. If this is not possible, ensure that it is regularly reviewed to monitor effectiveness, side-effects, misuse and dependency.

Short-term management

While treatment of borderline personality disorder should be considered to be a long-term process, various biological, psychological and social management strategies can be employed in the shorter term, with the aim of facilitating trust, building a positive relationship with health and social care services, and identifying and alleviating sources of distress.

Psychopharmacology

There are no medications that are currently licensed specifically (in the UK) for the treatment of borderline personality disorder. However, drugs can be useful to treat comorbid mental illness, or to manage cases of behavioural disturbance and suicidal behaviour during the more severe phases. Antipsychotics may be of some use in treating the pseudo-psychotic symptoms that are sometimes experienced. Antidepressants may be useful in treating depressive symptoms. SSRIs may help with obsessive-compulsive symptoms as well as impulsivity and self-harming behaviour. Mood stabilizers such as lithium, sodium valproate and lamotrigine may be useful in treating aggression, impulsivity and mood instability. Benzodiazepines should be used with caution due to the potential for abuse and dependence.

Psychosocial

Supportive psychotherapy provides patients with an authority figure during times of crisis. Regular contact with a healthcare professional can also provide the patient with a sense of containment. Members of the multidisciplinary team can provide psychoeducation, as well as facilitating development of coping strategies, relaxation, distraction techniques, improving disturbed relationships and development of skills and hobbies. In cooperation with social services, issues such as housing, finances and employment can be addressed.

Longer term management

The long-term management of patients with borderline personality disorder involves addressing and modifying maladaptive traits of personality. This generally involves a psychotherapeutic modality of treatment. Because traits and behaviours tend to be deeply engrained, this process can take many years. Around 40% of people with borderline personality disorder disengage with psychotherapy, and so it is important to build a trusting relationship and to be prepared for therapeutic change taking a long time.

There is evidence suggesting the efficacy of various modalities of psychotherapy in the treatment of borderline personality disorder. It may be that the consistency of therapy, the maintenance of boundaries and the empathic and non-judgemental stance of the therapist allows for the successful development of a therapeutic relationship, which may in itself be more important than the specific type of therapy. For more information on psychotherapy, see Chapter 3.

- Dialectical behaviour therapy (DBT) (see p. 31) uses a combination of cognitive and behavioural therapies, with some relaxation techniques from Zen Buddhism. It involves both individual and group therapy, and can be helpful in reducing self-harming and improving functioning.
- Mentalization-based therapy (MBT) (see p. 31) focuses on allowing patients to better understand what is going on in both their minds and in the minds of others. It can utilize both individual and group components, and can be effective in the treatment of borderline personality disorder.
- Cognitive behavioural therapy (CBT) (see p. 28) can be adapted for use in borderline personality disorder.

- Cognitive analytical therapy (CAT) (see p. 31) may be useful in the treatment of borderline personality disorder.
- Psychodynamic psychotherapy (see p. 26), as both individual and group therapy, can be effective in the treatment of borderline personality disorder.
- Therapeutic communities (see p.30) are a residential form of therapy, where the patient may stay for weeks or months. The community tends to run as a 'democracy', with patients often having as much say as the staff. Most of the therapeutic work is done in groups, and patients learn from getting on (or not getting on) with others. It differs from 'real life' in that any disagreements or upsets happen in a controlled and safe environment.

HINTS AND TIPS

Remember that personality disorders involve long-standing personality traits. While they are 'treatable', pharmacotherapy is not the mainstay, but is used to alleviate specific symptoms (e.g. comorbid depression, anxiety or impulsivity). Medications are unlikely to affect maladaptive personality traits. With appropriate psychosocial interventions, these may significantly improve with time. You may want to consider this when discussing management with patients.

Course and prognosis

The course of personality disorders, and the prognosis of sufferers, is not as dire as was once thought. Some 78–99% of patients with borderline personality disorder will show signs of sustained symptomatic remission at 16-year follow-up. Patients with antisocial personality may also improve with time, especially if they have formed a relationship with a therapist. Schizotypal and obsessive-compulsive personality disorders tend to be stable over time, although schizotypal patients may go on to develop schizophrenia.

Patients with personality disorder have a greater incidence of other mental illnesses such as depression, bipolar affective disorder, anxiety and schizophrenia. Furthermore, these tend to be more severe and have a worse prognosis than if the personality disorder was not present. Patients with personality disorder (especially cluster B) also have far higher rates of suicide and accidental death than the general population.

Eating disorders 23

● Objectives

After this chapter you should have an understanding of:
- The epidemiology of anorexia nervosa
- The difference between anorexia and bulimia nervosa
- The importance of family history and environmental factors in patients with anorexia and bulimia nervosa
- The role of antidepressants in the treatment of patients with anorexia and bulimia nervosa
- The treatments of choice in patients with anorexia
- The indications for hospitalization in patients with anorexia
- The poor prognostic factors associated with anorexia and bulimia nervosa

This chapter discusses the disorders associated with the presenting complaints in Chapter 17, which you might find helpful to read first.

ANOREXIA AND BULIMIA NERVOSA

Epidemiology

Eating disorders are approximately 10 times more common in females than males. As many as one female in 20 will have eating habits which give cause for concern, and most will be between the ages of 14 and 25 years old. The incidence rates of anorexia nervosa in the general population is 11 per 100 000 population. The exact incidence of bulimia nervosa is difficult to calculate, because many sufferers do not come to the attention of services. However, it is estimated that the incidence of bulimia nervosa is approximately five times that of anorexia nervosa. In terms of prevalence, between 0.5% and 1% of the female population are thought to suffer from bulimia nervosa. Eating disorders are far more common in certain occupations, specifically ballet dancers, gymnasts and athletes. Anorexia nervosa was previously considered to be more prevalent in higher socioeconomic classes; however, recent evidence has challenged this. Bulimia nervosa has an equal prevalence across all socioeconomic classes. Figure 23.1 summarizes the epidemiology of both anorexia and bulimia nervosa.

Aetiology

The cause of neither anorexia nor bulimia has been clarified, but both biological and psychosocial factors have been implicated.

Anorexia nervosa

Genetic/biological factors

Estimates from twin studies suggest that 58–76% of the variance in the liability to anorexia nervosa is due to genetic factors. There is a higher concordance rate for monozygotic (55%) than dizygotic twins (5%). Abnormalities of serotonin metabolism have been implicated. It is possible that the inherited liability might be mediated by certain personality traits, including inhibition, perfectionism, obsessionality and harmavoidance.

Environmental/psychological factors

In Western culture, the widely portrayed notion of the 'ideal body' influences perception of body image, meaning that unusual thinness is often valued more than natural curves. Relationship difficulties are often (but not always) found within families of patients with anorexia nervosa, including over-protectiveness, enmeshment (over-involvement, with lack of differentiation between parent and child), conflict avoidance, lack of conflict resolution and rigidity (resistance to change).

Bulimia nervosa

Genetic/biological factors

The genetic contribution to variance in liability to bulimia nervosa is 54–83%. Serotonin, noradrenaline (norepinephrine) and plasma endorphins have all been implicated, although many neurotransmitter abnormalities occur secondary to weight loss and purging. There is often a family history of depression and/or substance misuse.

Fig. 23.1	Epidemiology of anorexia and bulimia nervosa		
Disorder	**Prevalence**	**Age of onset**	**Sociodemographics**
Anorexia nervosa	0.3% of young women	More common in mid-adolescence	Initially thought to be more prevalent in higher socioeconomic classes; however, several studies do not support this (still debated). Much more prevalent in ballet dancers, gymnasts and athletes
Bulimia nervosa	1% of young women	More common in late adolescence and early adulthood	Equal socioeconomic class distribution

Environmental/psychological factors

Past exposure to dieting behaviour, which is more common in patients with a history of childhood obesity, parental obesity and early menarche, is usually present. Family relationships seem to be more conflictual than in patients with anorexia nervosa. The personality trait of perfectionism appears to be a risk factor, but to a lesser extent than in anorexia nervosa. Alcohol and substance abuse, personality disorders and depression are associated conditions.

Assessment, clinical features, investigations, complications and differential diagnosis

Discussed in Chapter 17.

HINTS AND TIPS

Although depression and obsessive-compulsive disorder may coexist with anorexia nervosa, these symptoms can also result from the effects of starvation. It may help to think 'what happened first?', and limit the use of drug treatment to symptoms that are particularly severe, or which do not improve with weight gain.

Management

Anorexia nervosa

Ambivalence towards treatment coupled with the psychological consequences of starvation (poor concentration, depression, lethargy) means that anorexia nervosa is often difficult to treat. Treatment should be collaborative, with an early aim of establishing a therapeutic alliance. Motivational interviewing and the application of the transtheoretical model of change (see Ch. 21, p.156) can be helpful for engaging patients and overcoming treatment resistance. The severity of the illness determines the level of care:

- Patients who simply diet excessively can be treated with education about nutrition and weight monitoring by a general practitioner (GP) or nurse. Voluntary organizations and self-help groups may also be helpful.
- Psychotherapy, preferably with familial involvement, is the treatment modality of choice for patients with anorexia nervosa. Weight should be monitored, and medical complications (see Fig. 17.3, p.129) actively sought. A multidisciplinary approach is required, involving the GP, a psychiatrist, a psychotherapist and possibly a member of the community mental health team. In young people, it may be beneficial to involve a paediatrician. Figure 23.2 summarizes the various forms of psychosocial therapeutic interventions.
- There should be a low threshold for referral to a specialist eating disorder service, especially in patients who are resistant to out-patient treatment, and those who have severe anorexia or poor prognostic factors (Fig. 23.3). Many areas have multidisciplinary intensive home treatment teams (see Ch. 5) specifically for patients with anorexia nervosa.
- Hospitalization is necessary in certain medical circumstances (e.g. body mass index less than 13.5 kg/m^2, rapid weight loss, severe electrolyte abnormalities, syncope) and psychiatric circumstances (risk of suicide, social crisis).
- In severe cases, patients can lose insight into the severity of their illness, by virtue of both the psychopathology of the illness and the neuropsychological effects of starvation. Where a patient lacks capacity to make decisions regarding their care and treatment, it may be necessary to use mental health legislation (see Ch. 4) to effect compulsory admission to hospital, and to initiate life-saving treatment.
- While mental health legislation in all UK countries only makes provision for the compulsory treatment of mental illness (not physical illness), food is considered to be treatment for mental illness because it

Fig. 23.2 Psychosocial therapy options for anorexia nervosa (see Ch. 3 for more information on psychological therapies)

Therapy type	Comments
Psychoeducation about nutrition and weight	Advice on balanced eating Education about the complications of excessive exercise, starvation, bingeing and purging Education about the nature of eating disorders (body image disturbance, starvation–hunger–bingeing relationship) Investigation results may be useful to aid motivation
Nutritional management and weight restoration	Negotiation of target weight Eating plan: amount of calories per day; three meals/day with snacks in between to avoid hunger Education on shopping and cooking skills if necessary
Cognitive-behavioural therapy (CBT)	20–24 sessions with 'top-up' as necessary May explore issues of control, low self-esteem and perfectionism
Interpersonal therapy (IPT)	Focus on improving social functioning and interpersonal skills
Family therapy	May be very effective for adolescents still living with parents, and when onset of illness occurs before adulthood May expose dysfunctional attachment patterns and interpersonal difficulties
Psychodynamic psychotherapy	Reserved for specialists in eating disorders

Fig. 23.3 Poor prognostic factors in anorexia nervosa

Long duration of illness
Late age of onset
Very low weight
Associated binge–purge symptoms
Personality difficulties
Difficult family relationships
Poor social adjustment

Fig. 23.4 Refeeding syndrome

Electrolyte abnormalities	Clinical manifestations
Hypophosphataemia	Muscle weakness
Hypokalaemia	Seizures
Hypomagnesaemia	Peripheral oedema
Hyponatraemia	Cardiac dysrhythmias
Metabolic acidosis	Hypotension
Thiamine deficiency	Delirium

leads to improvement in the psychological symptoms (impaired decision making) caused by starvation. Therefore, as a final resort, in certain cases patients may be force-fed under mental health legislation. In extreme cases, nasogastric or intravenous feeding may be necessary.

When a patient starts eating after a prolonged (more than 5 days) period of starvation, care must be taken to avoid the refeeding syndrome (Fig. 23.4), which is characterized by fluid and electrolyte disturbances. This can have potentially fatal consequences. Management hinges on replacement of fluid and electrolytes, which may need to be intravenous.

The use of psychotropic medication is limited, and should be instituted cautiously in patients who are underweight. SSRIs may be useful for treating comorbid depression and obsessive-compulsive disorder.

Bulimia nervosa

Patients with bulimia nervosa tend to be more motivated to address their eating difficulties, and are usually of a normal weight. Treatment is predominantly psychological, ranging from psychoeducation, self-help manuals and self-help groups in mild cases, to cognitive-behavioural therapy or interpersonal psychotherapy in more serious cases. Management by specialist eating disorder services may be necessary in severe cases. In-patient treatment is not usually required; however, it may be necessary for the treatment of electrolyte disturbances resultant from purging (which can be fatal), or for management of the risk of suicide or self-harm. Antidepressants (high-dose SSRIs) can be useful to reduce bingeing and purging behaviour. Comorbid substance abuse and depression is common and should be managed as indicated.

Prognosis

Anorexia

Although weight and menstrual functioning usually improve, eating habits and attitudes to body shape and weight often remain abnormal. Around a fifth of patients make a full recovery, a quarter develop bulimia nervosa, and a fifth remain severely unwell. The remainder tend to follow a relapsing-remitting course. The lifetime mortality from anorexia nervosa is about 15%: around half of these deaths are due to the complications of starvation, and around a third by suicide. Factors associated with a poorer prognosis are described in Figure 23.3, and indicate that poorer outcomes are seen in more severe illness.

Bulimia

The course of bulimia is also variable, although generally better than anorexia, with 50–70% of patients achieving either full or partial recovery after 5 years. It is thought that bulimia nervosa is not associated with increased mortality. However, there is a strong association with both depression and substance misuse, and higher mortality rates are associated with these conditions. Poor prognostic factors include severe bingeing and purging behaviour, low weight and comorbid depression.

Disorders relating to the menstrual cycle, pregnancy and the puerperium

24

● **Objectives**

After this chapter you should have an understanding of:
- The psychiatric symptoms and syndromes occurring in the premenstruum, pregnancy, the puerperium and the menopause
- The symptoms of premenstrual syndrome (PMS) and where they occur in the menstrual cycle
- Differences in the aetiology and management of postnatal blues, postnatal depression and puerperal psychosis
- How to manage the high risk of relapse of bipolar affective disorder during the puerperium
- The management of a woman with postnatal depression who wants to continue breast-feeding
- The factors on mental state examination that would concern you when assessing risk in a woman with puerperal psychosis
- Issues surrounding mental illness during the menopause

PREMENSTRUAL SYNDROME

Clinical features

The premenstrual syndrome (PMS) has been defined as the recurrence of symptoms during the premenstruum, with their absence in the postmenstruum. Symptoms tend to occur in the 10 days prior to menstruation and remit in the 2 weeks following. Psychological symptoms include low mood (71%), irritability (56%) and tiredness (35%). Physical symptoms such as headache (33%), abdominal bloating (31%) and breast tenderness (21%) are also fairly common.

Epidemiology/aetiology

Up to 40% of women report experiencing some symptoms of PMS and one study described recurrent cyclical symptoms in up to 80% of women. However, only about 5% of women experience symptoms of a severity sufficient to interfere with their work or lifestyle. The prevalence is higher in women over the age of 30 years, who are multiparous (prevalence increases with parity), who do not use oral contraception and who experience significant degrees of psychosocial stress. Genetic, hormonal/biological and psychosocial factors have been implicated in the aetiology (good relationships are thought to have a protective effect).

Management

Non-specific management of PMS includes reassurance, advice on healthy eating, stress-reduction, and exercise. Abstaining from caffeine or alcohol in the week before menstruation can also be helpful. Psychotherapeutic intervention may be beneficial, in the form of psychosocial counselling, stress management and cognitive-behavioural therapy (CBT). Pharmacological therapies may be helpful, specifically hormonal contraception (the combined pill, implants, patches), SSRIs, danazol (a testosterone analogue) and gonadotrophin-releasing hormone analogues.

MENOPAUSE

There is little evidence that the menopause itself leads to an increased incidence of mental illness. Psychological symptoms may understandably accompany the changes that occur with the menopause; however, it should be remembered that this is a time associated with other psychosocial stressors, such as children leaving home and a growing awareness of ageing. There is no clear psychiatric indication for hormone replacement therapy (HRT) and its use for psychological symptoms remains controversial. HRT should never substitute treatment with recognized antidepressants for the treatment of a depressive illness.

PSYCHIATRIC CONSIDERATIONS IN PREGNANCY

- The development of new psychiatric illnesses during pregnancy is no more common than in the general population. However, both psychosocial stressors and changing or stopping maintenance medications in women with a history of major mental illnesses carries a degree of risk, and the puerperium is a high-risk period for relapse in major mental illness, particularly bipolar affective disorder. Domestic violence is more common during pregnancy, and this can impair mental health and resilience.

- Women with a major mental illness (bipolar affective disorder, schizophrenia, severe depression) or history of puerperal psychosis who are pregnant or planning pregnancy should be referred to perinatal psychiatry services, even if they have been stable for some years. Figure 24.1 summarizes the indications for referral to a specialist perinatal mental health team.
- For patients prescribed psychotropic medication during pregnancy, a judgement needs to be made – in conjunction with the patient – regarding the risk of relapse against the risk of medication-induced teratogenic or adverse effects. Risks associated with various psychotropic medications are summarized in Figure 24.2. Decisions should be made prior to conception (if possible). Up-to-date information on the use of medications during pregnancy should always be sought.

- There is an increased incidence of adverse life events in the weeks prior to a spontaneous abortion (miscarriage).
- Following miscarriage and termination of pregnancy, there is an increased risk of adjustment and bereavement reactions (see Ch. 12). Also, the risk of puerperal psychosis remains.

Fig. 24.1 Indications for referral to perinatal mental health services

Preconceptual counselling (e.g. for women with bipolar disorder)
Pregnant women who are psychiatrically unwell
Pregnant women who are at high risk of significant puerperal illness
Women who are psychiatrically unwell and are the main carers of babies under 6 months old

---

HINTS AND TIPS

Pseudocyesis is the rare condition when a non-pregnant woman has the signs and symptoms of pregnancy (e.g. abdominal distension, breast enlargement, cessation of menses, enlargement of the uterus). Couvade syndrome describes the condition in which men develop typical pregnancy-related symptoms during their partner's pregnancy (e.g. morning sickness, vague abdominal pains, labour

---

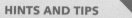

Fig. 24.2 Psychiatric medication during pregnancy and breast-feeding

Drug group	Pregnancy	Breast-feeding
Tricyclic antidepressants	Associated with neonatal hypoglycaemia, low APGAR score, neonatal jaundice and a mildly increased risk of fetal malformations	Low-dose amitriptyline appears safe, and clomipramine may be useful for obsessional phenomena. Avoid doxepin (accumulation of metabolite)
SSRIs	Can be associated with withdrawal symptoms in neonates, which are generally mild and self-limiting. Associated with persistent pulmonary hypertension. Paroxetine also associated with fetal heart defects, and is contraindicated during pregnancy	Paroxetine and sertraline: very small amounts excreted in breast milk; short half-life Fluoxetine and citalopram are excreted in relatively larger (but still small) amounts. Fluoxetine has a long half-life and thus may accumulate
Mood stabilizers	Associated with teratogenicity. Valproate carries the highest risk of fetal malformations, followed by carbamazepine, then lithium, then lamotrigine	Risk of neonatal lithium toxicity as breast milk contains 40% of maternal lithium concentration. Avoid if possible. Consider the use of valproate or carbamazepine if necessary, but bear in mind risk of infant hepatotoxicity
Antipsychotics	Most antipsychotics have no established teratogenic effects, but may cause self-limiting extrapyramidal side-effects in neonates. Olanzapine increases risk of gestational diabetes	Only small amounts excreted but possible effects on developing nervous system. Avoid high doses due to risk of lethargy in infant
Benzodiazepines and other hypnotics	Associated with floppy infant syndrome (hypotonia, breathing and feeding difficulties) and neonatal withdrawal syndrome	May cause lethargy in infant. Choose drugs with short half-lives (e.g. lorazepam) if necessary

pains). Both of these conditions are psychosomatic and should be distinguished from delusion of pregnancy. Pseudocyesis and delusion of pregnancy may occur together.

PUERPERAL DISORDERS

The incidence of psychiatric illness in the puerperium is exceptionally high. In primiparous women, there is up to a 35-fold increased risk of developing a psychotic illness and needing hospital admission in the first month following childbirth. This emphasizes the importance of close vigilance in the postpartum period, especially in women with a personal or family history of mental illness.

Postnatal 'blues'

Also known as 'maternity blues' and 'baby blues', this occurs in up to 50% of postpartum women. It presents within the first 10 days post-delivery, and symptoms peak between days 3 and 5. It is characterized by episodes of tearfulness, mild depression or emotional lability, anxiety and irritability. There appears to be no links with life events, demographic factors or obstetric events, which is suggestive of an underlying biological cause (e.g. a sudden fall in progesterone post-delivery). Postnatal blues is self-limiting, resolves spontaneously and usually only requires reassurance. However, an apparent bad case of postnatal blues may mark the onset of postnatal depression.

Postnatal depression

Clinical features

Postnatal depression (PND) usually develops within 3 months of delivery, and typically lasts between 2 and 6 months. The symptoms are similar to a non-puerperal depressive episode: low mood, loss of interest or pleasure, fatigability and suicidal ideation (although suicide is rare). Note that sleeping difficulties, weight loss and decreased libido can be normal for the first few months following delivery. Additional features of PND may include:

- Anxious preoccupation with the baby's health, often associated with feelings of guilt and inadequacy.

- Reduced affection for the baby with possible impaired bonding.
- Obsessional phenomena, typically involving recurrent and intrusive thoughts of harming the baby (it is crucial to ascertain whether these are regarded as distressing (ego-dystonic), as obsessions usually are, or whether they pose a potential risk).
- Infanticidal thoughts (thoughts of killing the baby), which are different from obsessions in that they are not experienced as distressing (ego-syntonic), may be seriously considered, and (worryingly) may involve planning. These symptoms necessitate urgent psychiatric assessment.

Epidemiology and aetiology

In the developed world, postnatal depression is the most common complication of childbirth, with rates of around 10%. There does not appear to be an association with socioeconomic class or parity. Evidence suggests that biological factors are not as important as they are in postnatal blues and puerperal psychosis. Psychosocial factors are strongly linked to the development of postnatal depression, with the lack of a close confiding relationship and young maternal age both implicated. A previous history of depression is an important risk factor. In women with a history of depression, obstetric complications during delivery are associated with an increased rate of postnatal depression.

Management

The diagnosis and management of postnatal depression is often undertaken within primary care. Psychological and social measures, such as mother-and-baby groups, relationship counselling and problem solving, are often helpful. Midwives and health visitors can be very helpful. For more severe illness, antidepressant medication is necessary. Antidepressants may be transmitted in small quantities to the baby via breast milk, and a judgement needs to be made, in conjunction with the patient, of the risks versus benefits of medication. It should be noted that (with the exception of doxepin) there has never been evidence to suggest that antidepressants transmitted via breast milk have caused harm to a baby, but there are significant risks for the baby's cognitive and emotional development if the mother has untreated depression. Figure 24.2 provides information on the use of psychotropic medication in breast-feeding mothers. Mothers with severe postnatal depression with suicidal/infanticidal ideation may require hospital admission, with admission with the baby to a mother-and-baby unit usually being preferable. Electroconvulsive therapy (ECT) may be indicated and usually results in a rapid improvement, which is important to allow the woman to resume contact with the baby as soon as possible. Remember that the assessment of the infant's well-being is an additional part of the comprehensive psychosocial and risk assessment.

HINTS AND TIPS

If a woman has been on an antidepressant during pregnancy, do not change after delivery to a different antidepressant that is 'better for breastfeeding'. Doing this means the child is exposed to two medications, instead of one. The fetus is exposed to far greater levels of antidepressant *in utero* than levels transmitted in breast milk, so if they are healthy at delivery they are unlikely to be harmed by further, lower, exposure.

Prognosis

Most women respond to standard treatment; however, some patients have a protracted illness and may require long-term treatment and follow-up. Woman who develop postnatal depression have around a 50% increased risk of developing a similar illness following childbirth in the future.

Postnatal depression is associated with disturbances in the mother–infant relationship, and this can lead to problems with the child's cognitive and emotional development.

HINTS AND TIPS

Despite the increased rate of depression, postnatal suicide is rare. The suicide rate in the year following childbirth is one-sixth the rate for a matched control group. However, note that suicide is far more common than infanticide, so if infanticidal thoughts are present the risk of suicide should be thoroughly explored.

Puerperal psychosis

Clinical features

The postpartum period is an extremely high-risk period for the development of a psychotic episode. These episodes characteristically have a rapid onset, usually between 4 days and 3 weeks post-delivery, and almost always within 8 weeks. They typically begin with insomnia, restlessness and perplexity, later progressing to suspiciousness and marked psychotic symptoms. The symptoms can be polymorphic, and frequently fluctuate dramatically in their nature and intensity over a short space of time. Patients often retain a degree of insight, and may not disclose certain bizarre delusions or suicidal/homicidal thoughts. There is some debate as to whether the puerperal psychoses represent a separate disease entity, a mood disorder with psychotic features, a schizophrenia-like episode, or a combination of these. In the majority of cases, the clinical presentation resembles a mood disorder (depression or mania) with delusions and hallucinations. Even when schizophrenia-like symptoms are present, patients often have associated mood symptoms; however, affective and psychotic symptoms may occur at separate times during the same illness.

Epidemiology and aetiology

Puerperal psychosis develops in about 1 in 500 childbirths. It occurs more frequently in primiparous women, and those who have a personal or family history of bipolar affective disorder or puerperal psychosis. If a close family member has bipolar affective disorder, the risk can be as high as 15 in 500 childbirths. Psychosocial factors seem less important, unlike in postnatal depression. Occasionally, a puerperal psychosis may be precipitated by an obstetric complication (e.g. pre-eclampsia, puerperal infection) or medication. Figure 24.3 summarizes the risk factors for puerperal psychosis.

Management

The assessment of the risk of infanticide and suicide is crucial. Concerning symptoms include:

- Thoughts of self-harm or harming the baby.
- Severe depressive delusions (e.g. belief that the baby is, or should be, dead).
- Command hallucinations instructing the mother to harm herself or her baby.

Hospitalization is invariably necessary, with joint admissions to a mother-and-baby unit being preferable when the mother is able to look after her infant under supervision. Detention under mental health legislation may be necessary. Depending on presentation, antipsychotics, antidepressants and mood-stabilizing medications may be necessary. Benzodiazepines may be

Fig. 24.3 Risk factors for puerperal psychosis
Previous puerperal psychosis
History of mood disorder (particularly bipolar affective disorder)
Family history of puerperal psychosis or bipolar affective disorder
Primiparous mother
Delivery associated with caesarean section or perinatal death

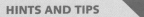

needed in cases of severe behavioural disturbance. All psychotropic drugs should be used with caution in breast-feeding mothers (see Fig. 24.2). ECT can be particularly effective in severe or treatment-resistant cases. Psychosocial interventions are similar to those for other psychotic episodes, but also include providing support for the father.

Prognosis

Most cases of puerperal psychosis will have recovered by 3 months (75% within 6 weeks). There is about a 60% chance of experiencing a recurrence after future childbirths. Women who have had both puerperal and non-puerperal depressive or manic episodes (i.e. have an established mood disorder) have up to an 85% chance of future puerperal psychotic episodes.

> **HINTS AND TIPS**
>
> The prevalence of postnatal blues, postnatal depression and puerperal psychosis is inversely related to their severity:
> • Postnatal blues develops after one in two childbirths.
> • Postnatal depression develops after one in eight childbirths.
> • Puerperal psychosis develops after about one in 500 childbirths.

Dementia and delirium (25)

This chapter discusses the disorders associated with the presenting complaints in Chapter 14, which you might find helpful to read first.

DEMENTIA

Epidemiology

The overall prevalence of dementia is approximately 1% of the total UK population, rising sharply with increasing age. Figure 25.1 illustrates the increasing prevalence of dementia with age. The prevalence in persons aged 65 or over is approximately 7%, in those over 80 about 20% and in those over 90 around 30%. Early onset dementia begins before age 65. Alzheimer's dementia is more common in women and vascular dementia more common in men.

Dementia is a syndrome due to various diseases, most commonly neurodegeneration or vascular damage as below:

- Alzheimer's disease, approximately 30–60% of cases.
- Vascular dementia, approximately 10–30%.
- Combined Alzheimer's and vascular ('mixed') dementia, approximately 10–30%.
- Dementia with Lewy bodies, approximately 5%.
- Frontotemporal dementia, approximately 2% (20% of early onset dementia).

Aetiopathology

Each type of dementia will be discussed separately.

Alzheimer's disease

Alzheimer's disease (AD) is classified as:

- Early onset (onset before age 65, usually familial, with relatives also affected before age 65).
- Late onset/sporadic (onset after age 65, either no family history or relatives affected after age 65).

At present, the cause of most cases of AD is unknown. It appears to be a combination of multifactorial genetic risk factors, vascular risk factors and other uncertain environmental factors. The characteristic pathological changes are:

1. Beta-amyloid **plaques** between neurones.
2. Neurofibrillary **tangles** of hyperphosphorylated tau inside neurones.

It is unclear whether either of these changes are a cause or a consequence of neuronal damage and death. The abnormalities generally begin in the medial temporal lobe (where key structures relating to memory are located) before becoming more diffuse, resulting in generalized cortical atrophy and compensatory ventricular enlargement. Degeneration of cholinergic neurons in the nucleus basalis of Meynert leads to a deficiency of acetylcholine which can be partially reversed by some anti-dementia medications (cholinesterase inhibitors). These drugs can temporarily slow the loss of cognitive function but not reverse or ultimately prevent it.

Genetic factors

Late-onset AD. There is a three-fold increased risk of developing AD in the first-degree relatives of sufferers. The most important gene associated with late-onset AD is the gene that codes a protein involved in cholesterol

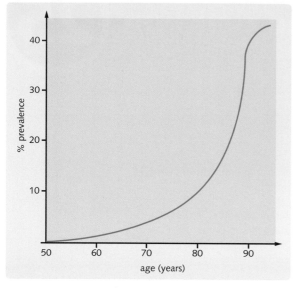

Fig. 25.1 Graph showing increasing prevalence of dementia with age

metabolism called apolipoprotein E (ApoE), which occurs in three different alleles (ε2, ε3 and ε4). Individuals who inherit one copy of the ApoE ε4 allele are at a roughly three-fold increased risk of developing AD, and those with two copies are at a roughly 10-fold increased risk. However, other environmental and genetic factors must be involved because having two ApoE ε4 alleles does not guarantee the development of AD, and many patients with AD have no copies of the allele. New genes which contribute a smaller risk are being discovered through whole genome analysis of large samples.

Early-onset AD. Some forms of early-onset familial AD are inherited in an autosomal dominant fashion. Three genes have been isolated so far:

- Amyloid precursor protein – chromosome 21.
- Presenilin-1 – chromosome 14.
- Presenilin-2 – chromosome 1.

These genes are all involved in metabolism of the amyloid protein. These autosomal dominant dementias present between the ages of 30 and 60 years, sometimes as early as age 28 when there is a mutation at presenilin 1.

Adults with trisomy 21 (Down's syndrome) invariably develop neuropathological changes similar to AD by middle age and many will develop dementia. This has been attributed to triplication and over-expression of the gene for amyloid precursor protein (APP).

> **HINTS AND TIPS**
>
> You should be aware of four genes in Alzheimer's disease (AD) – one in late-onset AD, and three in early-onset autosomal dominant AD:

- In late-onset AD, the ApoE ε4 allele increases an individual's susceptibility to develop AD.
- In early-onset AD, the possession of a mutated version of one of three genes, amyloid precursor protein, presenilin-1 and presenilin-2, virtually guarantees that an individual will develop AD. Late-onset sporadic AD accounts for the overwhelming majority of all AD cases.

Environmental factors

The main environmental risk factors for AD are vascular (Fig. 25.2). It is unclear whether vascular insufficiency in part causes the plaques and tangles seen in AD, or whether vascular damage reduces the brain's reserve, making a given amount of neurodegeneration more likely to manifest clinically. Head injury and low educational attainment are also risk factors.

> **HINTS AND TIPS**
>
> Neurodegeneration seems to be associated with misplaced proteins: Alzheimer's, dementia with Lewy bodies and frontotemporal dementia all involve the accumulation of degradation-resistant protein aggregates (see Fig. 25.3 for more detail).

Vascular dementia

The cause of vascular dementia is presumed to be multiple cortical infarctions or many small subcortical infarctions in white matter (Binswanger's disease) resulting from widespread cerebrovascular disease. On occasions, vascular dementia can arise from a single infarct. As with both Alzheimer's disease and cerebrovascular disease, vascular dementia is closely associated with increasing age. In rare cases, the disease is linked to *NOTCH3*, a gene on chromosome 19 involved in vascular smooth muscle cells response to injury (cerebral autosomal dominant arteriopathy with subcortical infarcts and leucoencephalopathy (CADASIL)). The risk

Fig. 25.2 Environmental risk factors for Alzheimer's and vascular dementia

Vascular	Both	Alzheimer's
Previous stroke Atrial fibrillation	Smoking Hypertension Diabetes Hypercholesterolaemia History of myocardial infarct Obesity	Head injury Low educational attainment

Fig. 25.3 Neuropathology of dementia

Dementia type	Abnormal protein(s)	Macroscopic findings	Microscopic findings
Alzheimer's disease	Beta amyloid Tau	Generalized cerebral atrophy, beginning in medial temporal lobes	Extracellular amyloid plaques Intracellular neurofibrillary tangles containing hyperphosphorylated tau and ubiquitin
Frontotemporal dementia (a heterogenous collection of dementias of which Pick's disease is one type)	Tau (most cases) Progranulin (some cases)	Atrophy of frontal and temporal lobes, particularly anteriorly	Intracellular aggregates of ubiquitin and tau, or ubiquitin and other abnormal proteins. Pick's disease features Pick bodies (tau-positive cytoplasmic protein aggregates)
Dementia with Lewy bodies	Alpha-synuclein	Mild atrophy frontal, parietal, occipital lobes	Lewy bodies (intracellular aggregates of alpha-synuclein and ubiquitin) in cortex
Parkinson's disease (30% develop dementia)	Alpha-synuclein	Atrophy of substantia nigra and locus coeruleus	Lewy bodies in brainstem nuclei
Huntington's disease	Huntingtin	Marked atrophy of basal ganglia and often frontal lobes	Intracellular aggregates of huntingtin and ubiquitin
Creutzfeldt–Jakob disease	Prion protein	Spongiform changes throughout cortex and subcortical nuclei	Extracellular prion protein plaques, particularly in cerebellum
Vascular dementia	None identified (in most cases)	Infarction – multiple small infarcts, or single large or strategic infarct	Infarcted grey and or white matter

factors for developing vascular dementia are the same as for cerebrovascular disease in general and are summarized in Figure 25.2.

Dementia with Lewy bodies

Dementia with Lewy bodies (DLB) is associated with Lewy bodies: neuronal inclusions composed of abnormally phosphorylated neurofilament proteins aggregated with ubiquitin and alpha-synuclein. Mutations in the gene coding for alpha-synuclein causes some familial cases of DLB, but the cause of sporadic cases is unclear. The Lewy bodies found in the paralimbic and neocortical structures of patients with DLB are identical to those found in the basal ganglia of patients with Parkinson's disease. Remember from Chapter 14 that parkinson-like motor features are a core feature of DLB. Lewy bodies are also found in the brains of patients with Alzheimer's disease and Down's syndrome, and sometimes in people without dementia.

Parkinson's disease with dementia

Idiopathic Parkinson's disease is due to neuronal death associated with Lewy bodies in the substantia nigra, the site of dopaminergic neurones in the basal ganglia.

However, there are often also diffuse Lewy bodies in many brain regions other than the basal ganglia. In around 30% of patients, damage to other brain regions leads to dementia with predominantly subcortical features. Mutations in genes coding for alpha-synuclein and proteins involved in the ubiquitin-proteasome system (e.g. parkin) lead to familial Parkinson's disease and suggest that abnormal protein degradation may be part of the pathophysiology of sporadic disease also. The syndrome of parkinsonism (as opposed to the specific disorder of idiopathic Parkinson's disease) can be due to any injury to the basal ganglia: cerebrovascular disease, head injury, carbon monoxide poisoning, dopamine antagonists (including antipsychotic medication), or other neurodegenerative disorders (e.g. 'Parkinson's plus' syndromes such as progressive supranuclear palsy).

Frontotemporal dementia

Frontotemporal dementias are a heterogeneous group of neurodegenerative disorders associated with degeneration of the anterior part of the brain. Their pathology and presentation overlap with motor neurone disease. Macroscopically, they are associated with bilateral atrophy of the frontal and anterior temporal lobes (atrophied paper-thin gyri known as 'knife-blade atrophy') and degeneration of the striatum. Microscopically, a range of intracellular inclusion bodies have been identified, grouping broadly into those which include mainly ubiquitin and tau (e.g. Pick's bodies) or, more commonly, those which include ubiquitin and other proteins. Mutations in genes coding for tau and progranulin (a protein involved in neuronal repair) cause familial frontotemporal dementias.

COMMUNICATION

Pick's disease is strictly a neuropathological diagnosis requiring the presence of Pick's bodies at post-mortem, but some clinicians use it to mean the clinical diagnosis of any type of frontotemporal dementia.

Huntington's disease

Huntington's disease has autosomal dominant inheritance with complete penetrance. It is caused by a gene on the short arm of chromosome 4 that contains an excessive number of trinucleotide (CAG) repeat sequences, usually more than 40, which results in production of the abnormal protein 'huntingtin'. The length of the abnormal trinucleotide repeat sequence is inversely correlated to the age of onset of the disease. This abnormal protein is associated with neuronal death, particularly in the basal ganglia, giving rise to the distressing motor signs of the disease.

Creutzfeldt–Jakob disease and other prion-related diseases

A prion is an infectious protein which can cause fatal neurodegeneration. All the prion-related disorders result in a spongiform degeneration of the brain in the absence of an inflammatory immune response, associated with the deposition of the prion protein (PrP) in the form of beta pleated sheets.

A number of prion diseases exist: kuru (prion transmitted by cannibalism of neural tissue, described in the highland tribes of New Guinea), Gerstmann–Sträussler syndrome (autosomal dominant condition caused by mutation of PrP gene on chromosome 20), scrapie in sheep and BSE (bovine spongiform encephalopathy) in cattle.

Most cases of Creutzfeldt–Jakob disease (CJD) appear to be sporadic, affecting people in their 50s, although it can be transmitted iatrogenically (e.g. via infected corneal transplants and surgical instruments). It presents with a rapidly progressing dementia with cerebellar ataxia and myoclonic jerks over a time course of 6–8 months. The electroencephalogram (EEG) characteristically shows stereotyped sharp wave complexes.

New variant CJD (nvCJD) is thought to be secondary to the ingestion of BSE-infected beef products. It typically presents in young adults with mild psychiatric symptoms such as depression and anxiety preceding the development of ataxia, dementia and finally death over a period of 18 months. There are no characteristic EEG changes, although nvCJD may have a characteristic MRI picture: a bilaterally evident high signal in the pulvinar (post-thalamic) region.

HIV-related dementia

Infection with the human immunodeficiency virus (HIV) is thought to cause direct damage to the brain in addition to the complications of HIV infection, such as opportunistic infections (cerebral cytomegalovirus infection, cryptococcosis, toxoplasmosis, tuberculosis, syphilis) and cerebral lymphoma. HIV encephalopathy presents clinically as a subcortical dementia and neuropathological examination shows diffuse multifocal destruction of the white matter and subcortical structures.

Assessment, clinical features, investigations and differential diagnosis

Discussed in Chapter 14.

Management

There is no cure for any of the neurodegenerative forms of dementia. Although the prognosis is invariably poor, considerable improvements in the quality of patients' lives are possible through a variety of psychosocial and pharmaceutical approaches. The principles of management are:

- Treating the underlying cause if possible (e.g. hypothyroidism, modifying vascular risk factors).
- Slowing down the rate of cognitive decline using anti-dementia drugs if indicated.
- Managing associated disorders or complications (e.g. aggression, depression, psychotic symptoms).
- Addressing functional problems that result (e.g. kitchen skills, financial management, social isolation).
- Providing advice and support for carers.
- Advising on legal measures to prepare for loss of capacity (e.g. Power of Attorney, Advance Statements).

Specific management strategies

Maintaining cognitive functioning

- Structured group cognitive stimulation programmes can be of benefit in mild to moderate dementia.

- The cholinesterase inhibitors, donepezil, rivastigmine and galantamine, are recommended by NICE (2010) for those patients with Alzheimer's dementia whose Mini-Mental State Examination score (MMSE) is above 10. Up to half the patients given these drugs will show a slower rate of cognitive decline and possible improvement in behavioural and psychological symptoms also. Cholinesterase inhibitors are probably also of benefit in vascular dementia, although the evidence is less strong. Rivastigmine has the best evidence of benefit in Lewy body dementia and dementia associated with Parkinson's disease. Medication is of little benefit in frontotemporal dementia.
- Memantine, an *N*-methyl-D-aspartate (NMDA) receptor antagonist, reduces excitotoxic damage by blocking NMDA receptors, preventing the influx of calcium. NICE (2010) recommends it for those with moderate to severe Alzheimer's disease or for those who cannot tolerate cholinesterase inhibitors.

Reducing behavioural and psychological symptoms of dementia

- Behavioural and psychological symptoms of dementia (BPSD) are the non-cognitive symptoms of dementia, including anxiety, agitation, delusions, hallucinations, aggression, wandering and sexual disinhibition (see p. 107).
- If a patient develops a BPSD, carefully assess for a change in their physical health, including pain. People with dementia may find it very difficult to communicate discomfort. Consider medication side-effects. Assess for depression. Consider also a change in the person's environment – are they troubled by noise, extremes of temperature, other patients?
- NICE (2010) recommends aromatherapy, massage, animal-assisted therapy, multi-sensory stimulation or therapeutic use of music or dancing for agitation.
- Pharmacological treatment can be considered for disturbed behaviour such as aggression or agitation that does not respond to non-pharmacological strategies and is causing significant distress or risk. Anxiolytic medication such as trazodone can be useful because of its relatively benign side-effect profile. Benzodiazepines should be avoided if at all possible because they worsen cognition, predispose to delirium, increase fall risk and may paradoxically disinhibit (and make more aggressive) those with dementia.
- Psychotic symptoms do not require treatment if they are not distressing to the patient nor causing risk to others. If there is felt to be significant distress a trial of an antipsychotic can be considered. Consider and document the increased risk of cerebrovascular accident. Discontinue if there is no benefit within 12 weeks.

- Depression in dementia is managed similarly to depression in older adults but with even more care taken to avoid anticholinergic drugs, which can worsen cognition.

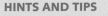

> **HINTS AND TIPS**
>
> Low doses of all medications are essential in older adults. In general, prescribe according to the rule 'start low and go slow'. This is particularly true when prescribing psychotropic medications for those with vulnerable brains (e.g. dementia) where doses a tenth of what would be used in a younger adult can be sufficient.

Legal issues

- People with dementia are likely in due course to lose the capacity to be able to make decisions about their welfare and financial affairs. It is advisable to arrange Power of Attorney as early as possible, before the person loses capacity to authorize this. They may also wish to consider an Advance Statement.
- People with dementia may not be safe to drive and they and their carers should be advised to notify the Driver and Vehicle Licensing Agency (DVLA) and their insurer of their diagnosis.

> **HINTS AND TIPS**
>
> •Benzodiazepines should be avoided if at all possible in most patients with dementia, as they are particularly vulnerable to their adverse effects such as sedation, falls and delirium.
>
> •Remember that 50% of patients with dementia with Lewy bodies (DLB) will have a catastrophic reaction to antipsychotics (even atypicals), precipitating potentially irreversible parkinsonism, impaired consciousness, severe autonomic symptoms and a two- to three-fold increase in mortality. Benzodiazepines and cholinesterase inhibitors are safer in this group of patients. This exemplifies the need to exercise caution when prescribing antipsychotics and the importance of differentiating the various types of dementia.

Course and prognosis

The course of dementia is invariably progressive. Around a third of people with dementia live in residential care. Dementia is a life-shortening illness directly and indirectly, because it reduces the ability to communicate and tolerate management of physical problems. A diagnosis of dementia roughly halves a person's remaining life expectancy. The average duration of survival from the time of diagnosis of a late onset dementia is 4 years, although there is a wide range.

DELIRIUM

Epidemiology

Most research into the epidemiology of delirium concentrates on the elderly, who, along with infants and young children, are more vulnerable to this disorder. The prevalence in hospitalized, medically ill patients ranges from 10% to 30%. Between 10% and 15% of patients over the age of 65 are delirious on admission and 10–40% develop a delirium during hospitalization. Patients with dementia are at an increased risk of developing a delirium; up to two-thirds of cases of delirium occur in patients with dementia.

Aetiology

Delirium is a final common pathway of disrupted homeostasis. In healthy individuals, a severe insult is required to cause it, e.g. head injury. In those with vulnerable brains, a minor insult is sufficient, e.g. constipation or a urinary tract infection. The commonest causes are medication (most commonly anticholinergics, opiates or benzodiazepines) or systemic illness, particularly infection. See Figure 14.4 for a fuller list. Sometimes no cause is found – this does not preclude the diagnosis.

The pathophysiological mechanism remains unclear, and may vary with cause. Suggested mechanisms include: aberrant stress response (neurotoxic effects of excess glucocorticoids), disrupted blood–brain barrier (allowing entry of toxins and cytokines to the brain) and impaired cholinergic neurotransmission.

Assessment, clinical features, investigations and differential diagnosis

Discussed in Chapter 14.

Management

Delirium can be highly distressing for patients and anxiety-provoking for medical ward staff who are less used to dealing with agitated patients. It can also be very distressing for the families and friends of the patient to see their loved one in this state. See Figure 25.4 for a management algorithm. General principles of management are as follows:

- Hospitalization is essential: delirium is a medical emergency.
- Vigorously investigate and treat any underlying medical condition.
- To limit confusion and foster trust, try to ensure that the patient is nursed by the same staff consistently.
- Merely the physical presence of a reassuring person is often enough to calm a distressed patient.
- Maximize visual acuity (e.g. glasses, appropriately lit environment) and hearing ability (e.g. hearing aid, quiet environment) to avoid misinterpretation of stimuli.
- Encourage a friend or family member to remain with the patient to help comfort and orientate them.
- Clocks, calendars and familiar objects may be helpful with orientation.
- Avoid medication unless the patient is causing a risk to themselves or others.
- Typical antipsychotics, especially low dose haloperidol, are generally effective in treating delirious symptoms, in part due to their sedative qualities, but perhaps also due to their effects on the dopamine–acetylcholine balance.
- Avoid benzodiazepines unless the patient is a risk and has not responded to haloperidol, as they tend to prolong delirium. The exception is alcohol- or substance-related delirium, in which they are highly effective.

The specific management of delirium tremens is outlined in Chapter 21.

> **HINTS AND TIPS**
>
> Remember that delirium indicates the presence of a medical condition that should be managed on a medical, not a psychiatric, ward.

Course and prognosis

The average duration of a delirium is 7 days, but delirium can be prolonged for weeks or months, even after the initial insult is treated. In-patients who develop delirium have an increased mortality, with around a third dying during that admission. This is unsurprising given that delirium is often a sign of severe systemic illness.

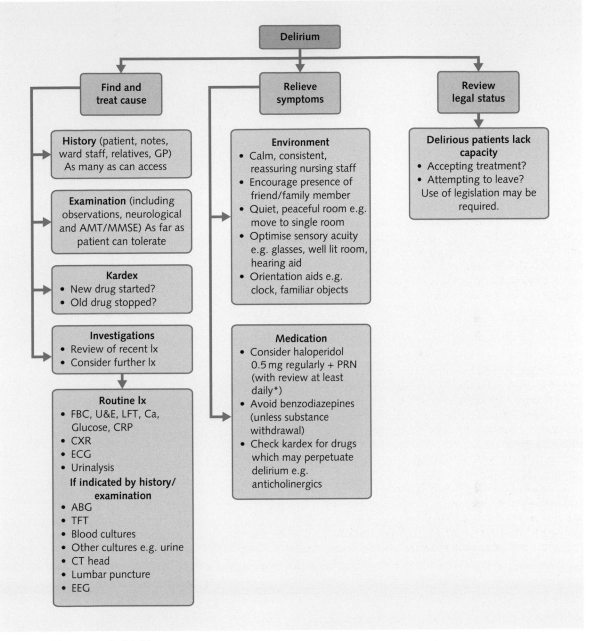

Fig. 25.4 Management of delirium
*Avoid in patients with Dementia with Lewy Bodies or Parkinson's Disease (see p. 177)

Older adult psychiatry (26)

● **Objectives**

After this chapter you should have an understanding of:
- The most prevalent psychiatric disorders in people over the age of 65
- Which features are particularly prominent in depression in older adults
- The dangers of prescribing tricyclic antidepressants to older adults
- How late-onset schizophrenia differs from early-onset schizophrenia
- The role of home assessments in older adult psychiatry
- Factors to consider before prescribing a benzodiazepine to an older adult

The most common psychiatric disorders in older adults are dementia and delirium (see Ch. 25). This chapter considers other psychiatric disorders in older adults.

Patients arbitrarily come under the care of older adult psychiatrists at the age of 65 years, as it is the average age of retirement. Services for older adults face a huge increase in demand over coming decades. Currently, one in six of the UK population is aged over 65 but by 2050 one in four people are projected to be over 65. The number of 'very old' (aged over 80) is set to almost triple by 2050.

Ageing is associated with an increased prevalence of both mental and physical health problems. Older adults may also face new social challenges such as coming to terms with retirement; income reduction; living alone or being separated from family; death of spouse, siblings and peers; and coping with deteriorating physical health and mobility.

MENTAL ILLNESS IN OLDER ADULTS

Epidemiology

The prevalence of all mental illness tends to increase with age and is about 25–30% in people over the age of 65. The prevalence of mental illness tends to be higher in residential homes. Figure 26.1 summarizes the prevalence of the individual psychiatric disorders in older adults.

Depressive disorders

Depression in older adults presents similarly to that in younger people, although certain features seem more prevalent:
- Severe psychomotor agitation or retardation.

- Cognitive impairment ('depressive pseudodementia').
- Poor concentration.
- Generalized anxiety.
- Excessive concerns about physical health (hypochondriasis).
- When psychotic, older adults are particularly likely to have hypochondriacal delusions, delusions of poverty and nihilistic delusions (see p. 69).

Depression is often under-diagnosed in older adults, so a high index of suspicion is needed. This is important considering that older adults are at high risk for completed suicide, even though the prevalence of self-harm in this group is lower than in younger adults.

> **HINTS AND TIPS**
>
> Self-harm in an older adult should be considered to be with suicidal intent until proven otherwise.

The principles of treatment are the same as for younger adults, although medication should be introduced cautiously as older adults have an increased risk of developing adverse side-effects and generally need lower doses. Tricyclic antidepressants should be avoided if possible as postural hypotension and cognitive impairment are very common side-effects in older adults. Response to antidepressants is often slower in older adults, with benefits taking 6–8 weeks to emerge.

Electroconvulsive therapy (ECT) is a very effective treatment for depression in this population group and should be considered for severe depression, suicidal ideation, severe psychomotor retardation, failure to respond to or tolerate medication and previous good response to ECT. Lithium augmentation may be used in treatment-resistant cases, although the dose is generally lower than that used in younger adults. Patients

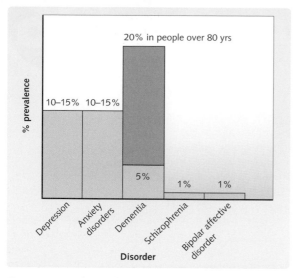

Fig. 26.1 Prevalence of mental illness in people over the age of 65

in this age group often need lifelong antidepressant treatment to reduce the chance of relapse. Psychosocial intervention in the form of social support and possibly cognitive-behavioural therapy are also important.

Poor prognostic factors include comorbid physical illness, late detection of illness and poor concordance with antidepressant medication. Depressed older adults have a higher mortality than the non-depressed do, even when physical illness is taken into account.

> **HINTS AND TIPS**
>
> Cotard's syndrome describes the presence of nihilistic and hypochondriacal delusions as part of a depressive psychosis and is typically seen in older adults.

Mania

Unlike depression, the incidence of bipolar affective disorder does not increase with age, although late onset cases seem to be less influenced by genetic factors (fewer of these patients have positive family histories for mood disorders). In a fifth of cases, mania is precipitated by an acute medical condition, e.g. stroke or myocardial infarction. The presentation and treatment is similar to that of younger adults.

Late-onset schizophrenia (late paraphrenia)

Older adult psychiatrists in the UK use the term *late-onset schizophrenia* or *late paraphrenia* to denote a group of patients who develop psychotic symptoms late in life, usually over the age of 60. Late-onset schizophrenia is characterized predominantly by delusional thinking, usually of a persecutory or grandiose nature. These delusions tend not to be as bizarre as they sometimes are in earlier onset schizophrenia (e.g. rather than believing that secret agents are monitoring them by satellite, a patient with paraphrenia may assert that the neighbours have been poisoning their water supply). Hallucinations may occur but disorganized thinking, inappropriate affect and catatonic features almost never feature.

The aetiology of late-onset schizophrenia seems different to early-onset schizophrenia in that sufferers are less likely to have a family history of schizophrenia. Also, late-onset schizophrenia is far more common in women than men – unlike early-onset schizophrenia, which is slightly more likely to arise in men. Sensory deprivation, particularly hearing loss and social isolation, is also implicated in its aetiology.

The treatment is with antipsychotics but some work is needed in building up a therapeutic relationship as these patients are often difficult to engage and poor concordance is associated with a poor treatment response. Note that although late-onset schizophrenia does seem to be a distinct entity, it is not a term used by the ICD-10 or DSM-IV; here, these patients would be classified as having schizophrenia or delusional disorder.

> **HINTS AND TIPS**
>
> Diogenes' syndrome, or 'senile squalor', is the term used to describe an elderly recluse who lives in a state of perpetual filth and gross self-neglect, often with the hoarding of rubbish. This is purely a descriptive term and may occur in individuals with alcohol abuse, frontal lobe dysfunction, personality disorder and chronic psychotic illness. It may also occur at a younger age.

ASSESSMENT CONSIDERATIONS IN OLDER ADULTS

- Home assessments are a very important part of older adult psychiatry. Patients can be assessed in their normal environment and collateral information can be obtained from family members. It is important to ascertain whether the patient can be managed at home (i.e. risk of harm to self and others; ability to carry out activities of daily living (ADL), drive, manage financial affairs, etc.), or whether additional community support or hospitalization is needed.
- Collateral information from the patient's general practitioner (GP), family and neighbours is an important part of history taking.
- Mental state examination follows the same format as for all adults, although extra consideration should be given to the assessment of cognitive functioning

and it is advisable to always do a standardized test, e.g. a Mini-Mental State Examination. (see Fig. 14.12 for alternatives).

- A thorough physical examination is very important. Do not forget to assess hearing and vision as well as tremors and involuntary movements.
- Routine investigations in the newly diagnosed or hospitalized older adult include: full blood count, urea and electrolytes, liver function tests, thyroid function tests, calcium, glucose, urinalysis (with mid-stream urine microscopy and culture if indicated), chest X-ray, electrocardiogram (ECG) and consideration of serum magnesium, phosphate, vitamin B_{12} and folate and a CT or MRI head. Remember that the chances of a physical illness causing or aggravating a mental deterioration are significant in older adults.

TREATMENT CONSIDERATIONS IN OLDER ADULTS

Physiological changes with ageing

There are a number of physiological changes that occur with ageing, which may affect the way the body handles certain drugs. Figure 26.2 describes the most important changes and their effects. The net result of these changes is that the tissue concentration of a drug may be increased by over 50%, especially in malnourished, dehydrated and debilitated patients. Therefore the adage, 'start low and go slow' applies especially to the use of psychotropic drugs in the older adult.

Polypharmacy

Those aged over 65 receive 45% of all prescriptions issued in the UK and many of these are for five drugs or more. This increases the risk of adverse reactions, drug interactions and poor concordance. Prescribing psychotropic drugs for common symptoms such as insomnia and headache should be avoided as they may lead to further non-specific symptoms, e.g. confusion, drowsiness and light-headedness. Medication should not be a substitute for adequate social care, the lack of which often underlies many of these symptoms.

Concordance

Concordance is often a problem in older adults, especially with those who are visually impaired, cognitively impaired, take numerous drugs and live alone. This may be improved by simplifying medication regimens, taking time to explain dosing schedules, using large font prescription labels or concordance aids such as dosette boxes. Organizing supervision of medication taking by a relative, friend or support worker may be necessary.

Psychosocial interventions

Psychological treatments, such as cognitive-behavioural therapy can be used with success in older adults as with younger adults. Reality orientation and reminiscence therapies have been used to reduce disorientation and stimulate remote memories in patients with dementia. Practical psychosocial interventions such as memory aids (e.g. notebooks, calendars) and assistance with mobility and daily activities by a support worker should not be underestimated. Occupational therapy assessment of activities of daily living (ADL), which assess skills such as washing, dressing, eating, shopping, etc., give carers an indication of patients' strengths and weaknesses and enable a care package to be tailored that caters specifically for these.

Fig. 26.2 Age-related changes in drug handling and effects	
Physiological changes	**Effects**
Reduction in renal clearance (glomerular filtration rate and tubular function)	Drugs excreted by filtration (e.g. lithium) need lower doses Drug concentrations may rise rapidly with dehydration, heart failure, etc.
Decreased lean body mass and total body water and increased body fat	Volume of distribution increases for lipid-soluble drugs (most psychotropic drugs), and reduces for water-soluble drugs (e.g. lithium). Half-life of lipid-soluble drugs prolonged
Decreased plasma albumin	Reduced drug binding resulting in increased physiologically active unbound fraction
Reduced hepatic metabolism and first-pass metabolism	May increase the bioavailability and elimination of some drugs
Increased sensitivity to central nervous system drugs	Sedating drugs may result in drowsiness, confusion, falls and delirium. Tricyclics more likely to be associated with anticholinergic and postural hypotensive effects. Antipsychotics more likely to be associated with parkinsonism and increased risk of cerebrovascular accident
Decreased total body mass	Lower doses of drugs needed (think in terms of mg/kg as opposed to standard dose for all)

Child and adolescent psychiatry (27)

After this chapter you should have an understanding of:
- How psychiatric disorders in children are classified
- The main characteristics of autism
- The difference between Rett's syndrome and childhood disintegrative disorder
- Differential diagnoses for attention deficit/hyperactivity disorder (ADHD)
- The pharmacological and psychosocial management of ADHD
- The difference between conduct disorder and oppositional defiant disorder
- The causes of school refusal and how it differs from truancy
- The types of tic that occur in Gilles de la Tourette's syndrome, and what conditions it is associated with
- The treatment of non-organic enuresis
- How depression may present in children
- The risk factors for child abuse, and what to do if you suspect a child is at risk

Children are often unable to explicitly verbalize psychological symptoms they might have. In fact, 'the problem' is usually brought to the psychiatrist's attention by someone else (e.g. parent, schoolteacher, paediatrician). Therefore the presenting problem is most commonly a complaint about the child's abnormal behaviour or performance rather than their psychological symptoms. This normally means that the clinician is presented with a non-specific presentation (e.g. 'being disruptive in the classroom').

Problems need to be considered in the context of a child's developmental stage; for example, 'temper tantrums' are normal for a 2-year-old child, but should have subsided by age 5.

CONSIDERATIONS IN THE ASSESSMENT OF CHILDREN

- Parents or carers usually accompany children and young adolescents. It is often useful to first interview them – with or without the child present – to obtain a full description of the current concerns, as well as a complete history (psychiatric, neurodevelopmental, educational and medical). An indirect evaluation of the parents' personalities, marital relationship and style of parenting often creates another perspective from which to understand the context of the presenting complaint.
- An interview with the child usually follows. The ability of youngsters to provide a candid account of their difficulties varies dramatically. To some degree, this varies with age. The assessment style should be tailored to the individual abilities of the child rather than to their age. In children who are unable to articulate their inner experiences (usually younger children), it is often necessary to observe them in play situations.
- The child's own understanding of their difficulties should (if possible) be taken into consideration, as this can affect their management (in terms of motivation to engage with psychosocial interventions, and their concordance with medication).
- The importance of obtaining collateral information cannot be overstated. This is extremely important in fully understanding the development of the presenting problem, and the child's premorbid functioning. It includes obtaining academic, educational or psychological reports as well as discussions with teachers and any other agencies involved. Remember to obtain consent from the parent/carer (and the child, if they are able).
- Further information can be obtained from structured and semi-structured interviews (e.g. Kiddie Schedule for Affective Disorders and Schizophrenia (K-SADS-P); Diagnostic Interview Schedule for Children (NIMH-DISC-IV)), objective assessment instruments (Autism Diagnostic Observation Schedule (ADOS)), and parent/teacher/self-rating scales (strengths and difficulties questionnaire (SDQ); Conners rating scale (CRS-R)).

CLASSIFICATION

The ICD-10 groups the psychiatric disorders in children and adolescents into four broad categories:

1. Intellectual disability (formerly referred to as mental retardation/learning disability) (see Ch. 28).
2. Developmental disorders (specific and pervasive).
3. Acquired disorders with onset usually in childhood or adolescence.
4. Acquired 'adult' disorders with onset in childhood or adolescence.

While these categories suggest obvious differences between 'developmental' and 'acquired' disorders, the reality of this division is less clear. Advances in genetic studies have shown that many 'acquired' disorders have a very strong genetic component, and that both genetic and environmental aetiological factors are likely to have a significant influence. Figure 27.1 provides an overview of the conceptual framework for the disorders of childhood and adolescence.

INTELLECTUAL DISABILITY

By their very nature, intellectual disabilities (formerly referred to as 'mental retardation' and 'learning disability') manifest at birth or during very early childhood. They pervade into adulthood, and (in the UK) are often diagnosed and managed by services separate from child

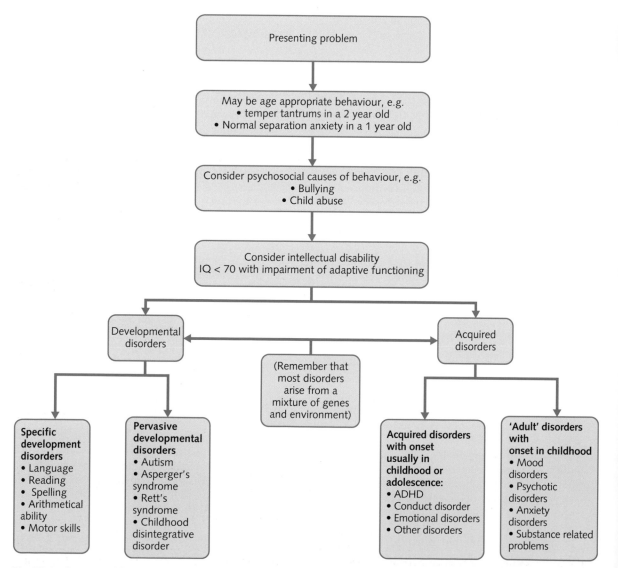

Fig. 27.1   Conceptual framework for the disorders of childhood and adolescence

and adolescent psychiatry. Although the division is somewhat arbitrary (and in practice involves a great degree of overlap with child and adolescent psychiatry), intellectual disability is covered separately in this book (Ch. 28).

DEVELOPMENTAL DISORDERS

The developmental disorders are a heterogeneous group of disorders whose defining characteristic is an impaired acquisition of expected cognitive, motor, social or adaptive skills, due to abnormalities in the development of the brain. The onset of these disorders is usually in infancy or early childhood and they tend to follow a chronic, steady course (see Fig. 27.1).

Specific developmental disorders

These disorders are characterized by the disturbed acquisition of a *specific* cognitive or motor function during a child's development (e.g. language, reading, spelling, arithmetical ability and motor skills). Other areas of cognitive functioning are normal, therefore a child may have a specific reading disorder (developmental dyslexia) but be of normal intelligence and have no problem with writing or mathematics. These disorders are thought to arise from a specific biological abnormality in cognitive processing, rather than a lack of opportunity to learn, sensory impairment or neurological disease. In some children, the consequences of the difficulty (e.g. school problems, teasing) might lead to secondary emotional or behavioural problems.

Pervasive developmental disorders

The pervasive developmental disorders are characterized by:

- Severe impairments in social interactions and communication skills.
- Restricted, stereotyped interests and behaviours.

These behavioural abnormalities pervade all areas of functioning and are usually evident within the first few years of life. While often associated with intellectual disabilities, this is not always the case. The diagnosis is made on the basis of abnormalities of behaviour, social interactions and communication skills rather than intellectual functioning. The pervasive developmental disorders include autism, Asperger's syndrome, Rett's syndrome and childhood disintegrative disorder. The term *autistic spectrum disorder* (ASD) is often used as an umbrella term to cover all pervasive developmental disorders including those that do not exactly meet diagnostic criteria. The use of the term ASD recognizes a continuum of disability, and that boundaries between different syndromes are often difficult to decipher.

Autism (childhood autism, autistic disorder)

Diagnosis and clinical features

The three characteristic features of autism manifest within the first 3 years of life and include:

1. *Impairment in social interaction* as evidenced by the poor use of non-verbal behaviours (e.g. eye contact, facial expression, gestures) and a failure to develop and share in the enjoyment of peer relationships.
2. *Impairment in communication* as evidenced by poor development of spoken language; extreme difficulty in initiating or sustaining conversation; repetitive use of idiosyncratic language and lack of imitative or make-believe play.
3. *Restricted, stereotyped interests and behaviours* as evidenced by intense preoccupations with interests such as dates, phone numbers and timetables; inflexible adherence to routines and rituals; repetitive, stereotyped motor movements such as clapping, rocking or twisting and an unusual interest in parts of hard or moving objects.

In addition to these diagnostic features, patients may also exhibit behavioural problems such as aggressiveness, impulsivity and self-injurious behaviour. Although autistic children can be of normal intelligence, 75% have significant intellectual disabilities. Epilepsy may develop in about 25–30% of cases.

Epidemiology and aetiology

- The prevalence of classical autism in the general population is about 1 per 1000 children.
- The male-to-female ratio is approximately 4:1.
- The exact cause of autism has not been clarified but genetic, prenatal, perinatal and immunological factors have been implicated. Phenylketonuria, tuberous sclerosis and congenital rubella are associated conditions.
- While autism remains a separate diagnostic entity to schizophrenia, social withdrawal, communication impairment and poor eye contact seen in autism are similar to the negative symptoms seen in schizophrenia. Evidence is currently emerging that the two disorders share a number of genetic factors. It may be clinically difficult to differentiate high-functioning autistic spectrum disorder from schizoid personality disorder or schizotypal disorder, which may also suggest a genetic link to schizophrenia.
- There is no good evidence to support the claim that the MMR vaccine (mumps, measles, rubella) results in autism.

Management and prognosis

- Prognosis is poor: only 1–2% achieve full independence; 20–30% achieve partial independence.
- Children with autism who have IQs above 70 and those who have good language development by age 5–7 have the best prognosis.
- Prognosis is improved if the home environment is supportive – family education and support are crucial.
- Management approaches are similar to those used in patients with intellectual disability (Ch. 28).

Asperger's syndrome

Asperger's syndrome is similar to autism in that there is impairment in reciprocal social interaction coupled with restricted, stereotyped interests and behaviours. However, there are no significant abnormalities in language acquisition and ability, or in cognitive development and intelligence. Indeed, IQ and language may be superior in some cases. Abnormalities may be more obvious in the early years, and difficulties in later childhood and adolescence tend to be in the domain of social interaction. Asperger's syndrome is far more prevalent in males. Due to under-recognition, prevalence may be as high as 3 in 1000. Family history of autism and mild motor clumsiness may be present.

Figure 27.2 summarizes the differences between autism and Asperger's syndrome.

Rett's syndrome (disorder)

Rett's syndrome, which has almost only been seen in girls, is caused by mutations in the gene *MECP2* located on the X chromosome, and can arise sporadically or from germline mutations. It is initially characterized by an apparently normal antenatal development with a normal head circumference at birth, followed by an apparently normal psychomotor development in the first 5 months after birth. From 6 months to 2 years of age, a progressive and destructive encephalopathy results in a deceleration of head growth; loss or lack of development of language, and loss of purposeful hand movements and fine motor skills, with subsequent development of stereotyped hand movements (e.g. midline hand-wringing). After a decade, most girls are bound to a wheelchair with incontinence, muscle wasting and rigidity and almost no language ability.

Childhood disintegrative disorder (Heller's syndrome)

This disorder, which is more common in boys, is characterized by about 2 years of normal development, followed by a loss of previously acquired skills (language, social and adaptive skills, play, bowel and bladder control and motor skills) before age 10. It is also associated with an autism-like impairment of social interaction as well as repetitive, stereotyped interests and mannerisms. Thus, after the deterioration, these children may resemble autistic children.

ACQUIRED DISORDERS

The *acquired disorders* of childhood are illnesses 'superimposed' on a relatively normally developing child, implying that if the illness were 'removed', a more or less normally developed child would remain. They tend to follow a fluctuating course and are often amenable to treatment. Acquired disorders can further be divided into those disorders developing specifically in childhood and the 'adult' psychiatric disorders that have their onset in childhood (see Fig. 27.1).

Acquired disorders with onset usually in childhood or adolescence

Attention deficit/hyperactivity disorder (hyperkinetic disorder)

Diagnosis and clinical features

Attention deficit/hyperactivity disorder (ADHD) is described in the DSM-IV. Hyperkinetic disorder is similarly described in ICD-10. Although it is described as an acquired disorder in current classification systems, ADHD is now considered by most to be a highly heritable neurodevelopmental disorder with a genetic

Fig. 27.2 Some differences between autism and Asperger's syndrome (from Ghaziuddin M, Mental health aspects of Autism and Asperger's syndrome. Jessica Kingsley Publishers, 2005)

	Autism	Asperger's syndrome
Onset/recognition	Before the age of 3 years	After the age of 5 years
Social deficits	Severe	Mild
Type of interaction	Aloof or passive	Active but odd
Speech	Usually not pedantic	Usually pedantic
Intellectual profile	Low verbal IQ	High verbal IQ
Focused interests	Intense	Intense; usually more sophisticated
Clumsiness	Present	Present but less severe

contribution to variance in liability of around 76%. It usually manifests before the age of 7 and is characterized by: (1) *impaired attention;* (2) *hyperactivity and/or impulsivity:*

1. Impaired attention includes: difficulty sustaining attention in work or play tasks; not listening when being spoken to; being highly distractible – moving from one activity to another; reluctance to engage in activities that require a sustained mental effort (e.g. schoolwork); and being forgetful or regularly losing things.

2. Hyperactivity includes: restlessness; incessant fidgeting; running and jumping around in inappropriate situations; excessive talkativeness or noisiness; and difficulty engaging in quiet activities. Impulsivity includes: difficulty awaiting turn; interrupting others' conversations or games; and prematurely blurting out answers to questions.

These symptoms should be evident in more than one situation (e.g. at school and at home), and should have been present for at least 6 months.

It is important to distinguish ADHD from:

- Age-appropriate behaviours in young active children. ADHD is usually not recognized until the child has started school because of the normal variation of behaviours in preschool children. However, ADHD is diagnosed and treated in clear cases in young children.
- Children placed in academic settings inappropriate to their intellectual ability. This includes children with intellectual disabilities and highly intelligent children in an under-stimulating environment.
- Other mental illnesses (e.g. pervasive developmental disorders, depression, etc.).

Diagnosis should only be made by a specialist psychiatrist, paediatrician or other professional with expertise in the diagnosis of ADHD. This diagnosis should be based on a full clinical and psychosocial assessment, including developmental history, assessment of impairment, observer reports and mental state examination.

probably due to the narrower diagnostic criteria of the ICD-10's hyperkinetic disorder.

- The male-to-female ratio is approximately 3:1.
- Genetic studies have shown that ADHD has one of the highest heritabilities of all psychiatric illnesses. Manifestation of symptoms is likely to be due to gene–environment interactions, with pre- and peri-natal factors, and psychosocial factors (prolonged emotional deprivation, diet) also implicated.

Management and prognosis

Pharmacological management is indicated as first-line treatment in school-age children with severe ADHD. The central nervous system (CNS) stimulant methylphenidate (Ritalin®, Concerta®, Equasym®) is normally tried in the first instance. Atomoxetine (Strattera®) and dexamfetamine are also licensed in the UK for the management of ADHD: these tend to be used in cases where methylphenidate is ineffective or poorly tolerated. The use of stimulant medication can be helpful in up to three-quarters of cases, improving ability to sustain attention and academic efficiency. In treatment resistant cases, the (unlicensed) use of bupropion, clonidine, modafinil and imipramine may be considered; however, this should only be done following referral to a tertiary centre. Antipsychotics are not recommended for the management of ADHD.

Psychosocial interventions are recommended in all cases, and are used first-line in children with mild to moderate ADHD, and in all preschool children. The choice of treatment naturally depends on the developmental stage of the child or adolescent. Useful strategies may include: parental education or training; cognitive-behavioural therapy; and social skills training.

Improvement usually occurs with development, and remission of symptoms often occurs between the ages of 12 and 20. Unstable family dynamics and coexisting conduct disorder are associated with a worse prognosis. Around 15% of patients have symptoms persisting into later life and may require ongoing management from adult mental health services.

HINTS AND TIPS

Restlessness, overactivity, impaired concentration and inattention may also arise in children with agitated depression or anxiety. ADHD should not be diagnosed in these cases unless there is clear evidence that these symptoms were present before, or persist after the resolution of, the depression or anxiety.

COMMUNICATION

Parents' concerns need to be addressed as well as the patient's. Treatment of ADHD has received much media interest, especially potential side-effects – be aware of this. Methylphenidate is associated with growth suppression with prolonged use. It is only prescribed in specialist settings with regular weight and height monitoring. Drug holidays can be used to allow children to make up growth gains.

Epidemiology and aetiology

- The prevalence of ADHD in the USA is 3–7% in school-age children. It is about 1% in the UK,

Conduct disorder

The onset of conduct disorder is usually before the age of 18. Most affected boys meet the criteria by age 10–12 years and most affected girls by age 14–16 years. The disorder is characterized by a repetitive and persistent pattern of: aggression to people and animals; destruction of property (including fire-setting); deceitfulness or theft; and major violations of age-appropriate societal expectations or rules (e.g. truancy, staying out at night, running away from home). Prevalence estimates vary from 1% to 10%; however, rates among populations in young offenders institutions have been estimated to be as high as 87%. The male-to-female ratio is approximately 4:1. Aetiological factors include genetics, parental psychopathology (mental illness, substance abuse, antisocial personality traits), child abuse and neglect, poor socioeconomic status and educational impairment. Many adolescents improve by adulthood; however, a substantial proportion go on to develop antisocial personality disorder and substance-related problems, especially those with an early age of onset. Management strategies include behaviour, cognitive, family and group therapy.

Oppositional defiant disorder describes a persistent pattern of negativistic, defiant, hostile and disruptive behaviour *in the absence of* behaviour that violates the law or the basic rights of others as occurs in conduct disorder (e.g. theft, cruelty, bullying, assault). Children with this disorder deliberately defy requests or rules, are angry and resentful and annoy others on purpose.

HINTS AND TIPS

It helps to remember that family histories should relate to both genetic lineage and factors that influence psychological development: the risk of developing conduct disorder is increased if a first-degree relative suffers from it, but also if there is a history of antisocial personality disorder in a close family member, regardless of whether they are a biological relative.

Emotional disorders

The emotional disorders in childhood are often thought to be exaggerations of normal developmental trends rather than discrete illnesses in themselves. They rarely persist into adulthood, and tend to have a good prognosis. The treatment of these disorders is focused on behavioural and family therapy.

Separation anxiety disorder

Normal separation anxiety usually occurs in children from 6 months to 2 years. However, some children experience inappropriate and excessive anxiety about separation from attachment figures. This disorder is only diagnosed when the anxiety is of such a severity that it is markedly different from other children of a similar age or when it persists beyond the usual age period (e.g. a 6-year-old girl becoming incredibly distressed when her mother drops her off at school).

Phobic anxiety disorder

Minor phobic symptoms are common in childhood, and the object of the phobia varies with developmental stage (e.g. fear of animals or monsters in preschool children). Phobic anxiety disorder is diagnosed when the phobic object is age-inappropriate (e.g. a 9-year-old boy who is afraid of monsters under the bed), or where levels of anxiety are clinically abnormal. Non-developmental phobias (e.g. agoraphobia) do not fall under this category, but under the adult phobia category (see Chs. 10 and 20).

Social anxiety disorder

Normal stranger anxiety occurs in well-adjusted children from 8 months to 1 year. Social anxiety disorder is a persistent and recurrent fear and/or avoidance of strangers. This disorder is only diagnosed when the anxiety is of such a severity that it is markedly different from other children of a similar age or when it persists beyond the usual age period.

Sibling rivalry disorder

Minor emotional disturbance or jealousy is normal after the birth of a sibling. However, when the levels of jealousy or rivalry become excessive or persistent, sibling rivalry disorder can be diagnosed.

HINTS AND TIPS

School refusal is the refusal to go to school because of anxiety in spite of parental pressure. It may be caused by separation anxiety (younger children), another mental illness (e.g. depression, social phobia), or negative psychosocial factors (e.g. bullying, teasing). Truancy, on the other hand, is an absence from school by choice and is associated with conduct disorder, poor academic performance, family history of antisocial behaviour and large family size.

Other disorders with onset usually in childhood or adolescence

Elective mutism (selective mutism)

Elective mutism is a selectivity in vocal communication depending on the social circumstances. The child speaks normally in some situations (e.g. at home), but is mute in others (e.g. at school). These children have adequately developed language comprehension and ability (although a minority may have slight speech delay or articulation problems). It usually presents before the age of 5, is slightly more common in girls, and is associated with psychological stress, social anxiety and oppositional behaviour.

Tic disorders

Tics are sudden, repetitive, non-rhythmic motor movements or vocalizations. They are involuntary; however, they can be voluntarily suppressed (although this can be very difficult). Tics often become more prominent during times of stress. Tics are divided into:

- Simple motor tics (e.g. eye-blinking, neck-jerking, facial grimacing).
- Simple vocal tics (e.g. grunting, coughing, barking, sniffing).
- Complex motor tics (e.g. jumping, touching self, copropraxia (use of obscene gestures)).
- Complex vocal tics (senseless repetition of words, coprolalia (use of obscene words or phrases)).

Gilles de la Tourette's syndrome

More commonly known simply as 'Tourette's syndrome', this is characterized by the presence of both multiple motor tics and one or more vocal tics for more than 1 year. The motor tics usually present by age 7 years, although tics can present as early as 2 years of age. Obsessions and compulsions (OCD) and attention difficulties and impulsivity (ADHD) are associated conditions (see p. 87 and 188). Drug treatment is not always required: cognitive behavioural therapy and other psychosocial interventions can be used to help manage the anxiety that aggravates tics, and treatment of comorbid ADHD or OCD (with medication and/or psychotherapy) can be effective. However, if tics persist, dopamine antagonists can be helpful (haloperidol is licensed, but pimozide, clonidine and sulpiride have been effective). Risk of side-effects should always be balanced against benefits on an individual basis.

Non-organic enuresis

This condition is characterized by the involuntary voiding of urine in children who, according to their developmental stage, should have established consistent bladder control (therefore ordinarily not diagnosed before the age of 5). It may occur during the day or night and is not directly caused by any medical condition (e.g. seizures, diabetes, urinary tract infection, structural abnormalities of the urinary tract) or use of a substance (e.g. diuretic). Two types of enuresis have been described: primary enuresis means that urinary continence has never been established; and secondary enuresis means that continence has been achieved in the past. Non-organic enuresis occurs in around 7% of 5-year-olds; 4% of 10-year-olds; and around 1% of adolescents older than the age of 15 years. Gender distribution is equal in younger patients; however, cases that persist into adolescence tend to be males. Aetiological factors include genetics, developmental delays, psychosocial stressors (moving house, birth of a sibling, start or change of school, divorce, bereavement) and inadequate toilet training. About 75% of children with non-organic enuresis have a first-degree biological relative who has had the same problem. Management involves exclusion of physical cause, parental education about toilet training (especially in primary enuresis), behavioural therapy (pad and buzzer apparatus, star chart, bladder training), and – as a last resort – pharmacotherapy (imipramine, nasal desmopressin). Most cases of non-organic enuresis resolve by adolescence.

Non-organic encopresis

This condition is characterized by the deposition of normal faeces (i.e. not diarrhoea) in inappropriate places, in children who – according to their developmental stage – should have established consistent bowel control (therefore ordinarily not diagnosed before the age of 4). It may be due to unsuccessful toilet training where bowel control has never been achieved (primary encopresis), or may occur after a period of normal bowel control (secondary encopresis). Encopresis may result from a developmental delay, coercive or punitive potty training, emotional, physical or sexual abuse, a disturbed parent–child relationship, parental marital conflict, or can feature as a symptom of another psychiatric disturbance (e.g. autism). About 1% of 5-year-olds have the condition and it is more common in males. Management includes ruling out an organic cause (constipation with overflow incontinence, anal fissure, gastrointestinal infection), assessing and treating disturbed family dynamics (ruling out child abuse), parental guidance regarding toilet training and behaviour therapy (e.g. star chart). Stool softeners may be used for constipation. The prognosis is good with 90% of cases improving within a year.

'Adult' disorders with onset in childhood

All psychiatric disorders that usually present in adulthood can also develop in childhood (e.g. affective disorders, psychotic disorders, anxiety disorders, substance-related problems), although many (such as schizophrenia) are much rarer in childhood than adulthood. The diagnostic criteria are essentially the same as for adults (see relevant chapters).

COMMUNICATION

It is useful to broaden the frame of questions used when taking a history from (or about) a child. For example, depression may present with irritability and failure to meet expected weight and growth gains rather than with low mood and weight loss.

CHILD ABUSE

Child abuse includes the overlapping concepts of physical, sexual and emotional mistreatment, as well as neglect or deprivation of the child. Figure 27.3 lists the risk factors associated with child abuse. In addition to the physical manifestations, victims of abuse may present with failure to thrive and symptoms of depression, anxiety, aggression, age-inappropriate sexual behaviour and self-harm. They are also at an increased risk for the development of a substantial range of psychiatric problems in later life.

All NHS Trusts in the UK have specific child protection guidelines which should be easily accessible and consulted before they are needed. All healthcare staff (not just child psychiatrists and paediatricians) have a duty to protect children from harm, and the safety of a child should always take priority. If a child discloses abuse (of any sort), or if you suspect that they are being abused or neglected, confidentiality cannot be maintained, and this should (if appropriate) be explained to the child. Comprehensive notes should be kept, and care taken to allow the child to make the disclosure in their own words without suggestion from others (either family or healthcare staff). Concerns should be reported as soon as practically possible. While local procedures vary slightly, the police, social work, and the duty paediatrician should be able to offer guidance. In some cases, the child may be in imminent danger (e.g. being taken home by the alleged perpetrator). It may be necessary to involve the police to prevent further harm and to remove the child to a place of safety.

Fig. 27.3 Risk factors for child abuse

Parent/environmental factors	Child factors
Parents who were abused	Low birth weight or prematurity
Parental substance abuse	Early maternal separation
Parental mental illness (intellectual disability, depression, schizophrenia, personality disorders)	Unwanted child
	Intellectual or physical disability
	Challenging behaviour
Step-parent	Hyperactivity
	Excessive crying
Young, immature parents	
Parental criminality	
Poor socioeconomic status and overcrowding	

After this chapter you should have an understanding of:
- The nomenclature of intellectual disability
- The definition of intellectual disability, and its classification and diagnosis
- Epidemiology and the aetiological factors associated with intellectual disabilities
- Clinical features of intellectual disability
- Management strategies for patients with intellectual disabilities, including the role of prevention, psychosocial care and medication

Many terms have been used in the past to describe people with significantly lower than average intelligence. Initially, terms such as 'idiot' and 'imbecile' were used. Subsequently, a number of further terms have been adopted, and superseded after they have crept into colloquial language and gained negative connotations. While both the ICD-10 and DSM-IV use the term 'mental retardation' to describe people with intellectual impairment, this term is now considered to be dated. Until recently, the term 'learning disability' was preferred in the UK, although this has recently been superseded by the term 'intellectual disability'. The latter term will be used for the purposes of this chapter.

INTELLECTUAL DISABILITY (MENTAL RETARDATION/ LEARNING DISABILITY)

Definition and diagnosis

Intellectual disability is an umbrella term used to describe diverse afflictions which manifest as significant intellectual impairment associated with an impaired ability to adapt to the normal demands of daily living, with onset prior to the age of 18 years (but normally in the very early years). These disorders are generally caused by an interruption in the normal development of the brain, from various causes. Intellectual disability is a lifelong condition.

Adaptive functioning is a measure of how patients cope with activities of living such as communication, self-care, social skills, and academic and vocational skills. This is assessed by a thorough developmental, psychiatric and medical history from the patient's parents and other care providers.

Intellectual functioning is usually defined by the intelligence quotient (IQ). This can be assessed by standardized intelligence tests (e.g. Wechsler Intelligence Scales for Children – WISC). An IQ of 70 or below, which is two standard deviations below the mean (IQ $= 100$), is said to represent sub-average intellectual functioning. It is important to remember the limitations of using standardized testing instruments. Many standardized tests tend to be aimed at people of (or around) average intelligence, and therefore may be unsuitable for patients with more severe difficulties. Also, differences in native language and background, as well as sensory, motor or communication difficulties may lead to patients obtaining falsely low IQ scores. Therefore, patients obtaining IQ scores lower than 70 should not be diagnosed as having intellectual disability if there is no evidence of significant impairments in adaptive functioning.

HINTS AND TIPS

Whereas dementia describes a loss of cognitive ability already acquired, intellectual disability describes the failure to develop a normal level of cognitive functioning in the first place. Note, however, that individuals with Down's syndrome are also at very high risk for developing Alzheimer's disease in later life.

COMMUNICATION

The terms intellectual disability and learning difficulty are often confused. A learning difficulty refers in general to any condition that impairs learning and is most often not associated with a global reduction in IQ. A specific learning difficulty is one particular problem which impairs learning (e.g. dyslexia, dyscalculia). Intellectual disabilities are often associated with learning difficulties.

Classification and clinical features

The ICD-10 specifies intellectual disabilities (under the term 'mental retardation') as mild, moderate, severe and profound, according to the degree of intellectual and adaptive impairment. Figure 28.1 summarizes the clinical features of the degrees of intellectual disabilities; however, note that this is simplified and that difficulties experienced can vary from person to person. In addition to the impairment of adaptive functioning, patients may have clinical features associated with the specific cause of their intellectual disability (e.g. Down's syndrome: epicanthic folds with oblique palpebral fissures, broad hands with single transverse palmar crease, flattened occiput, cardiac septal defects). Other features associated with intellectual disabilities include aggression, self-injurious behaviours, repetitive stereotypical motor movements and poor impulse control. Up to a third of people with an intellectual disability have a comorbid psychiatric illness, most commonly schizophrenia (4%), which occurs at a higher rate in individuals with learning disabilities than in the population in general.

Epidemiology and aetiology

The prevalence of intellectual disabilities in the general population is about 1–2%, with a male-to-female ratio of approximately 3:2. Around 85% of all cases are considered to be mild (see Fig. 28.1), and many of these individuals may live alone with varying degrees of support. No clear aetiology can be determined in at least a third of patients with mild intellectual disabilities, and this may suggest that they represent the lower end of a normal distribution curve for intellectual functioning. Specific causes, however, are more likely to be found in patients with severe or profound intellectual disabilities. Remember that intellectual disability is a descriptive term and can still be used regardless of whether patients have a specific psychiatric or physical cause for their intellectual impairment or not (e.g. autism, Down's syndrome). Figure 28.2 lists the potential identifiable causes of intellectual disability.

HINTS AND TIPS

The DSM-IV uses a multi-axial diagnostic system that separates Axis I conditions (major mental illnesses, e.g. psychotic and mood disorders), Axis II conditions (personality disorders and intellectual disabilities – referred to as 'mental retardation') and Axis III conditions (general medical conditions), so that all three areas potentially requiring clinical attention are considered.

Management and prognosis

Prevention and detection

Primary prevention includes genetic screening and counselling for higher risk groups, prenatal testing (e.g. amniocentesis, rhesus incompatibility), improved

Fig. 28.1 Degrees of intellectual disability		
Degree of intellectual disability	Intelligence quotient (IQ) range	Adaptive functioning
Mild (85% of cases)	50–69	Difficulties may be subtle and difficult to identify Often only identified at a later age Difficulties in academic work (reading and writing) but greatly helped by educational programmes Usually capable of unskilled or semi-skilled manual labour May be able to live independently or with minimal support
Moderate (10% of cases)	35–49	Language and comprehension limited Self-care and motor skills impaired, may need supervision May be able to do simple practical work with supervision Rarely able to live completely independently
Severe (3–4% of cases)	20–34	Marked degree of motor impairment Little or no speech during early childhood; may learn to talk in school-age period Capable of only elementary self-care skills May be able to perform simple tasks under close supervision
Profound (1–2% of cases)	< 20	Severely limited in ability to communicate their needs Often severe motor impairment with restricted mobility and incontinence Little or no self-care Often require residential care

Fig. 28.2	Causes of mental retardation (intellectual disability)
Genetic	Chromosomal: e.g. Down's syndrome, fragile X syndrome, Prader–Willi syndrome Other: e.g. phenylketonuria, neurofibromatosis, tuberous sclerosis, Lesch–Nyhan syndrome, Tay–Sachs disease, other enzyme deficiency diseases
Prenatal	Congenital infections: e.g. TORCH infections (toxoplasmosis, rubella, cytomegalovirus, herpes simples and zoster (chicken pox)), also syphilis and acquired immune deficiency syndrome (AIDS) Substance use during pregnancy: e.g. fetal alcohol syndrome, prescribed drugs with teratogenic effects Complications of pregnancy: e.g. pre-eclampsia, intrauterine growth retardation, antepartum haemorrhage
Perinatal	Birth trauma: e.g. intracranial haemorrhage, hypoxia Prematurity: e.g. intraventricular haemorrhage, hyperbilirubinaemia (kernicterus), infections
Environmental	Neglect, malnutrition (e.g. iodine deficiency in developing countries), poor linguistic and social stimulation
Neuropsychiatric conditions	Pervasive developmental disorders (e.g. autism, Rett's syndrome)
Medical conditions in childhood	Infections: e.g. meningitis, encephalitis Head injury Toxins (e.g. lead, other heavy metals)

perinatal and neonatal care, and early detection of metabolic abnormalities that may contribute to intellectual impairment (e.g. phenylketonuria, neonatal hypothyroidism). Milder intellectual disabilities may be less obvious, and early detection requires the ability of teachers and family doctors to be able to identify difficulties as soon as possible. Secondary prevention aims to prevent the progression of disability, by providing compensatory education and early attempts to reduce behavioural problems. If you suspect a child has an intellectual disability, this should be discussed with either a paediatrician or a child and adolescent mental health specialist, who will be able to provide guidance on local services. If you suspect an adult has an undiagnosed mild intellectual disability, this should be discussed with the local intellectual disabilities team, who may suggest an initial referral for neuropsychological assessment.

Help for families

Families require information, advice, and both psychological and practical support from the time that the diagnosis is first made. Adequate time should be devoted to this, and should aim to involve the parents in helping their child achieve their full potential. Support should be ongoing, and should focus on education, practical matters and psychological support. This may need to be increased at the more challenging times, such as puberty, starting or leaving school, times of stress (e.g. bereavement or illness), and the transition to adult services.

Education, training and occupation

If the needs of a child with intellectual disability can be met by mainstream education, this should be encouraged due to the benefits of societal integration and mutual understanding. However, many children with intellectual disabilities have complex needs that are best addressed in specialist schools. Later, vocational guidance should be offered: most people with mild intellectual disabilities are able to take mainstream or supported employment (e.g. Remploy).

Housing and social support

Most people with mild intellectual disabilities are able to live independently, with varying degrees of social and familial support. Assessment of tasks of daily living will be necessary to ensure that people are appropriately placed. For people with more severe difficulties, residential care may be necessary. In such cases, development of social skills should be encouraged as far as is practical.

Medical care

People with intellectual disabilities should have the same access to medical services as everyone else, although communication difficulties and false attribution of symptoms to the intellectual disability (diagnostic overshadowing) mean care is often suboptimal. See Figure 28.3 for considerations of aspects of communication when assessing an individual with an intellectual disability. Extra medical care is often required due to comorbidities

Fig. 28.3 Communication considerations in intellectual disability
Allow extra time
Speak first to the person with the intellectual disability, not their carer
Assess their understanding early and involve them as much as possible
Ask short, simple questions
Use literal, direct language, not abstract or medical terms (e.g. 'Does it hurt when you pee?', rather than 'How are your waterworks?', or 'Do you experience dysuria?')

such as physical disability or epilepsy. Many general hospitals have specialist nurses who are experienced in the management of individuals with intellectual disabilities admitted for medical treatment or surgery.

Psychiatric care

Given the higher prevalence of comorbid mental illness in this group, people with intellectual disabilities should have access to specialist care (usually on an out-patient, community or day-patient basis) as and when required. Because the assessment and management of psychiatric illness and behavioural disturbances in individuals with intellectual disability can be difficult, most areas have multidisciplinary specialist teams. These teams can address not only major mental illnesses (e.g. schizophrenia, bipolar affective disorder, depression), but can also help manage autism and challenging behaviours. Psychotropic medication may be indicated; however, given the common difficulties with unusual presentations, polypharmacy, comorbidities and sensitivity to medication, there should be a low threshold for seeking advice from, or referral to, a specialist doctor. Behavioural therapy may be useful in the management of maladaptive or otherwise difficult behaviours (e.g. self-injury, aggression, destructiveness).

HINTS AND TIPS

Epilepsy is a common comorbidity in individuals with intellectual disabilities, and can often complicate assessment and management. Remember that a number of different psychotropic medications can lower seizure threshold, and that 'mood stabilizers' (with the exception of lithium) are antiepileptic medications.

COMMUNICATION

Collateral histories are invaluable when assessing someone with an intellectual disability. When a change in behaviour occurs, it is useful to ask about what else has changed in the patient's life or their daily routine. However, the prevalence of other psychiatric disorders is three to four times higher and so these must be excluded.

Forensic psychiatry (29)

Objectives

After this chapter you should have an understanding of:
- The association between mental illness and crime
- Which psychiatric disorders are associated with violent crime
- The similarities and differences between antisocial personality disorder, dissocial personality disorder and psychopathy
- The methods used to predict violence
- Factors associated with a future risk of violence
- The link between mental disorders, culpability for alleged offences and associated legal defences

Forensic psychiatry, in its narrowest sense, is concerned with assessment and treatment of mentally disordered offenders as well as the assessment of the dangerousness of individuals who may not yet have committed an offence. In practice, forensic psychiatric services tend to assess and manage those who pose a high risk to the safety of others. Some patients may be managed in the community; however, others may require treatment and rehabilitation in a secure environment. Levels of security can vary from a locked ward in a psychiatric hospital to a maximum security 'special hospital' (Broadmoor, Rampton or Ashworth Hospital, or The State Hospital in Scotland).

HINTS AND TIPS

Mental disorders associated with violent crime (personality disorders, alcohol and substance dependence, and paranoid psychotic disorders) have a multiplicative effect for the risk of future violence when they occur in combination.

HINTS AND TIPS

Delusional jealousy (Othello's syndrome) is often associated with alcohol abuse and linked to violent crime such as assault and homicide.

MENTAL DISORDER AND CRIME

The vast majority of patients suffering from a mental illness have never committed an offence, and most offences are not committed by people with a mental illness. Indeed, a recent study showed that patients with mental disorders were four times more likely to fall victim to violence than members of the general population. However, there is a significantly higher prevalence of mental disorders among prisoners than in the general population: in the UK, it is estimated that 66% of prisoners have a personality disorder; 45% are dependent on illicit drugs; 30% are dependent on alcohol; and 45% have a neurotic disorder (depression or anxiety). Around 10% of prisoners may have some form of psychotic disorder, and between 20% and 30% are thought to have an intellectual disability that adversely affects their ability to cope with incarceration. Figure 29.1 describes the crimes associated with these disorders.

Personality disorder and crime

The German clinician Koch first used the term 'psychopathy' in 1891. At that time, it included all forms of personality disorder. However, the term was later used to describe individuals who exhibited antisocial behaviour. Unfortunately, the term 'psychopathic personality' and the related term 'psychopath' have been misused in both the medical and tabloid press. They were, for the most part, superseded by the term sociopathic personality disorder for a time and subsequently by the favoured, and currently used term, antisocial personality disorder (see Ch. 16). However, it should be noted that the DSM-IV criteria for antisocial personality disorder is largely based on past behaviour. ICD-10's dissocial personality disorder includes more cognitive factors (e.g. lack of guilt, callousness, inability to learn from punishment), with psychopathy possibly representing an extreme

Fig. 29.1 Mental disorders associated with crime

Mental disorder	Associations with crime
Personality disorder	Associated with violent crime, especially antisocial personality disorder. Antisocial and borderline personality disorders are frequently diagnosed in forensic settings, often in association with comorbid substance abuse
Alcohol and substance use	Substance misuse is one of the key factors that significantly increases the risk of violence, especially in those with comorbid mental illnesses (e.g. schizophrenia). Alcohol intoxication may also lead to driving offences and public drunkenness, and offences may be committed to fund drug habits
Schizophrenia	Schizophrenia increases the risk of violent acts by a factor of four. Many offences committed by people with schizophrenia are minor and are manifestations of impaired social skills. More people with schizophrenia are victims of crime than perpetrators
Mood disorders	Depression is associated with shoplifting and, in rare cases, homicide. These cases are usually due to mood-congruent delusions (e.g. everyone would be better off dead) and are often followed by suicide. Postnatal depression is sometimes a cause of maternal filicide. Offences by manic patients usually reflect financial irresponsibility or acts of aggression, which are usually not serious
Intellectual disabilities	There is an association between intellectual disabilities and sexual offences (especially indecent exposure), as well as arson

subtype of this. It may therefore be useful to think of these diagnoses as being an overlapping continuum, with antisocial personality at the milder end and psychopathy at the more severe end.

Psychopathy is now narrowly defined by the Hare Psychopathy Checklist – Revised (PCL-R), and is not a recognized diagnosis in either DSM-IV or ICD-10. It is characterized, in part, by antisocial behaviour and emotional impairment, such as the diminished capacity for guilt or remorse. Psychopathy is not synonymous with antisocial personality disorder as only a third of individuals diagnosed with antisocial personality disorder meet the criteria for psychopathy.

The prevalence of borderline personality disorder in offenders and prison populations is significantly higher than the general population, with around 14% of male and 20% of female prisoners meeting diagnostic criteria. Reasons may include the impulsiveness characteristic of borderline personality disorder, the presence of comorbid antisocial personality disorder and the high prevalence of substance misuse disorders in these patients.

> **HINTS AND TIPS**
>
> The term 'dangerous severe personality disorder' (DSPD) is a political (rather than a clinical) term to describe 'individuals from whom the public at present are not properly protected, and who are restrained effectively neither by the criminal law, nor by the provisions of the Mental Health Act'. DSPD is a controversial concept, about which a number of psychiatrists have expressed concern.

ASSESSING AND MANAGING RISK OF VIOLENCE

The key principle in assessing the risk of violence that a patient with a mental disorder poses to others poses an ethical conflict between protecting the community from a potentially violent offender and respecting the human rights of the individual in question (see Ch. 4). This is often a very difficult balance to achieve. Forensic multidisciplinary teams in the UK have moved from simply trying to predict the risk of future violence (generally unsuccessful), to looking at the evidence-based risk factors present in an individual patient. This enables a formulation of scenarios in which future violence would be more likely to occur, facilitating the creation of management plans which will decrease the risk in a proactive fashion. Approaches to assessment include:

- **Unaided clinical risk assessment**: this involves drawing on the experience of the clinician involved. This has been demonstrated to be associated with a less effective and less accurate risk assessment than evidence-based methods.
- **Actuarial methods**: assessment using predetermined static actuarial or statistical variables (e.g. demographic factors). These methods do not take into account the specific factors of the case, and – used in isolation – can be misleading.
- **Structured clinical judgement**: assessment utilizing both empirical actuarial knowledge and clinical expertise. The Historical/Clinical/Risk Management 20-item (HCR-20) scale is by far the predominant

Fig. 29.2 Some factors associated with risk of violence (HCR-20 items, from HCR-20 © 1997 by the Mental Health, Law, and Policy Institute, Simon Fraser University. Reprinted with permission of the copyright owner)

Historical (past)	Clinical (present)	Risk management (future)
Previous violence	Lack of insight	Plans lack feasibility
Young age at first violent incident	Negative attitudes	Exposure to destabilizers
Relationship instability	Active symptoms of major mental illness	Lack of personal support
Employment problems	Impulsivity	Non-compliance with remediation attempts
Substance use problems	Unresponsive to treatment	Stress
Major mental illness		
Psychopathy		
Early maladjustment		
Personality disorder		
Prior supervision failure		

mode of risk assessment used in the UK, and is particularly useful in assisting with risk management. Some newer tools have been developed that take protective factors significantly into account.

Figure 29.2 summarizes some of the factors that have been associated with the risk of violence.

A clinician confronted with an individual who poses a serious risk of violent behaviour will need to discuss the case with colleagues, including social workers and forensic mental health specialists. Compulsory hospitalization may be required in some cases. Clinicians have a duty to breach confidentiality to warn potential victims of serious threats that have been made (in consultation with the police), as per the Tarasoff ruling.

> **COMMUNICATION**
>
> A past history of violent behaviour is the best predictor of future violent behaviour. It is important to both ask the patient about this, and to seek verification from other sources (police, social work, medical records).

CONSIDERATIONS IN COURT PROCEEDINGS

Where there are grounds to believe that the accused may have been suffering (or is currently suffering) from a mental disorder, a psychiatric defence may be used. A psychiatric defence means that the presence of mental disorder may have been a mitigating factor in the offence or may interfere with court proceedings. Throughout the UK, this is mainly based on case law rather than legislation. The role of the forensic psychiatrist is to act as an expert witness to the court. While the psychiatrist can

make recommendations, the ultimate decision comes from the court.

Fitness to plead

Individuals with mental disorder are not exempt from taking responsibility for their actions. However, defendants should be competent to stand trial and mount a defence against their charges. The term 'fitness to plead' is used in English law to describe this capacity. Using psychiatric and/or psychological evidence, the court determines this by assessing whether the accused can:

- Understand the difference between a plea of guilty and not guilty.
- Understand the nature of the charge.
- Instruct counsel (legal representation).
- Follow the evidence brought before the court.
- Challenge a juror.

Criminal responsibility

Before a defendant can be convicted, criminal responsibility needs to be determined. It should be determined whether, at the time of the offence, the person was able to control their own behaviour and choose whether to commit an unlawful act or not. Integral to this process is the concept of *mens rea* ('guilty intent' or 'guilty mind'), which means that the individual realized the nature of, and intended to commit the unlawful act. Varying levels of *mens rea* are recognized, known as 'modes of culpability'. *Actus reus* ('guilty act' or 'crime') means the person is guilty of committing the act, whatever their intent. A defendant may be deemed to have decreased criminal culpability due to:

- Age: in England and Wales, children are only deemed legally responsible for their actions after the age of 14 years. Children under the age of 10 years are deemed incapable of criminal intent *(dolci incapax)*. Children aged 10–14 years are not considered criminally responsible unless the prosecution can prove *mens rea*.

- Reason of insanity: in English law, legal insanity (not a psychiatric term) is defined in terms of the M'Naghten Rules, which state that: *'at the time of committing the act, the party accused was labouring under such a defect of reason, from disease of the mind, as to not know the nature and quality of the act he was doing, or, if he did know it, that he did not know what he was doing was wrong.'* It is a defence that is rarely successful due to the high threshold of the legal definition of insanity.
- Diminished responsibility: in English law, a defence of diminished responsibility is only available in relation to charges for murder. If successful, this will lead to the accused being found guilty of manslaughter rather than murder, which allows for flexible sentencing (murder carries a mandatory life sentence). It depends upon the presence of: *'an abnormality of mind (whether arising from a condition of arrested or retarded development of mind or any inherent causes or induced by disease or injury)'*. An 'abnormality of mind' is not a psychiatric term and is open to wide interpretation, leading to successful defences such as 'emotional immaturity' and 'premenstrual tension'.

- Automatism: an act committed without presence of mind (e.g. during sleepwalking or epileptic seizure) may warrant this rare defence.

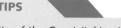

HINTS AND TIPS

Self-induced ('voluntary') intoxication with alcohol or other drugs cannot be used as a defence on the grounds of insanity or diminished responsibility.

HINTS AND TIPS

It is the responsibility of the Court (taking into consideration advice from expert witnesses) to decide upon sentencing or 'disposal' (i.e. what happens to the individual after trial). In cases where psychiatric defences are successfully used, the Court may utilize mental health legislation to transfer the individual to a secure hospital. In other cases, the Court may decide to impose a custodial sentence, or to place conditions upon the individual (e.g. to adhere to a drug treatment programme).

The sleep disorders (30)

Objectives

After this chapter you should have an understanding of:
- The differences between slow wave (stages 3 and 4) and REM sleep and their associated parasomnias
- The three main causes of secondary sleep disorders
- What non-pharmacological strategies may be used to treat primary insomnia
- The role of benzodiazepines in treating primary insomnia
- The four characteristic symptoms of narcolepsy
- How circadian rhythm sleep disorders cause hypersomnia
- The risk factors for obstructive sleep apnoea syndrome
- How to distinguish between nightmares and night terrors (sleep terrors)

Sleeping is intimately related to mental health. Not only can psychiatric illnesses such as depression and schizophrenia disturb the quantity and quality of sleep, but certain psychiatric drugs can also have the same effect. Furthermore, persistent primary sleep disturbances, which are common, can result in significant psychological consequences in an otherwise mentally healthy individual.

DEFINITIONS AND CLASSIFICATION

Sleep is divided into five distinct stages as measured by polysomnography (see later): four stages of non-rapid eye movement (stages 1, 2, 3 and 4) and a rapid eye movement stage (REM). Figure 30.1 summarizes the key characteristics of the stages of sleep.

The DSM-IV organizes the sleep disorders into four sections according to their causes:

1. Primary sleep disorders.
2. Sleep disorders secondary to another mental illness.
3. Sleep disorders secondary to another medical condition.
4. Sleep disorders secondary to the use of a substance.

This chapter will focus principally on primary sleep disorders, which are not caused by another medical condition (e.g. arthritis) or mental illness (e.g. depression), and do not occur secondary to the use of a substance (e.g. alcohol). These disorders are presumed to arise from some defect of an individual's endogenous sleeping mechanism (the reticular activating system) coupled with unhelpful learned behaviours (e.g. worrying about not sleeping). The primary sleep disorders, in turn, are divided into the dyssomnias and the parasomnias:

1. The dyssomnias are characterized by abnormalities in the amount, quality or timing of sleep. They include primary insomnia, primary hypersomnia, narcolepsy, circadian rhythm sleep disorders and breathing-related sleep disorders.
2. The parasomnias are characterized by abnormal episodes that occur during sleep or sleep-wake transitions. They include nightmares, night terrors and sleepwalking.

Insomnia

Insomnia describes sleep of insufficient quantity or poor quality due to:

- Difficulty falling asleep.
- Frequent awakening during the course of sleep.
- Early morning awakening with subsequent difficulty getting back to sleep.
- Sleep that is not refreshing despite being adequate in length.

In addition to daytime tiredness, persistent insomnia can have significant effects on mood, behaviour and performance. It has been shown that insomnia can also lead to an impairment of health-related quality of life similar to congestive cardiac failure or depression.

HINTS AND TIPS

You may find it useful to think in terms of 'altered sleep patterns' rather than of insomnia per se. While common in depression, it is only early morning wakening that is part of the somatic syndrome (see p. 50) and 20% will have atypical symptoms e.g. weight gain, increased appetite and hypersomnia

Stage of sleep	Duration spent in this phase during night	Characteristics and electroencephalogram (EEG) findings
Stage 1	5%	• Transition from wakefulness to sleep **EEG: theta waves** Theta waves: low amplitude, spike-like waves, 4–7Hz
Stage 2	45%	**EEG: sleep spindles and K-complexes** Sleep spindles: short rhythmic waveform clusters of 12–14Hz K-complex: sharp negative wave followed by a slower positive component
Stage 3 and 4 (Slow wave sleep)	25%	• Deep sleep • Unusual arousal characteristics: disorientation, sleep terrors, sleepwalking • Occur in first third to half of night **EEG: delta waves** *Stage 3 – delta waves <50%* *Stage 4 – delta waves >50%* Delta waves: high amplitude, low frequency (<4Hz)
REM	25%	• Occurs cyclically through the night, every 90 minutes alternating with non-REM sleep • Each episode increases in duration – most episodes occur in last third of night • Features penile erection, skeletal muscle paralysis, and surreal dreaming (including nightmares) **EEG: low amplitude, high frequency, with saw-tooth waves** Saw-tooth pattern

Fig. 30.1 Stages of sleep

Primary insomnia is diagnosed when present for at least a month, and not attributable to medical or psychiatric illness, substance misuse, or other dyssomnia or parasomnia. The numerous causes of insomnia as summarized in Figure 30.2 include primary sleep disorders, medical and psychiatric illness and substance use.

Assessment of insomnia

Assessment involves excluding a medical, psychiatric or substance-related cause of insomnia. Many cases of primary insomnia are related to poor sleep hygiene (see Fig. 30.3). Therefore it is essential to enquire about sleeping times and patterns, and caffeine consumption.

> **Fig. 30.2** Common causes of insomnia
>
> **Primary sleep disorders**
> - Dyssomnias
>   a. Primary insomnia
>   b. Circadian rhythm sleep disorders (jet-lag, shift work)
>   c. Breathing-related sleep disorders (sleep apnoea syndromes)
> - Parasomnias (all)
>
> **Psychiatric**
> - Anxiety
> - Depression
> - Mania
> - Schizophrenia
>
> **Medical**
> - Painful conditions (malignancies, arthritis, reflux disease)
> - Cardiorespiratory discomfort (dyspnoea, coughing, palpitations)
> - Nocturia (prostatism, urinary tract infections)
> - Metabolic or endocrine conditions (thyroid disease, renal or liver failure)
> - Central nervous system lesion (especially brainstem and hypothalamus)
>
> **Substances**
> - Caffeine and other stimulants
> - Alcohol
> - Prescribed drugs (e.g. SSRIs, some antipsychotics)
> - Substance withdrawal syndrome

It is also useful to obtain collateral information from the patient's sleeping partner regarding sleeping patterns, snoring and movements during the night.

The following questions might be helpful in eliciting the key symptoms of insomnia:

- Do you fall asleep quickly or do you find yourself tossing and turning for some time before dropping off?

> **Fig. 30.3** Correct sleep hygiene
>
> - Avoid sleeping during the day
> - Exercise during the day and maintain a healthy diet
> - Eliminate the use of stimulants (e.g. caffeine, nicotine, alcohol), especially around bedtime
> - Condition the brain by only using the bed for sleeping and sex – not for reading, watching TV, etc.
> - Go to bed and awaken at the same time each day
> - Avoid stimulating activities before bedtime (e.g. television, games). Instead, engage in relaxation techniques or reading
> - Try having a hot bath or drinking a cup of warm milk near bedtime
> - Avoid large meals near bedtime
> - Ensure that the bed is comfortable and that the bedroom is quiet
> - Do not lie in bed awake for longer than 15 minutes. Get up and do another relaxing activity and try sleeping later

- Do you wake up repeatedly in the night or can you sleep through once you have managed to get to sleep?
- Do you sometimes awaken too early in the morning and then find that you are unable to get back to sleep?
- Is your sleep refreshing or do you still feel tired in the morning?

In treatment-resistant cases it might be necessary to refer the patient to a sleep specialist for further investigation. Polysomnography is the simultaneous process of monitoring various physical parameters during sleep, including electroencephalogram (EEG), electrocardiogram (ECG), electromyogram, electrooculogram (eye movement), blood oxygen saturation, chest and abdominal excursion, mouth and nose air entry rates and the loudness of snoring.

> **COMMUNICATION**
>
> When considering insomnia, ask what the normal amount of sleep is for the patient in order for them to feel refreshed in the morning and what time they normally wake up. There is significant individual variation.

Management of primary insomnia

The most important aspect of management is providing education about correct sleep hygiene (Fig. 30.3).

There is a limited role for medication in the treatment of primary insomnia. Hypnotics may help in the short term, but the development of tolerance to their effects (usually within 2 weeks), possible dependence, and their propensity to cause rebound insomnia limit their use. Therefore, they should only be prescribed on a time-limited basis, ideally for use on alternate or occasional nights rather than every night. Drugs with a long half-life should be avoided, to prevent leaving patients feeling drowsy the next day (the 'chemical hangover'), and to avoid accumulation with repeated doses. Commonly used agents include the 'Z-drugs' (zopiclone, zolpidem, zaleplon) and benzodiazepines with a short half-life (such as temazepam). It may be useful to consider the use of other sedative medications (e.g. sedating antihistamines) with less potential for dependence or misuse.

Hypersomnia and narcolepsy

Hypersomnia describes excessive sleepiness that manifests as either a prolonged period of sleep or sleep episodes that occur during normal waking hours.

Primary hypersomnia is diagnosed when patients present with hypersomnia for at least a month not attributable to a medical or psychiatric condition, substance use, or other dyssomnia (especially narcolepsy and sleep apnoea) or parasomnia.

Narcolepsy is due to an abnormality of the REM-inhibiting mechanism and is characterized by a tetrad of:

1. Irresistible attacks of refreshing sleep that may occur at inappropriate times (e.g. driving).
2. Cataplexy (sudden, bilateral loss of muscle tone usually precipitated by intense emotion leading to collapse, and lasting for seconds to minutes).
3. Hypnagogic or hypnopompic hallucinations (see p. 67).
4. Sleep paralysis at the beginning or end of sleep episodes.

All four symptoms occur in less than 50% of cases and the diagnosis is usually made with evidence of sleep attacks and cataplexy. Patients usually have 2–6 episodes of sleep per day which usually last 10–20 minutes each. Hypnagogic/hypnopompic hallucinations and the paralysis of voluntary muscles occur as a result of elements of REM sleep intruding into the transition between sleep and wakefulness. Other features may include persistent tiredness, and problems with memory and concentration.

The numerous causes of hypersomnia as summarized in Figure 30.4 include primary sleep disorders, medical and psychiatric illness, substance use and sleep deprivation.

The treatment of primary hypersomnia is usually with stimulants such as dexamphetamine, methylphenidate and modafinil. The treatment of narcolepsy

includes taking forced naps at regular times. In some cases, stimulants are needed to reduce daytime sleepiness; tricyclic antidepressants increase muscle tone and may help to control cataplexy and sleep paralysis.

Circadian rhythm sleep disorders

Circadian rhythm sleep disorder (sleep–wake schedule disorder) is characterized by a lack of synchrony between an individual's endogenous circadian rhythm for sleep and that demanded by their environment, resulting in their being tired when they should be awake (hypersomnia) and being awake when they should be sleeping (insomnia). This disorder results from either a malfunction of the internal 'biological clock' that regulates sleep or from an unnatural environmental change (e.g. jet lag, night-shift work).

Breathing-related sleep disorders

Abnormalities of ventilation during sleep can cause repeated disruptions to sleep. This results in unrefreshing sleep and excessive sleepiness during the day. Obstructive sleep apnoea syndrome, the most common breathing-related sleep disorder, is characterized by obstruction of the upper airways during sleep, in spite of an adequate respiratory effort. Typically, an individual will have noisy breathing during sleep with loud snoring interspersed with apnoeic episodes lasting from 20 to 90 seconds, sometimes associated with cyanosis. It is not an uncommon condition, affecting 4% of middle-aged men, 2% of adult women and 1% of children. The prevalence is much higher in obese, elderly or hypertensive individuals and is also prominent in some patients with intellectual disabilities. This illness has significant cardiovascular and neuropsychiatric morbidity and should be actively excluded when an at-risk patient presents with hypersomnia, impairment of concentration and memory or other psychiatric symptoms. Collateral history from a bed-partner, who is often aware of the sleeping difficulties, is extremely useful.

Fig. 30.4 Common causes of hypersomnia

Primary sleep disorders
- Dyssomnias
  a. Primary insomnia
  b. Narcolepsy
  c. Breathing-related sleep disorders (sleep apnoea syndromes)
  d. Circadian rhythm sleep disorders (jet-lag, shift work)
- Parasomnias (all)

Psychiatric
- Depression with atypical features

Medical
- Encephalitis and meningitis
- Stroke, head injury, space occupying lesion
- Degenerative neurological conditions
- Toxic, metabolic or endocrine abnormalities
- Kleine–Levin syndrome

Substances
- Alcohol
- Prescribed drugs (e.g. antipsychotics, benzodiazepines, tricyclic antidepressants)
- Substance withdrawal syndrome

Secondary to insomnia or sleep deprivation

COMMUNICATION

Insomnia occurs in a variety of physical conditions. It is not uncommon for patients with poor sleep to be treated for depression before their obstructive sleep apnoea is correctly diagnosed. You may find it useful to have a list of possible diagnoses in your mind.

Sleep terrors (night terrors)

Sleep terrors are episodes that feature an individual (usually a child) abruptly waking from sleep, usually with a scream, appearing to be in a state of extreme fear. These episodes are associated with:

- Autonomic arousal, e.g. tachycardia, dilated pupils, sweating and rapid breathing.
- A relative unresponsiveness to the efforts of others to comfort the person, who appears confused and disorientated.

Upon full awakening, there is amnesia for the episode and no recall of any dream or nightmare. Sleep terrors last from 1 to 10 minutes, and usually occur during slow wave sleep (stage 3 and 4) and are therefore predominantly in the first third of the night. Sleep terrors are seen in up to 6% of children aged 4–12 and usually resolve by adolescence. Sleepwalking and sleep terrors seem to be related conditions as they share clinical and aetiological similarities. Sleep terrors should be distinguished from nightmares, panic attacks, and epileptic seizures. Panic attacks tend not to be associated with confusion, and amnesia is uncommon.

Nightmares

Between 10% and 50% of children aged 3–5 experience repeated nightmares, although they occur occasionally in up to 50% of adults. Nightmares are characterized by an individual waking from sleep due to an intensely frightening dream involving threats to survival, security or self-esteem. Nightmares are distinguished from sleep terrors by the observation that not only is the individual alert and orientated immediately after awakening, but is able to recall the bad dream in vivid detail. Furthermore, nightmares tend to occur during the second half of the night because they arise almost exclusively during REM sleep, which tends to be longer and have more intense, surreal dreaming during the latter part of the night.

Sleepwalking (somnambulism)

Sleepwalking is characterized by an unusual state of consciousness in which complex motor behaviour occurs during sleep. While sleepwalking, the individual has a blank staring face, is relatively unresponsive to communication from others, and is difficult to waken. When sleepwalkers do wake up, either during an episode or the following morning, they have no recollection of the event ever having occurred. Sleepwalking is not associated with impairment of cognition or behaviour, although there may be an initial brief period of disorientation subsequent to waking up from a sleepwalking episode. Sleepwalking usually occurs during slow wave sleep (stage 3 and 4) and is therefore predominant in the first third of the night. The peak prevalence of sleepwalking occurs at the age of 12, with an onset between the age of 4 and 8 years. About 2–3% of children and about 0.5% of adults have regular episodes. Sleepwalking runs in families with 80% of sleepwalkers having a positive family history for sleepwalking or sleep terrors.

After this chapter you should have an understanding of:
- How sexual dysfunction is classified in relation to the four-phase sexual response cycle
- The three most common sexual dysfunctions in men and women respectively
- How age, physical and relationship health and educational achievement affect sexual functioning
- How antidepressants worsen and improve sexual functioning
- The principles of sex therapy and which type of couples are most suitable
- Which techniques may be useful in treating premature ejaculation
- Which biological treatments may be effective in erectile dysfunction
- Which sexual dysfunctions have the best prognosis
- Which paraphilias are most often seen in forensic settings and how they differ in terms of their classification
- Which interventions have limited efficacy in the treatment of paraphilias
- The management options for gender dysphoria

Healthy sexual functioning requires a healthy body and, perhaps more importantly, a healthy mind and relationship. Physical or psychological problems (or a combination of the two) can cause a wide variety of sexual problems. Mental health workers may be consulted about sexual problems that are largely due to psychological difficulties (not predominantly due to a biological problem) – i.e. psychosexual problems.

The psychosexual disorders can be classified into three groups:

- Sexual dysfunction.
- Disorders of sexual preference (paraphilias).
- Gender identity disorders.

SEXUAL DYSFUNCTION

Clinical features

The DSM-IV describes the sequence of psychological and physiological responses to sexual stimulation in a four-phase sexual response cycle, which is summarized in Figure 31.1.

Sexual dysfunction describes pain associated with intercourse or abnormalities of the sexual response cycle that lead to difficulties in participating in sexual activities. Although this chapter is focused on psychogenic dysfunction, the sexual response cycle consists of both psychological and biological processes and it is rarely possible to identify cases of sexual dysfunction with a purely physiological or purely psychogenic aetiology. Nevertheless, both the ICD-10 and the DSM-IV stipulate that a sexual dysfunction disorder should only be diagnosed when there is a suspected psychogenic component to the problem (i.e. not due exclusively to a medical condition or use of a substance). Figure 31.2 summarizes the sexual dysfunction disorders.

> **HINTS AND TIPS**
>
> Women have a large inter-individual variability in the type and duration of stimulation that results in orgasm. The diagnosis of female orgasmic disorder should only be made if the ability to achieve orgasm is less than would be reasonably expected for a woman's age, sexual experience and quality of sexual activity – and then only if the orgasmic dysfunction results in marked distress or relationship difficulties.

Epidemiology

Sexual dysfunction is very common, with a prevalence of about 43% in women and 31% in men. The reported frequency of specific sexual dysfunction is shown in Figure 31.3. The evidence suggests that:

- The prevalence of sexual problems in women tends to decrease with increasing age, except for those who report trouble lubricating.

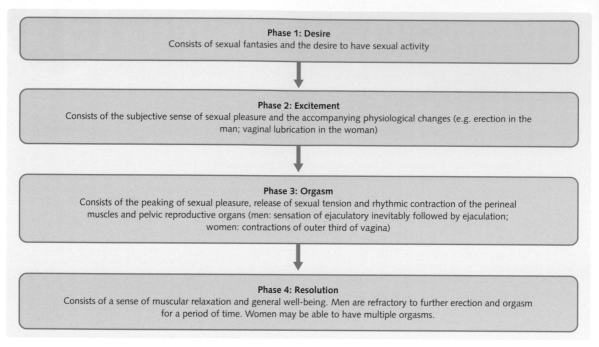

Fig. 31.1 The four-phase sexual response cycle

- Men, in contrast, have an increased prevalence of erectile problems and lack of interest in sex with increasing age.
- Sexual dysfunction is more likely among people with poor physical and emotional health.

- Sexual dysfunction is highly associated with negative experiences in sexual relationships.
- Married individuals and those with high educational attainment are at a lower risk of experiencing sexual dysfunction.

Fig. 31.2 Sexual dysfunction disorders

Phase of cycle	Dysfunction*	Description
Desire	Lack or loss of sexual desire [Hypoactive sexual desire disorder] Sexual aversion and lack of sexual enjoyment [Sexual aversion disorder]	Loss of desire to have, or to fantasize about sex – not due to other sexual dysfunction (e.g. erectile dysfunction, dyspareunia) Avoidance of sex due to negative feelings (fear, anxiety, repulsion), or lack of enjoyment
Excitement	Failure of genital response [Male erectile disorder; Female sexual arousal disorder]	Inability to attain or maintain sexual intercourse due to an inadequate erection in men, or poor lubrication–swelling response in women
Orgasm	Orgasmic dysfunction [Male/female orgasmic disorder] Premature ejaculation [Premature ejaculation]	Recurrent absence, or delay, of orgasm or ejaculation despite adequate sexual stimulation Recurrent ejaculation with minimal sexual stimulation before the man wishes
Sexual pain	Nonorganic dyspareunia [Dyspareunia not due to a general medical condition] Vaginismus [Vaginismus not due to a general medical condition]	Genital pain during sex in men or women – not due to other sexual dysfunction (e.g. poor lubrication–swelling response, vaginismus) or medical condition (e.g. atrophic vaginitis) Recurrent, involuntary spasm of the muscles that surround the outer third of the vagina, causing occlusion of the vaginal opening

*The DSM-IV terms are in square brackets; the ICD-10 terms are not.

Fig. 31.3 Reported frequency of sexual dysfunction in Americans aged 18–59 years (data from Laumann EO et al 1999 Sexual dysfunction in the United States: prevalence and predictors. JAMA 281: 537–544)

Reported frequency of sexual dysfunction in Americans aged 18–59 years		
Men	Premature ejaculation	31%
	Lack of sexual interest	15%
	Erectile difficulties	10%
	Unable to achieve orgasm	10%
Women	Lack of sexual interest	32%
	Unable to achieve orgasm	26%
	Trouble lubricating	21%
	Dyspareunia	16%

Fig. 31.4 Prescribed and recreational drugs associated with sexual dysfunction

Psychiatric drugs
- Antidepressants (tricyclics, SSRIs and MAOIs)
- Antipsychotics (especially first generation antipsychotics)
- Benzodiazepines
- Lithium

Recreational drugs
- Alcohol
- Amphetamines
- Cannabis
- Cocaine
- Opiates

Medical drugs
- Anticonvulsants
- Antihistamines
- Antihypertensives (including beta-blockers)
- Digoxin
- Diuretics

SSRI, selective serotonin reuptake inhibitor; MAOI, monoamine oxidase inhibitor.

Aetiology

There are many, often interrelated, psychosocial factors that may result in psychogenic sexual dysfunction:

- Ambivalent attitude about sex or intimacy (e.g. anxiety, fear, guilt, shame).
- History of rape or childhood sexual abuse.
- Fears of consequences of sex (e.g. impregnation, sexually transmitted diseases).
- A poor or deteriorating relationship (e.g. feeling undesirable, finding the partner undesirable, lack of trust, feelings of resentment or hostility, lack of respect, fear of rejection).
- Anxiety about sexual performance or physical attractiveness.
- Fatigue, stress or difficult psychosocial circumstances.

Frequently, there is more than one psychosocial problem that can affect more than one of the phases of the sexual response cycle. For example, the belief that sex is inherently sinful, in the context of an abusive relationship may lead to a lack of desire, a poor lubrication–swelling response and difficulty in reaching orgasm.

Differential diagnosis

Other causes of sexual dysfunction should be excluded when assessing a patient with sexual dysfunction. These include:

- Medical conditions (e.g. diabetes mellitus, vascular disease, vaginitis, endometriosis, spinal cord injuries, pelvic fractures, prostatectomy, multiple sclerosis, thyroid disease, hyperprolactinaemia).
- Prescribed or illicit drugs (see Fig. 31.4).
- Psychiatric illness: mental disorders such as depression, anxiety and alcohol dependence are frequently associated with sexual dysfunction. In addition, psychiatric medication often results in sexual dysfunction as a side-effect. However, sexual functioning frequently improves as the patient's mental

illness (e.g. depression) improves, even though the medication (e.g. antidepressants) may have adverse sexual effects.

> **HINTS AND TIPS**
>
> The clear presence of a biological cause of sexual dysfunction does not rule out a psychogenic sexual dysfunction, as the two are often interrelated. For example, a 55-year-old man with diabetes and advanced atherosclerosis notices a weakened erection; he subsequently becomes anxious during sex, fearing that he is losing his virility. This leads to a complete loss of his erectile potency.

Assessment considerations

- The wide differential diagnosis requires a comprehensive history including medical, psychiatric, sexual and relationship histories as well as current medication and recreational substance use. Questions regarding sexual matters outside the problematic context (e.g. morning erections, masturbatory activities) can be very helpful.
- A thorough physical examination, including genitalia, should be conducted. In addition, gynaecological examination may be needed for cases of dyspareunia or vaginismus in women.
- In addition to blood tests (e.g. thyroid functions, fasting glucose, liver and renal functions, prolactin,

testosterone), further investigations may be necessary to exclude medical causes of sexual dysfunction (e.g. monitoring of nocturnal penile tumescence (excludes physiological causes of impotence if able to have erection during REM sleep) and monitoring penile blood flow with Doppler ultrasonography).

COMMUNICATION

Taking a sexual history can be embarrassing for both patients and doctors, and basic communication skills are very important. Privacy should be ensured, and non-verbal aspects of communication utilized (e.g. body language, use of silence). Appropriate terminology should be used (e.g. 'vagina', rather than 'down below'; 'condom', rather than 'protection'). Reassurance and acknowledgement of discomfort (e.g. 'I can see how difficult this is for you to talk about') can be very helpful.

Management considerations

- Many patients may need no more than reassurance, advice and sexual education. Furthermore, patients who have significant relationship difficulties may be advised to engage in relationship counselling before attempting specific treatment for sexual dysfunction.
- Some couples with minor problems benefit from self-help materials, particularly those with no major relationship difficulties.
- Urology clinics deal mainly with physiological sexual dysfunction, particularly erectile problems.
- Sexual dysfunction clinics have multidisciplinary teams that focus on both psychological and physical aspects of sexual dysfunction and are best equipped to deal with cases that do not respond to non-specific measures.
- Some couples benefit from sex therapy, in which partners are treated together and are taught to communicate openly about sex, in addition to receiving education about sexual anatomy and the physiology of the sexual response cycle. They also take part in graded assignments, beginning with caressing of their partner's body, without genital contact, for their own and then their partner's pleasure. These behavioural tasks progress through a number of stages with increasing sexual intimacy, with the focus remaining on pleasurable physical contact as opposed to the monitoring of sexual arousal or the preoccupation with achieving orgasm. Couples suitable for sex therapy include those with a significant psychological component to their problem, those with reasonable motivation and those with a reasonably harmonious relationship.

Fig. 31.5 Specific exercises useful in sexual dysfunction

Sexual dysfunction	Exercise
Female orgasmic disorder	Exercises in sexual fantasy and masturbation, sometimes with a vibrator or dildo
Premature ejaculation	Squeeze technique: woman squeezes the glans of her partner's penis for a few seconds when he feels that he is about to ejaculate Start–stop method: stimulation is halted and arousal is allowed to subside when the man feels that ejaculation is imminent. The process is then repeated Quiet vagina: man keeps penis motionless in vagina for increasing periods before ejaculating
Vaginismus	Desensitization, first by finger insertion followed by dilators of increasing size

- Figure 31.5 summarizes some of the specific exercises often used in the context of sex therapy that may be helpful with particular problems.
- Biological treatments may be very effective, especially for erectile problems (e.g. oral sildenafil (Viagra®), intracavernosal injections, vacuum devices, prosthetic implants and surgery for venous leakage). Testosterone may increase sexual drive in patients with low levels. For difficulties with premature ejaculation, SSRIs may delay ejaculation, but this is rarely a long-term solution.

Prognosis

Vaginismus has an excellent prognosis. Premature ejaculation and psychogenic erectile dysfunction also respond fairly well to treatment. Problems associated with poor sexual desire, especially in men, seem more resistant to treatment.

DISORDERS OF SEXUAL PREFERENCE (PARAPHILIAS)

The essential features of a paraphilia are recurrent sexually arousing fantasies, sexual urges or behaviours involving: (1) non-human objects; (2) the suffering or humiliation of oneself or one's partner; or (3) children or other non-consenting individuals. It is useful to divide the paraphilias into two groups:

1. Abnormalities of the object of sexual interest (e.g. paedophilia, fetishism, transvestic fetishism).

Fig. 31.6 The paraphilias	
Abnormalities of the object of sexual interest	
Paedophilia	Sexual fantasies, urges or behaviours involving children
Fetishism	Sexual fantasies, urges or behaviours involving inanimate objects or parts of the body that are not directly erogenous
Transvestic fetishism	Sexual fantasies, urges or behaviours involving cross-dressing (wearing of clothes of the opposite sex). Rare in women
Zoophilia (bestiality)	Sexual fantasies, urges or behaviours involving animals
Necrophilia	Sexual fantasies, urges or behaviours involving corpses
Abnormalities of the sexual act	
Exhibitionism	Sexual fantasies, urges or behaviours involving the exposure of genitals to unsuspecting strangers
Voyeurism	Sexual fantasies, urges or behaviours involving the act of observing unsuspecting people engaging in sexual activity or undressing
Sexual sadism	Sexual fantasies, urges or behaviours involving the infliction of acts of physical or psychological suffering or humiliation on others
Sexual masochism	Sexual fantasies, urges or behaviours involving the infliction of acts of humiliation or suffering on oneself

2. Abnormalities of the sexual act (e.g. exhibitionism, voyeurism, sexual sadism, sexual masochism).

Figure 31.6 summarizes the specific paraphilias.

The paraphilias are mainly confined to men (with the exception of sexual masochism) and usually begin in late adolescence or early adulthood. Paedophilia and exhibitionism are frequently seen in a forensic setting and account for the majority of sexual offenders referred for a psychiatric opinion (see Ch. 29).

The aetiology is unknown, but there is often an impaired capacity for affectionate sexual activity and patients with paraphilia often have personality disorders.

Management options include behaviour therapy (covert sensitization, where patients attempt to pair paraphilic thoughts with humiliating consequences) and aversion therapy (pairing paraphilic thoughts with a noxious stimulus such as an unpleasant odour or taste). Individual psychodynamic and group therapies are also used. Cognitive-behavioural therapy programmes and anti-androgens (e.g. cyproterone acetate) have shown some efficacy in the treatment of some paedophiles and exhibitionists; however, there is little evidence that any treatment is consistently effective in either of these conditions. It should be noted that, dependent on risk of offending, management within a forensic setting may be required (see Ch. 29).

Paraphilias associated with a young age of onset, a high frequency of acts, no remorse about acts and a lack of motivation for change have a particularly poor prognosis.

GENDER IDENTITY

Gender identity describes an individual's inner sense of being male or female. This usually corresponds to the person's sexual identity which comprises all their biological and anatomical sexual characteristics (i.e. external and internal genitalia, chromosomes, sex hormones and secondary sex characteristics). Gender identity is thought to be fully formed by the age of 3 years.

There has been considerable debate over the years as to whether gender identity disorder (transsexualism) is a mental disorder. Many do not regard cross-gender feelings and behaviours as a 'disorder', and instead question what constitutes a normal gender identity or gender role. The DSM-V (due to supersede the DSM-IV in mid-2013) has replaced the term with the (less stigmatizing) term 'gender dysphoria'.

Many areas provide multidisciplinary clinics for people whose biological gender is inconsistent with their gender identity. The role of the psychiatrist is to exclude the presence of mental disorder as a cause of gender dysphoria, and to assess and treat comorbid mental disorders which may be present.

Patients who are committed to gender change can be helped with hormones and surgery, usually after they have completed a 'real life test', which involves living as the opposite sex for at least a year.

> **HINTS AND TIPS**
>
> Transsexualism (gender dysphoria) and transvestism are not the same. Transsexualism describes a refusal to live as the gender assigned at birth, while transvestism describes dressing in clothes intended for members of the opposite sex. Questions you may find useful to differentiate between the two include: do they wish to be accepted as the opposite sex? Are they content with their gender? Does cross-dressing cause sexual arousal? The latter would suggest transvestic fetishism.

SELF-ASSESSMENT

Best of fives questions (BOFs)   215

Extended-matching questions (EMQs)   233

BOF Answers   255

EMQ Answers   271

Best of fives questions (BOFs)

Chapter 2 Pharmacological therapy and electroconvulsive therapy

1. Nurses ask for urgent review of a 24-year-old man who is a psychiatric in-patient and is hypertensive, tachycardic and pyrexial. He is very drowsy and has rigid limbs. What action will most help distinguish between neuroleptic malignant syndrome and serotonin syndrome?
   A. Checking serum creatinine kinase levels
   B. Looking at his drug kardex
   C. Checking his past medical history
   D. Formally assessing his cognition
   E. Monitoring his condition over time

2. Nurses ask for urgent review of a 24-year-old man who is a psychiatric in-patient and is hypertensive, tachycardic and pyrexial. He is very drowsy and has rigid limbs. He was admitted a week ago with a first episode psychosis and has received large doses of haloperidol since. What management step should be done first?
   A. Discontinue all antipsychotics
   B. Work up for ECT
   C. Give dantrolene
   D. Give bromocriptine
   E. Assess ABC

3. A 37-year-old woman with treatment resistant schizophrenia is considering commencing clozapine. What should she be advised about the monitoring required initially?
   A. Weekly blood pressure checks
   B. Weekly liver function tests
   C. Weekly full blood counts
   D. Weekly lipid profiles
   E. Weekly fasting glucose assays

4. A 45-year-old woman has recently started phenelzine. She is out for lunch with her friend who is a doctor. She asks her friend what she can eat from the menu.
   A. Broccoli and stilton soup
   B. Pickled herring on a bed of salad
   C. Marmite and sesame toast
   D. Smoked mackerel paté
   E. Egg mayonnaise toastie

5. A 37-year-old woman who takes lithium for bipolar affective disorder has recently completed a course of ibuprofen for a knee injury. She now feels very tired and weak. She is unsteady on her feet and has a coarse tremor. A random lithium level is sent. What is the lowest result that could explain her symptoms?
   A. 0.2 mmol/L
   B. 0.4 mmol/L
   C. 0.8 mmol/L
   D. 1.0 mmol/L
   E. 1.8 mmol/L

6. A 42-year-old woman with bipolar affective disorder recently commenced lamotrigine for prophylaxis of depressive episodes. Three days ago she developed a maculopapular rash. This morning she noticed concentric circles of erythematous and pale skin on her hands, and she has a blister on her lip. What is the best management option?
   A. Gradually withdraw lamotrigine
   B. Discontinue lamotrigine
   C. Screen for Wegener's granulomatosis
   D. Screen for HIV
   E. Start oral aciclovir

Chapter 3 Psychological therapy

1. A 49-year-old man has been struggling to move on with his life after his son died in a car accident 6 months ago. Which ONE of the following would be the most appropriate psychological therapy in the first instance?
   A. Psychodynamic therapy
   B. Cognitive-behavioural therapy
   C. Person-centred counselling
   D. Exposure and response prevention
   E. Mindfulness-based cognitive therapy

2. A 22-year-old woman with a diagnosis of borderline personality disorder has been given information about various types of psychotherapy. Which ONE of the following is most accurate?
   A. Classical psychoanalysis is the best treatment for borderline personality disorder
   B. The modality of therapy is less important than the therapeutic alliance between the patient and their therapist
   C. Good quality psychodynamic interpretations are a curative factor in borderline personality disorder
   D. Group therapy should be reserved for the more disturbed patients
   E. Family therapy is frequently used in the treatment of borderline personality disorder in the UK

3. A 35-year-old man is undergoing psychodynamic psychotherapy, and a letter from his therapist describes the 'transference'. Which of the following is the most accurate description of transference?
   A. The level of trust in the patient–therapist relationship

B. Good eye contact throughout sessions
C. Patient response towards the therapist based on previous relationships
D. The level of empathy in the patient–therapist relationship
E. Therapist attitude towards the patient based on previous relationships

4. A 30-year-old woman asks for psychological therapy to help with her phobia of cats. Which of the following is NOT associated with graded exposure?
A. Assertiveness training
B. Construction of hierarchy
C. Empathic therapeutic attitude
D. Desensitization of the stimulus
E. Gradual exposure to more anxiety-provoking situations

5. A 25-year-old male student has a history of depression, and has been referred to cognitive-behavioural therapy. He reports that 'my life is over because I failed my final exams'. Which ONE of the following most accurately describes this cognitive distortion?
A. Emotional reasoning
B. Fortune telling
C. Personalization
D. Labelling
E. Magnification

6. A 57-year-old housewife describes that she feels better after completing a course of interpersonal therapy. In which of the following conditions has interpersonal therapy proven to be of benefit?
A. Alzheimer's disease
B. Moderate depression
C. Generalized anxiety disorder
D. Paranoid schizophrenia
E. Panic disorder

Chapter 4 Mental health and the law

1. Which patient is most likely to have capacity for the decision required?
A. A 23-year-old man who has suffered a head injury in a road traffic accident and has a Glasgow Coma Scale score of 8. The decision is whether he should be ventilated or not.
B. A 59-year-old man who suffered Wernicke's encephalopathy and now cannot remember any new information. The decision is which accommodation option he should choose.
C. A 34-year-old woman experiencing a manic episode with psychotic features. She broke her leg jumping off a bus shelter but denies the need for surgery as she thinks she can heal her leg herself. The decision is whether she needs surgery or not.
D. A 26-year-old woman with a severe intellectual disability. The decision is whether she should use oral contraception or not.

E. A 55-year-old man with schizophrenia with chronic auditory hallucinations and negative symptoms. The decision is whether he start a statin or not.

2. A 72-year-old woman has recently been diagnosed with dementia. She continues to drive and gets shopping for her and her partner every week. He says there are no problems with her driving. Which ONE of the following should be advised?
A. She should stop driving immediately
B. She should stop driving once she feels her driving is less good than it used to be
C. She should stop driving once her partner feels her driving is less good than it used to be
D. She should notify the DVLA
E. Her GP will notify the DVLA

Chapter 5 Mental health service provision

1. Which patient is LEAST likely to need secondary mental health services?
A. A 34-year-old woman with a first episode of depression, responding well to cognitive-behavioural therapy
B. A 34-year-old woman with a first episode of depression, who has not responded to cognitive-behavioural therapy or two antidepressants
C. A 34-year-old woman with a first episode of hypomania and previous episode of depression
D. A 34-year-old woman with a first episode of depression who recently took an overdose
E. A 34-year-old woman who says she has been depressed for years but objectively seems euthymic

2. A 21-year-old man with no past history is experiencing odd beliefs that he has some special power and that things around him are of special significance. He struggles to explain these beliefs further and says they cannot be true. He has stopped going out with his friends and his personal hygiene has deteriorated. He has no thoughts of harm to himself or others. Which team is best placed to manage him?
A. Community mental health team
B. Early intervention in psychosis team
C. Assertive outreach team
D. Home treatment team
E. In-patient unit

Chapter 6 The patient with thoughts of suicide or self-harm

1. You diagnose a 27-year-old man with depression. Which ONE of the following symptoms of depression has the strongest association with suicide?
A. A patient who reports loss of enjoyment in all activities

B. A patient who feels they have no energy
C. A patient who is no longer interested in sex
D. A patient who finds it difficult to fall asleep and wakes early
E. A patient who walks slowly into the room and pauses for a long time between words

2. A 15-year-old tells you that she has been self-harming by inflicting lacerations on her forearms. Which ONE of the following is the most common motive given by young people to explain their reason for self-cutting?
A. Escape from a terrible state of mind
B. Pressure from peer group
C. Demonstration of desperation
D. Attention-seeking
E. Wanted to frighten someone

3. A 23-year-old woman presents at the A&E department stating that she is feeling suicidal and has taken an overdose of paracetamol several hours ago. She is requesting help. Which ONE of the following aspects of her clinical care should take priority?
A. History of circumstances leading to overdose
B. Mental state examination
C. Measurement of serum paracetamol levels
D. Determination of suicidal intent
E. Evaluation of current social supports

4. You are taking an occupational history from a 44-year-old man who has self-harmed. He tells you that he tried to kill himself. Which ONE of the following professions is most associated with completed suicide?
A. Gas plumbers
B. Rock musicians
C. General practitioners
D. Investment bankers
E. Veterinary surgeons

5. A 45-year-old policeman, with a history of self-harm, depression, and alcohol dependence, discloses that he has been thinking about ways of killing himself since his wife left him a month ago. Which ONE of the following preparatory measures would suggest strong suicidal intent?
A. Internet research
B. Contacting the Samaritans
C. Telling his ex-wife of his plans
D. Making a will and paying bills
E. Visiting GP for a check-up

6. A 29-year-old builder with a diagnosis of depression states that he is considering various methods of suicide. Which ONE of the following is the most common method of completed suicide in England and Wales?
A. Jumping from height
B. Paracetamol overdose
C. Suspension hanging
D. Firearm wound
E. Carbon monoxide poisoning

Chapter 7 The patient with low mood

1. A 40-year-old woman who was started on a new medication a month ago presents with a 4-week history of depression. Which of the following medications might account for her presentation?
A. Paracetamol
B. Omeprazole
C. Salbutamol
D. Verapamil
E. Prednisolone

2. A 35-year-old woman presents with mild depression. On examination you notice a midline neck swelling. What is the most appropriate next step?
A. Refer to psychiatry
B. Check thyroid function
C. Start an antidepressant
D. Request a neck ultrasound
E. Advise her to return if the symptoms persist

3. A 55-year-old man with no previous psychiatric history presents with low mood, anhedonia and fatigue. He has come for help as he believes his organs are rotting away. What is the most likely diagnosis?
A. Bipolar affective disorder
B. Schizoaffective disorder
C. Schizophrenia
D. Depression with psychotic features
E. Severe depression

4. A 25-year-old student turns up late for her appointment. She gives a 1-month history of low mood, anhedonia and fatigue. What is the most important area to cover in what remains of the appointment time?
A. Presence of biological symptoms of depression
B. Drug history
C. Family history of mood disorder
D. Suicidal ideation
E. Past medical history

5. A 19-year-old shop-assistant presents in tears because her boyfriend broke up with her the day before. She did not sleep well last night and did not feel like having breakfast. She feels hopeless about the future and thinks she will never meet anyone else. She says she feels really depressed. What is the best management?
A. Start an antidepressant
B. Refer to psychiatry
C. Ask her to complete a mood diary
D. Watchful waiting
E. Check FBC, U&E, LFT and TFT

Chapter 8 The patient with elevated or irritable mood

1. A 34-year-old man with bipolar affective disorder attends for review. What is the commonest mood in mania?
A. Euphoria

B. Delusional
C. Lability
D. Depression
E. Irritability

2. Reception staff ask the GP to see a 29-year-old man with a past history of bipolar affective disorder who is standing at the front desk gesticulating angrily at the computer. He is speaking very quickly and no one can understand what he is trying to say. What is the most likely cause?
   A. Thought disorder due to mania
   B. Dysarthria due to Bell's palsy
   C. Malingering
   D. Partial seizure
   E. Dysphasia due to cerebrovascular accident involving Broca's area

3. A 55-year-old man has had several admissions to hospital with elated episodes when he believes he is Jesus Christ, but has never been depressed. What is the diagnosis?
   A. Recurrent hypomania
   B. Bipolar affective disorder
   C. Schizoaffective disorder
   D. Cyclothymia
   E. Recurrent mania

4. A 25-year-old farmer is brought to A&E by the police after he tried to steal a tractor. He is agitated, but shows no remorse, stating loudly that it rightfully belongs to him as he is the King of Tractors. He has no past psychiatric history, past medical history or previous criminal offences. Which investigation will be most important diagnostically?
   A. CT head
   B. EEG
   C. Full blood count
   D. Urine drug screen
   E. Thyroid function

5. A 24-year-old unemployed woman presents to her GP asking to be treated for bipolar disorder. She has looked it up on the internet and thinks it may explain why she is always losing her temper with people. Her mood swings frequently, sometimes several times in a day. She often does things she later regrets, and has never managed to maintain a long-term relationship or job. She has had these mood swings from when she was a little girl. What is the most likely diagnosis?
   A. Bipolar affective disorder
   B. Dysthymia
   C. Cyclothymia
   D. Emotionally unstable personality disorder
   E. Multiple sclerosis

Chapter 9 The psychotic patient

1. A 78-year-old widow with macular degeneration is brought to her GP by her daughter who is concerned that her mother has been asking her to move

nonexistent dogs and cats off her couch. Her mother is otherwise alert, orientated, and in good health. What is the most likely diagnosis?
   A. Schizophrenia
   B. Charles Bonnet syndrome
   C. Delirium
   D. Brain tumour
   E. Dementia

2. A 62-year-old man with schizophrenia attends his GP. He is dishevelled and smells strongly of tobacco. He reports feeling that someone is pressing on his chest, particularly when he approaches the church at the top of the hill. He wonders if it is the devil. What is the most likely cause of the sensation in his chest?
   A. Tactile hallucination
   B. Delusion of control
   C. Persecutory delusion
   D. Thought disorder
   E. Ischaemic heart disease

3. A 43-year-old man tells his GP he thinks his wife is having an affair. She has frequently been coming home late from work and 2 weeks ago he thinks he saw her kissing another man. He is very upset by this and determined to get conclusive evidence to confront her with. He has quit his job in order to follow her and taken out a personal loan to purchase cameras to place in her car, workplace and handbag. What is the psychopathology described here?
   A. Delusion
   B. Obsession
   C. Hallucination
   D. Over-valued idea
   E. Erotomania

4. A 19-year-old man is brought to A&E by his flatmates because for the last fortnight he has been complaining the neighbours are talking about him and tonight stated 'enough was enough' and picked up his cricket bat to go and confront them. His friends cannot hear the neighbours. The man has smoked cannabis every day for the last 6 months and has recently been experimenting with some 'legal highs'. What is the most likely diagnosis?
   A. Schizophrenia
   B. Schizophrenia-like psychotic disorder
   C. Delusional disorder
   D. Depressive episode, severe, with psychotic features
   E. Psychosis secondary to psychoactive substance use

5. A 16-year-old boy is referred to psychiatry because he has not been able to attend school for 3 months and has lost contact with his friends. He is very difficult to understand because his words do not seem to follow on from each other. Sometimes he laughs or grimaces for no discernible reason. What subtype of schizophrenia does he have?
   A. Paranoid
   B. Simple

C. Catatonic
D. Undifferentiated
E. Hebephrenic

Chapter 10 The patient with anxiety, fear or avoidance

1. A 21-year-old student calls an ambulance for the fourth time in a month because of chest pain, shortness of breath and a feeling she is about to die. This settles by the time she reaches A&E. On all occasions, her examination, ECG and cardiac enzymes are normal. She has her final exams in a fortnight and admits she is very worried. What is the most likely diagnosis?
   A. Acute coronary syndrome
   B. Thyrotoxicosis
   C. Hypoglycaemia
   D. Panic attack
   E. Hypertrophic obstructive cardiomyopathy

2. A 57-year-old obese man keeps cancelling appointments with the practice nurse to have bloods taken for cholesterol and glucose. Although he is normally very cheerful and relaxed, he becomes pale, sweaty and tremulous when you offer to take his bloods during the consultation. What is the most likely diagnosis?
   A. Myocardial infarction
   B. Depressive episode
   C. Blood–injection–injury phobia
   D. Panic disorder
   E. Hypochondriasis

3. A 63-year-old woman with a past history of depression presents to A&E and tells you she has a dry mouth, a choking sensation, butterflies in her stomach, palpitations and shortness of breath. What is the most appropriate first step in management?
   A. ECG
   B. Observations
   C. Psychiatry referral
   D. Bloods: FBC, U&Es, LFTs and troponin
   E. Arterial blood gas

4. A 24-year-old man who was recently diagnosed with type 1 diabetes attends his GP. Over the last month he has experienced recurrent attacks of anxiety associated with sweating and tachycardia. The episodes do not seem to have any triggers, last for about 20 minutes, and resolve when he sits down with his girlfriend and has a cup of tea and a biscuit. What should the GP advise the patient to do next time it happens?
   A. Deep breathing exercises
   B. Note it in a diary along with what else happened that day
   C. Take diazepam
   D. See a counsellor
   E. Check blood sugar

5. A 44-year-old businessman presents to his GP because for the last month he has felt anxious, sweaty and shaky in the mornings. He feels better when he has lunch, and generally his mood is good. He admits to drinking a bottle of red wine every night, and usually having champagne during business lunches. What is the most likely diagnosis?
   A. Depressive episode
   B. Diabetes
   C. Panic disorder
   D. Alcohol withdrawal
   E. Work phobia

Chapter 11 The patient with obsessions and compulsions

1. A 29-year-old woman mentions she is obsessed with a TV talent show. She watches each episode multiple times and has pictures of all the contestants on her bedroom wall. She called in sick the day of the final as her shift clashed with the showing. She enjoys watching and thinking about the show, and thinks she might audition next year. What is the most likely diagnosis?
   A. No mental illness
   B. Social phobia
   C. Impulse control disorder
   D. Obsessive-compulsive disorder
   E. Delusional disorder

2. A 36-year-old man keeps thinking about his own death. He sees repetitive images of his body in a coffin. He tries to distract himself but it does not work. The images started about 3 months ago, around the time he started to feel low in mood associated with fatigue, less pleasure in life, insomnia and anorexia. What is the most likely diagnosis?
   A. Obsessive-compulsive disorder
   B. Generalized anxiety disorder
   C. Depressive episode
   D. Hypochondriacal disorder
   E. Nihilistic delusion

3. A 44-year-old man has had intrusive thoughts regarding security for several years. He keeps thinking his house is unlocked and has developed a routine of checking every door and window nine times before leaving the premises. This means he has to get up half an hour early and sometimes come home from work early to recheck. This has caused friction with a new manager and over the last month he has noticed his mood is lower. He no longer enjoys playing football, is very tired all the time, and is struggling to concentrate at work. What is the most likely diagnosis?
   A. Depressive episode
   B. Obsessive-compulsive disorder
   C. Obsessive-compulsive disorder with sub-syndromal depressive symptoms

D. Obsessive-compulsive disorder with comorbid depressive episode
E. Obsessive-compulsive (anankastic) personality disorder

4. A 33-year-old graphic designer is driven to produce perfect images. She has always been very conscientious, even at primary school. The thought of a mistake in one of her designs makes her feel so anxious she often stays late at work checking them through. She is proud of the quality of work, and feels her colleagues are sloppy and should work harder. She had to leave her last company because she told the manager this. What is the most likely diagnosis?
A. Obsessive-compulsive disorder
B. Obsessive-compulsive (anankastic) personality disorder
C. No mental illness
D. Autistic spectrum disorder
E. Obsessive-compulsive disorder with sub-syndromal depressive symptoms

5. A 23-year-old woman reports a voice inside her head telling her to harm herself. She is not sure where it comes from as no one is around when she hears it. What is the psychopathology she displays?
A. Obsession
B. Pseudohallucination
C. Rumination
D. Thought insertion
E. Hallucination

Chapter 12 The patient with a reaction to a stressful event or bereavement

1. A 23-year-old man with a history of schizophrenia appears confused and withdrawn the morning after he was severely assaulted by a group of youths in the local park. He has no recollection of the event. Which ONE of the following diagnoses should be initially considered?
A. Acute stress reaction
B. Adjustment disorder
C. Relapse of schizophrenia
D. Intracranial haemorrhage
E. Post-traumatic stress disorder

2. A 57-year-old lady has been referred urgently by her GP for symptoms of low mood, weight loss and insomnia. These have been troublesome for the past 10 weeks, since she watched her husband drown while on a yachting holiday. Which ONE of the following would be suggestive of a diagnosis of depression rather than a normal bereavement reaction?
A. Thinking that she would be better off dead
B. Difficulty concentrating on watching the television

C. Inability to tend to her self-care or get out of bed
D. Extreme guilt for not making her late husband wear a lifejacket
E. Hearing the voice of her late husband while lying alone in bed

3. A 28-year-old woman was signed off her job in a call centre with 'work-related stress' 2 weeks ago, a month after she was promoted to a supervisory position in a new department. She has no psychiatric history and denies substance misuse. At interview, she tells you she feels 'unable to cope' with the demands of her new role. She is sleeping well, and continues to enjoy jogging on a daily basis. Which of the following would be the most appropriate diagnosis?
A. Depressive disorder
B. Adjustment disorder
C. Conversion disorder
D. Acute stress reaction
E. No mental illness

4. Which of the following disorders would be LEAST likely to occur comorbidly with post-traumatic stress disorder in a previously well 34-year-old male soldier, who has recently returned from a difficult tour of duty in Afghanistan?
A. Acute and transient psychotic disorder
B. Paranoid schizophrenia
C. Alcohol dependence
D. Panic disorder
E. Depression, moderate severity

5. A 19-year-old female asylum seeker is brought to hospital by a social worker regarding concerns with her memory. She recalls her entire life until 3 months ago when she received news that government militia were coming towards her former hometown in Sierra Leone. She has memory of the last 4 weeks of her life in the UK, and is able to tell you about her current address, social circle and circumstances. You see from her medical notes that she had a termination of pregnancy 6 weeks ago; however, she has no recollection of either the conception or the procedure. Physical examination and investigations reveal no abnormalities, and she seems indifferent to her difficulties. Which ONE of the following is the most likely diagnosis?
A. Dissociative amnesia
B. Anterograde amnesia following head trauma
C. Transient global amnesia
D. Post-traumatic stress disorder
E. Wernicke–Korsakoff syndrome

6. A 21-year-old hairdresser described feeling 'worthless' and suicidal since she was voted out of the semi-final of a TV singing competition. You consider making a diagnosis of adjustment disorder. Which ONE of the following is a necessary criterion for such a diagnosis to be made?
A. Meets criteria for diagnosis of comorbid anxiety disorder
B. Onset of symptoms within 3 months of original stressor

C. Significantly increased consumption of alcohol
D. The initial stressor must be severe
E. Suicidal ideation must be present

Chapter 13 The patient with medically unexplained physical symptoms

1. A 26-year-old male teacher attends his GP requesting tests to confirm that he is suffering from multiple sclerosis. He thinks that he has this because he had some stabbing pain in his upper arm last week. The pain has now resolved and examination is unremarkable. Which ONE of the following should the GP do?
   A. Watchful waiting
   B. Refer for urgent neurology appointment
   C. Organize MRI scan and lumbar puncture
   D. Tell the patient that he is worrying too much
   E. Organize another appointment in 3 days

2. A 25-year-old woman insists that she wants plastic surgery on her nose, as she feels it is crooked and deformed. She has stopped leaving the house for fear of other people noticing. She tells you that she cannot stop thinking about how ugly it is, and this often keeps her awake at night. On examination, her nose is entirely normal and she does appear slightly reassured when you tell her this. Which ONE of the following is the most likely diagnosis?
   A. Somatic delusional disorder
   B. Factitious disorder
   C. Malingering
   D. Body dysmorphic disorder
   E. Hypochondriacal disorder

3. A 19-year-old female office assistant complained of intermittent bloating, abdominal pain, constipation and profuse diarrhoea. After thorough investigation, no physical abnormalities were found and a diagnosis of irritable bowel syndrome was made. Which of the following would be the most appropriate description of irritable bowel syndrome?
   A. A somatization disorder
   B. A hypochondriacal disorder
   C. A somatoform pain disorder
   D. A factitious disorder
   E. A somatoform autonomic dysfunction

4. A 44-year-old man is angry at being referred to a psychiatrist for his multiple and varied physical health complaints, for which no structural cause has ever been found. Which of the following would preclude (ICD-10 criteria) diagnosis of somatization disorder?
   A. Multiple and varied physical symptoms
   B. Preoccupation with the symptoms
   C. Persistent refusal to accept medical reassurances
   D. Symptoms present for 1 year
   E. Repeated consultations

5. A 32-year-old former nurse complains of pelvic pain. Despite the apparent severity of the pain and the presence of multiple abdominal surgical scars, her physical appearance, examination and basic investigations are entirely normal. She tells you in great detail about her previous diagnoses and invasive investigations, and demands pethidine and a diagnostic laparoscopy. She claims to be visiting from a distant town. Which of the following should be the next step in her management?
   A. Arrange an urgent diagnostic laparoscopy
   B. Prescribe pethidine at her request
   C. Tell her that she is lying
   D. Contact previous centres of care for further information
   E. Refer to psychiatry

6. A 72-year-old man is referred to psychiatry because of dyspnoea and stabbing pain in his chest. He has not seen a GP for years, and examination and routine blood tests are normal. The medical doctor feels that he has panic attacks. Which ONE of the following should be the next step in his management?
   A. Cognitive-behavioural therapy
   B. Further physical investigations
   C. Explanation of functional illness
   D. Antidepressant medication
   E. Watchful waiting

7. A 41-year-old woman is a frequent visitor to her GP. She has had numerous special investigations over several years for a multitude of physical symptoms, including abdominal pain, dysmenorrhoea, dysuria and difficulty swallowing. She refuses to accept her GP's explanation that there is no physical cause for her symptoms. She is now requesting a referral to a neurologist because she has a persistent tingling sensation in her legs. Which of the following is the likely diagnosis?
   A. Somatoform pain disorder
   B. Factitious disorder
   C. Briquet's syndrome
   D. Hypochondriacal disorder
   E. Undifferentiated somatoform disorder

Chapter 14 The patient with impairment of consciousness, memory or cognition

1. An 82-year-old woman is brought to A&E by her family. They are concerned that over the last couple of days she has been very suspicious of them, has mentioned seeing wolves in her kitchen and has been pacing her sitting room all night. She scores 4/10 on the Abbreviated Mental Test. She normally functions well, living alone with no carers. What is the most likely diagnosis?
   A. Late onset schizophrenia
   B. Lewy body dementia
   C. Alzheimer's dementia
   D. Delirium
   E. Charles Bonnet syndrome

2. A woman brings her 62-year-old father to register at a new GP practice as he has recently moved to the area to be closer to her. He tells the GP about an exciting and varied personal and past medical history but his daughter says none of this is true, and that for some months now he has a very poor memory for both old and new information. He can spell 'WORLD' backwards and draw a clock face without difficulty. He used to be a heavy drinker. What is the most likely diagnosis?
   A. Amnesic syndrome
   B. Dementia
   C. Alcohol excess
   D. Malingering
   E. Fugue state

3. A 75-year-old retired fisherman presents to his GP with a 12-month history of gradual onset, gradually worsening memory impairment confirmed by his wife. He is no longer able to cook or help mend nets like he used to. MMSE is 22/30. He has a past medical history of hypertension and is an ex-smoker. Physical examination is normal. He has had normal full blood count, U&Es, calcium, glucose and thyroid function in the last month. What further investigations should this man receive?
   A. CT head
   B. Vitamin B_{12} and folate level
   C. Syphilis and HIV serology
   D. CT head and vitamin B_{12} and folate level
   E. Syphilis and HIV serology and vitamin B_{12} and folate level

4. A 77-year-old woman is an in-patient on a general medical ward. She was admitted 2 weeks ago with a severe urinary tract infection requiring intravenous antibiotics. In A&E her AMT was 2/10. Since admission she has been disorientated and hallucinating. Her antibiotics finished a week ago and her inflammatory markers returned to normal. Four days ago she was almost discharged, but became very confused and agitated the night before going. Repeat AMT was 4/10. Prior to admission she functioned well and was cognitively normal. What is the most likely diagnosis?
   A. Delirium
   B. Late onset schizophrenia
   C. Lewy body dementia
   D. Alzheimer's dementia
   E. Charles Bonnet syndrome

5. A 74-year-old man is admitted to hospital because he has acute cognitive impairment and is hypervigilant and agitated. Past medical history is of insomnia and ischaemic heart disease. His medications are amitriptyline 50 mg every night, aspirin 75 mg every morning, simvastatin 20 mg every night. His daughter thinks he has recently started a new medication. Physical examination, blood tests, ECG, CXR and CT head are normal. What is the most likely cause of his presentation?
   A. Acute renal failure
   B. Acute myocardial infarction
   C. Acute subdural haematoma
   D. Pneumonia
   E. Anticholinergic medication

Chapter 15 The patient with alcohol or substance use problems

1. A 54-year-old man reports consuming a litre of vodka per day. Which of the following symptoms is NOT one of the Edwards and Gross criteria for alcohol dependence?
   A. Subjective awareness of compulsion to drink
   B. Withdrawal symptoms
   C. Narrowing of the drinking repertoire
   D. An acquired tolerance to alcohol
   E. Increased use of other substances (e.g. nicotine)

2. A 45-year-old woman described auditory hallucinations telling her that she was evil. These started a week ago, after several months of heavy use of alcohol. Her concentration and memory were normal. Other than slightly abnormal liver function tests, physical examination and investigations were normal, and breath alcohol was undetected. Which ONE of the following is the most likely diagnosis?
   A. Delirium tremens
   B. Late-onset schizophrenia
   C. Hepatic encephalopathy
   D. Alcoholic hallucinosis
   E. Wernicke–Korsakoff syndrome

3. A 62-year-old salesman is admitted to an orthopaedic ward for an elective surgical repair of his anterior cruciate ligament. Two days later (before his surgery), he appears shaky, confused, disorientated, and tells you that he can see a small horse on the table. His wife discloses that he had been drinking a bottle of whisky per day in the 3 months prior to admission. Which of the following aspects of his management should be delayed?
   A. Benzodiazepines
   B. Parenteral thiamine
   C. Exclusion of other causes of delirium
   D. Anterior cruciate ligament surgery
   E. Intensive nursing care

4. A 27-year-old man comes to your out-patient clinic and tells you that he has been injecting heroin on a daily basis for several months and wants you to restart his methadone to help him stop. Which ONE of the following should be done in the first instance?
   A. Prescribe his previous dose of methadone
   B. Give him some dihydrocodeine to use first
   C. Obtain a urine sample for drug testing
   D. Refer him to the drug counselling service
   E. Give him advice on harm minimization

5. A 35-year-old lady asks you about 'safe' limits for drinking alcohol. You know the answer is 14 units per week; however, she asks you to explain this in terms of how many drinks she can safely take. Which ONE of the following would you tell her?
   A. Six pints (568 mL) of continental lager (5.3% ABV) per week
   B. A 'half bottle' (350 mL) of premium gin (40% ABV) per week
   C. Two bottles (2 × 750 mL) of red wine (12.5% ABV) per week
   D. A large (3 L) bottle of strong white cider (8.4%) per week
   E. Six bottles (6 × 330 mL) of 'alco-pops' (4.9% ABV) per week

6. A 24-year-old accountant confides in you that he has tried cocaine on a work night out. He wants to know more about the effects of cocaine. Which ONE of the following is NOT a common effect of cocaine intoxication?
   A. Euphoria
   B. Tachycardia
   C. Hyperthermia
   D. Haptic hallucinations
   E. Hypotension

Chapter 16 The patient with personality problems

1. A 20-year-old woman has a diagnosis of borderline personality disorder. According to DSM-IV, which of the following is a diagnostic criterion?
   A. Chronic feelings of emptiness
   B. Callous unconcern for the feelings of others
   C. Perfectionism that interferes with task completion
   D. Seeking others to make most of one's important life decisions
   E. Takes pleasure in few, if any, activities

2. A 45-year-old male, single and living alone, seems indifferent to praise or criticism, appears aloof, and prefers his own company. He is not depressed, and there has been little change in his situation since he left school. Which ONE of the following personality disorders is most likely?
   A. Narcissistic personality disorder
   B. Antisocial personality disorder
   C. Avoidant personality disorder
   D. Schizoid personality disorder
   E. Paranoid personality disorder

3. A 25-year-old male prisoner hospitalized a fellow inmate by throwing him down the stairs. He states that he feels no guilt, as the man 'was asking for it' after looking at him strangely. Which ONE of the following personality disorders is most likely?
   A. Borderline personality disorder
   B. Schizoid personality disorder
   C. Antisocial personality disorder
   D. Paranoid personality disorder
   E. Anankastic personality disorder

4. You consider diagnosing a 26-year-old hairdresser with histrionic personality disorder. Which ONE of the following is most accurate regarding personality disorder?
   A. Maladaptive personality traits occur only at times of stress
   B. Interpersonal relationships are not generally affected
   C. Onset of difficulties generally occurs in adolescence or early adulthood
   D. Development of psychiatric illness invalidates the diagnosis
   E. Emotional distress is not genuine

5. A 19-year-old man has lacerated the name of his ex-partner on his chest. He reported feeling incredibly depressed since she separated from him yesterday, and kicked him out of the house. He is crying and tells you that he wants to die. He is intoxicated with alcohol. Which ONE of the following is the most likely diagnosis?
   A. Acute severe depression
   B. Emotionally unstable personality disorder – borderline type
   C. Adjustment reaction
   D. No mental illness or personality disorder
   E. Unable to say

6. A 54-year-old history teacher is brought to you by his wife for assessment of lifelong obsession with orderliness and perfection. He apparently spends most of his spare time rewriting school reports to ensure he is happy with his grammar. He does not feel there is a problem. Which of the following is FALSE regarding obsessive-compulsive personality disorder?
   A. Sigmund Freud previously described it as 'anal retentive character'
   B. Rigidity of attitude often places great strain on interpersonal relationships
   C. DSM-IV calls it 'anankastic personality disorder'
   D. Obsessions are ego-dystonic and distressing
   E. It is approximately twice as common in males than females

7. A 22-year-old man has a long history of self-harm, explosive outbursts of anger, impulsive reckless behaviour, feelings of emptiness, and quickly forming intense and volatile 'love–hate' relationships. He reports hearing the voice of his uncle, who sexually abused him as a child, inside his head when he is feeling stressed. He has no axis I mental illness. Which ONE of the following would be the most appropriate diagnosis?
   A. Borderline personality disorder
   B. Schizoid personality disorder
   C. Dependent personality disorder
   D. Paranoid personality disorder
   E. Antisocial personality disorder

Chapter 17 The patient with eating or weight problems

1. A 22-year-old female medical student is brought to your clinic by her mother, who discovered she was making herself vomit after meals. Which ONE of the following is suggestive of a diagnosis of anorexia nervosa rather than bulimia nervosa?
   A. Body weight at least 15% below expected for height
   B. A dread of fatness and a distorted image of being too fat
   C. Use of herbal dieting medications
   D. A tendency to exercise excessively
   E. A preoccupation with being thin

2. The weight of a 13-year-old boy is significantly lower than expected, and as a result he has not started puberty. He reports that he eats well, and denies any concerns regarding body image. Which ONE of the following should you do next?
   A. Refer for senior psychiatric assessment
   B. Make a diagnosis of anorexia nervosa
   C. Consider physical causes for weight loss
   D. Try to establish rapport to facilitate assessment
   E. Ask him to keep a food diary

3. A 32-year-old barmaid has lost a great deal of weight recently. She describes feeling tired all the time, and having no appetite. Physical examination and investigations reveal no abnormalities. Which ONE of the following psychiatric causes of weight loss should be considered first?
   A. Bulimia nervosa
   B. Acute depressive disorder
   C. Obsessive-compulsive disorder
   D. Anorexia nervosa
   E. Alcohol or substance misuse

4. A 25-year-old female lawyer has a diagnosis of anorexia nervosa (purging type), with a BMI of 14.5 kg/m^2. Which ONE of the following investigation results would you NOT expect to see?
   A. Hypoglycaemia
   B. Normocytic normochromic anaemia
   C. Hypocholesterolaemia
   D. Hypophosphataemia
   E. Hypokalaemia

5. A 19-year-old female accountant describes a dread of fatness, and feels that she is overweight despite having a BMI of 13.6 kg/m^2. She describes a 1-year history of severely restricting her dietary intake. She reports amenorrhoea (secondary) and has 'lanugo' hair. Which of the following is the most likely diagnosis?
   A. Major depressive disorder
   B. Bulimia nervosa
   C. Paranoid schizophrenia
   D. Anorexia nervosa
   E. Obsessive-compulsive disorder

Chapter 18 The mood (affective) disorders

1. Which of the following patients with depression would not be considered for ECT?
   A. A 47-year-old woman who is not eating or drinking
   B. A 52-year-old man who believes he is already dead, so there is no point taking medication
   C. A 36-year-old woman who has experienced no benefit from two antidepressants
   D. A 55-year-old man who has benefited from ECT in the past
   E. A 29-year-old woman who has experienced no benefit from several antidepressants but does not want ECT

2. A 24-year-old man is brought to A&E by the police. He has a 1-week history of irritable mood, insomnia and grandiose delusions that he has super powers. The police found him about to jump off some scaffolding to prove he is invincible. He does not believe he is unwell and says there is no way he is coming into hospital. What is the best management option?
   A. Appointment with GP later that day
   B. Informal admission
   C. Admission under mental health legislation
   D. Urgent out-patient psychiatric review
   E. Police custody after arrest for breach of the peace

3. A 45-year-old man is admitted to hospital with a 6-week history of low mood. He plans to kill himself at the first opportunity because he believes the world is going to end soon and wants to die quickly. He is not currently on any medication. What would be the best management option?
   A. Citalopram
   B. Amitriptyline
   C. Quetiapine
   D. Citalopram and quetiapine
   E. Amitriptyline and quetiapine

4. A 37-year-old married bank clerk whose mother, sister and grandfather have depression is recovering from her third depressive episode. She asks why she keeps getting depressed?
   A. She probably has genes that make her vulnerable
   B. She suffers chronic pain
   C. She is socially isolated
   D. She is unemployed
   E. She has young children to care for

5. A 29-year-old postgraduate student with a diagnosis of bipolar affective disorder is admitted with a manic episode after stopping medication. She is very agitated on the ward, pacing, being verbally aggressive to staff and fellow patients, and punching her wardrobe. What is the best medication to commence?
   A. Lithium
   B. Olanzapine

C. Citalopram
D. Valproate
E. Lamotrigine

6. A 36-year-old lecturer with moderate to severe depression wants to try a psychological therapy for depression. Which of the following should be offered?
   A. Self-help CBT
   B. Structured group physical activity
   C. Individual CBT
   D. Dialectical behaviour therapy
   E. Graded exposure therapy

Chapter 19 The psychotic disorders: schizophrenia

1. A pregnant woman with schizophrenia asks how likely her child is to develop schizophrenia? Her partner does not have a mental illness.
   A. 1%
   B. 12.5%
   C. 25%
   D. 37.5%
   E. 50%

2. A pregnant woman with schizophrenia asks how likely her child is to develop schizophrenia? Her partner also has schizophrenia.
   A. 1%
   B. 12.5%
   C. 25%
   D. 37.5%
   E. 50%

3. A 22-year-old man was started on olanzapine 4 months ago for a first episode of schizophrenia. He is now symptom free, but troubled by weight gain. He asks how long in total he needs to stay on the antipsychotic?
   A. 6 months
   B. 9 months
   C. 1–2 years
   D. 3–5 years
   E. Lifelong

4. A 27-year-old woman has developed schizophrenia. She is interested in talking therapies. What type of psychological therapy does NICE (2009) recommend is offered to all patients with schizophrenia?
   A. Psychodynamic psychotherapy
   B. Interpersonal therapy
   C. Dynamic behavioural therapy
   D. Cognitive-behavioural therapy
   E. Cognitive analytic therapy

5. A 35-year-old woman experiencing a manic episode with psychotic features had been attempting to make the voices go away by repeatedly banging her head against her sink. De-escalation techniques had not worked and she had refused oral medication, so in view of the

significant risk to herself she received intramuscular rapid tranquillization. She has no past medical history. What monitoring does she now require?
   A. No monitoring is required
   B. Temperature, pulse, blood pressure and respiratory rate every hour
   C. Temperature, pulse, blood pressure and respiratory rate every half hour
   D. Temperature, pulse, blood pressure and respiratory rate every 5–10 minutes
   E. Continuous monitoring of pulse, blood pressure and respiratory rate with regular temperatures

6. A 35-year-old woman has received intramuscular rapid tranquillization. Which of the following is she NOT now at increased risk of?
   A. Respiratory depression
   B. Inability to protect her own airway
   C. Hypoglycaemia
   D. Acute arrhythmia
   E. Life-threatening hypotension

Chapter 20 The anxiety and somatoform disorders

1. A 25-year-old male plumber presents with anxiety. Which of the following anxiety disorders are as common in men as women?
   A. Generalized anxiety disorder
   B. Panic disorder
   C. Specific phobia
   D. Social phobia
   E. Post-traumatic stress disorder

2. A 25-year-old male plumber presents with anxiety. Which of the following anxiety disorders is LEAST likely to persist into his 30s?
   A. Generalized anxiety disorder
   B. Panic disorder
   C. Obsessive compulsive disorder
   D. Social phobia
   E. Post-traumatic stress disorder

3. A 25-year-old male plumber presents with anxiety. He is unable to go to work because of his symptoms, and would rather try medication than a talking therapy. For which of the following anxiety disorders is an SSRI NOT first line?
   A. Generalized anxiety disorder
   B. Panic disorder
   C. Obsessive-compulsive disorder
   D. Social phobia
   E. Specific phobia

4. A 35-year-old woman has been recently diagnosed with somatization disorder. How should this diagnosis change her management by her GP?
   A. She should not be allowed access to urgent appointment slots

B. She should be seen on a planned, regular schedule
C. She should not be investigated for physical complaints
D. She should never be prescribed benzodiazepines
E. She should be confronted with the fact that her symptoms are only in her mind

5. A 17-year-old school pupil has a phobia of bodily fluids but aspires to be a nurse. What treatment can she be offered?
   A. None – she should change her career plans
   B. CBT with desensitization
   C. CBT focused on trauma
   D. PRN diazepam – to be taken before any possible contact with bodily fluids
   E. SSRI

6. A 29-year-old chemist has OCD regarding orderliness. She has been tidying up her colleagues' lab benches and spoilt some experiments. She has been threatened with dismissal. She does not want to try any talking therapies. What treatment can she be offered?
   A. Clomipramine
   B. Mirtazapine
   C. SSRI
   D. Pregabalin
   E. Self-help

Chapter 21 Alcohol and substance-related disorders

1. A 29-year-old man with alcohol dependence syndrome. He tells you that he wants to give up drinking, but is worried that he will lose all his friends from the pub. At which stage of the Prochaska and DiClemente Transtheoretical Model of Change would you consider him to be?
   A. Pre-contemplation of change
   B. Contemplation of change
   C. Preparation for change
   D. Action for change
   E. Maintenance of change

2. A 21-year-old homeless woman tells you that she uses £20 of heroin per day via intravenous injection. She is keen to be prescribed methadone. Which ONE of the following measures would be essential prior to titration to an adequate dose?
   A. History from a friend to corroborate her usage
   B. Viral serology for HIV and hepatitis C
   C. Thorough physical examination with focus on injection sites
   D. Admission to psychiatric hospital
   E. Urine drug test to confirm presence of opiates

3. A teenager is telling his GP some things that his friends have told him about the legal status of drugs. Which of the following is true regarding the Misuse of Drugs Act 1971?

A. As of 2012, cannabis is considered to be a Class C drug
B. Knowingly allowing the use of drugs in your home is not an offence
C. Legislation is different in Scotland, and the Act does not apply
D. Giving prescribed Ritalin to friends can attract a 14-year prison sentence
E. Possession of heroin is illegal, even if prescribed by a doctor

4. A 45-year-old man is being treated by the alcohol problems team. He has successfully been 'detoxified' using chlordiazepoxide. Which ONE of the following is true regarding his future pharmacological treatment?
   A. Trazodone can be prescribed to treat his alcohol dependence
   B. Long-term, low-dose chlordiazepoxide is the treatment of choice
   C. Naltrexone can be helpful even if he relapses back to drinking
   D. Acamprosate causes an unpleasant reaction when taken with alcohol
   E. Disulfiram should control his cravings for alcohol

5. An 18-year-old man tells you that he is injecting heroin. He does not want to stop. However, he is concerned about HIV, and requests information on the local 'needle exchange'. Which ONE of the following strategies best describes a 'needle exchange' service?
   A. Harm-reduction
   B. Substitution therapy
   C. Therapeutic community
   D. Motivational therapy
   E. Safe injection centre

6. A 26-year-old woman asks you for help with her heroin dependence. She does not want to receive methadone, as she feels this is more addictive than heroin. Which ONE of the following drugs could be used for 'substitution therapy'?
   A. Lofexidine
   B. Diazepam
   C. Buprenorphine
   D. Clonidine
   E. Naltrexone

Chapter 22 The personality disorders

1. A 22-year-old lady reports that she feels depressed and suicidal. She has a diagnosis of borderline personality disorder. In comparison to unipolar depressive disorders, which ONE of the following is TRUE of patients with a diagnosis of borderline personality disorder?
   A. Lower lifetime risk of suicide
   B. Easier to engage with psychotherapy
   C. More responsive to antidepressant treatment
   D. Costlier and longer treatment
   E. Less likely to misuse substances

2. A charming and pleasant 41-year-old man has an established diagnosis of antisocial personality disorder. Which ONE of the following factors would predict a negative response to therapy?
   A. Recent self-harm
   B. Quasi-psychotic symptoms
   C. Diagnosis of depression
   D. History of violence to others
   E. Presence of anxiety

3. A 19-year-old hairdresser has a diagnosis of borderline personality disorder, and requests information on drug treatment that may be beneficial. According to the 2010 Cochrane systematic review, which ONE of the following is TRUE regarding pharmacotherapy for borderline personality disorder?
   A. Semisodium valproate is ineffective for reducing interpersonal problems
   B. Omega-3 fatty acids are effective in reducing impulsivity
   C. Aripiprazole is ineffective for reducing anger
   D. Amitriptyline is more effective than haloperidol in treating low mood
   E. Flupentixol decanoate is effective in reducing suicidal behaviour

4. A 34-year-old man has a diagnosis of borderline personality disorder, and requests information on different types of psychotherapy that may be beneficial. Which ONE of the following is FALSE regarding psychotherapy for borderline personality disorder?
   A. Dialectical behavioural therapy involves group therapy
   B. Mentalization-based therapy increases awareness of mental state
   C. Psychodynamic therapists set an agenda at the start of sessions
   D. Cognitive-analytical therapy usually lasts between 16 and 24 sessions
   E. Therapeutic communities involve 'residential' group therapy

5. A 27-year-old female postgraduate student has a diagnosis of borderline personality disorder. She reported low mood and insomnia for the past month, and has subsequently been absent from university (which is unusual for her). Normally, she is easily angered, but relatively cheerful. Which ONE of the following is TRUE regarding the management of comorbid depression in patients with borderline personality disorder?
   A. Psychological therapies are not helpful during periods of acute illness
   B. Patients should be encouraged to adhere to their current care plan
   C. Diazepam or lorazepam should be prescribed
   D. Admission to an acute psychiatric ward is preferable
   E. Consideration should be given to 'weekly dispensing' of medication

6. A 29-year-old man has a diagnosis of antisocial personality disorder. He coldly tells his psychiatrist of his intention to kill his landlord following an argument about rent arrears, before describing a detailed plan on how he would stab him in the throat. Which ONE of the following is TRUE?
   A. He would not be held criminally responsible for his actions
   B. Confidentiality should be maintained at all times
   C. The police and the intended victim should be immediately warned
   D. The man should be detained and transferred to a psychiatric hospital
   E. Specific details of the threat should not be recorded for medicolegal reasons

Chapter 23 Eating disorders

1. An 18-year-old student has a diagnosis of anorexia nervosa, restrictive type. She asks for information about how common eating disorders are. Which ONE of the following statements is most accurate?
   A. Anorexia nervosa is about five times more common in females than males
   B. About 4% of the general population have a diagnosis of bulimia nervosa
   C. Anorexia nervosa is more prevalent in higher socioeconomic classes
   D. About 5% of the female population have eating habits that cause concern
   E. Eating disorders are less common in professional gymnasts

2. A 25-year-old male nurse reported a 7-year history of bingeing and purging, associated with a distorted body image and a fear of fatness. He is of normal weight. He is diagnosed with bulimia nervosa. Which ONE of the following is most accurate regarding the aetiology of bulimia nervosa?
   A. The role of genetics is thought to be insignificant
   B. A long history of dieting behaviour is common
   C. Family 'enmeshment' is more common than in anorexia nervosa
   D. Substance misuse is a rare comorbidity in bulimia nervosa
   E. History of sexual abuse is more common than in other mental illnesses

3. A 20-year-old law student has a diagnosis of anorexia nervosa, and is undergoing psychotherapy for this. Her therapist is curious to explore various traits of her personality. Which ONE of the following personality traits is NOT commonly seen in individuals with anorexia nervosa?
   A. Novelty-seeking
   B. Perfectionism
   C. Harm-avoidance
   D. Inhibition
   E. Obsessionality

4. A 17-year-old boy has a BMI of 16, wears baggy clothes, and states that he is worried about being overweight. He is diagnosed with anorexia nervosa, although he does not feel that he has a problem. However, he is agreeable to meeting a therapist, mainly to please his mother. Which ONE of the following modalities of psychotherapy would be useful in the first instance?
   A. Cognitive-analytical therapy
   B. Systemic family therapy
   C. Psychodynamic psychotherapy
   D. Cognitive-behavioural therapy
   E. Motivational interviewing

5. A 29-year-old female actuary is diagnosed with anorexia nervosa. Which ONE of the following factors is associated with a poor prognosis?
   A. Early age of onset
   B. Rapid weight loss
   C. Binge–purge symptoms
   D. Family history of anorexia
   E. Slow to engage with psychotherapy

Chapter 24 Disorders relating to the menstrual cycle, pregnancy and the puerperium

1. A 27-year-old schoolteacher reports increased irritability in the week prior to menstruation. This quickly resolves within a day of starting her period. Which ONE of the following symptoms is NOT suggestive of a diagnosis of premenstrual syndrome?
   A. Low mood
   B. Tearfulness
   C. Elevated mood
   D. Tiredness
   E. Insomnia

2. A 53-year-old housewife reports low mood, increased fatigability and early morning wakening for the past 2 months, accompanied by increased suicidal thoughts. She attributes this to her menopause. With regards to the case, which ONE of the following statements is TRUE?
   A. HRT should be prescribed in the first instance
   B. Dietary and lifestyle advice is unlikely to be helpful
   C. There is good evidence to suggest the use of omega-3 fish oils
   D. HRT can be used as an alternative to antidepressants for major depression
   E. Psychological therapies and social support may be helpful

3. A 25-year-old artist has a history of bipolar affective disorder. She has been taking lithium and has been well for the past 3 years. She wants to start a family with her partner, and has heard that lithium can cause problems with fetal malformations. Which ONE of the following is most appropriate?
   A. Her medication should be switched to semisodium valproate
   B. Discussing risk vs benefit can facilitate the woman's informed choice
   C. Lithium is teratogenic and should be discontinued
   D. It should be the doctor's decision whether or not the lithium is continued
   E. If continued, it is unlikely that the dose of lithium will need changed

4. A 33-year-old woman previously experienced a protracted episode of postnatal depression following the birth of her first child, which necessitated admission to a mother and baby unit. The episode responded well to antidepressant medication. She has recently become pregnant and is incredibly anxious that she will become unwell again postnatally. Which ONE of the following would be an appropriate first line management strategy?
   A. Reassurance that becoming unwell would be unlikely
   B. Restart antidepressant treatment immediately
   C. Referral to psychologist to identify relapse signature
   D. Watchful waiting
   E. Referral to perinatal mental health team

5. A 22-year-old lady is found by the police. She was knee-deep in a river with her 2-week-old baby boy. She reported that the infant was possessed by the devil, and that she needed to drown him to save humanity. At interview, she appears perplexed and is openly responding to auditory hallucinations. Which ONE of the following is NOT considered to be a risk factor for the development of puerperal psychosis?
   A. Primiparous mother
   B. Family history of bipolar affective disorder
   C. Having a caesarean section
   D. Unsupportive interpersonal relationship
   E. Pre-eclampsia

Chapter 25 Dementia and delirium

1. A 91-year-old nursing home resident with severe Alzheimer's dementia frequently shouts unintelligible words. Physical examination and investigations are normal, and she does not seem low in mood. Staff can detect no pattern or triggers to her shouting. She appears mildly distressed by it. What option should be tried first to reduce her shouting?
   A. Aromatherapy
   B. Antipsychotic
   C. Antidepressant
   D. Cholinesterase inhibitor
   E. Referral to speech and language therapy

2. A 74-year-old woman has type 2 diabetes, is obese and has hypercholesterolaemia. She attends her GP with memory loss. What type of dementia is she at increased risk of?
   A. Vascular dementia
   B. Alzheimer's dementia
   C. Vascular and Alzheimer's dementia
   D. Lewy body dementia
   E. Frontotemporal dementia

3. A 75-year-old man has Lewy body dementia. His carers are worried that he is not eating well.
   He tells his GP that he is certain his carers are trying to poison him. What management strategy should be avoided?
   A. Antipsychotics
   B. Nutritional supplements
   C. Cholinesterase inhibitors
   D. Antibiotics
   E. Antidepressants

4. A 77-year-old man was admitted 3 days ago with abdominal pain of uncertain aetiology. Initially he was cognitively normal but nurses are concerned that he is now acutely disorientated and agitated. Which medication is most likely to explain his presentation?
   A. Paracetamol
   B. Metoclopramide
   C. Co-codamol
   D. Omeprazole
   E. Cyclizine

5. A GP is asked to visit a 71-year-old woman in her home. She is disorientated in time, does not recognize the GP (whom she has known for years) and is very drowsy. She is plucking at her bed clothes and refuses to let the GP examine her because she thinks he wants to hurt her. Her husband states she was fine until 2 days ago, but now he cannot cope with her. Where should the GP manage this lady with acute onset psychotic symptoms?
   A. Her own home
   B. Day hospital
   C. Emergency respite via social work
   D. Acute medical ward
   E. Acute psychiatric ward

Chapter 26 Older adult psychiatry

1. A 74-year-old woman gives a 6-month history of low mood, anhedonia and fatigue associated with difficulty concentrating and remembering. Neighbours have noticed she is forgetting to put her bins out and no longer cooks meals for herself. ACE-R is 72/100. What is the best management option?
   A. Antidepressant
   B. Cholinesterase inhibitor
   C. Memantine
   D. Refer for aromatherapy and massage
   E. Refer for counselling

2. A 72-year-old widow has presented to her GP 20 times in the last month with minor physical concerns. Previously she attended infrequently. During consultations she is restless, wrings her hands and seems to struggle to remember advice given to her. Her friends are struggling to cope as she telephones them throughout the night to check they are alright. MMSE is 28/30. What is the most likely diagnosis?
   A. Mild cognitive impairment
   B. Generalized anxiety disorder
   C. Depressive episode
   D. Late onset schizophrenia
   E. Hypochondriacal disorder

3. A 71-year-old widower has a 3-month history of low mood, fatigue and anhedonia associated with anorexia. He was admitted 4 weeks ago after an episode of acute kidney injury precipitated by poor oral intake. He has been commenced on an antidepressant but is poorly concordant and his presentation has changed little. His kidney function has not returned to baseline as he continues to drink little fluid. What is the best management option?
   A. ECT
   B. Continue current oral antidepressant
   C. Commence depot medication with antidepressant properties
   D. Change to an alternative oral antidepressant
   E. Change to lithium

4. A psychiatrist is asked to visit a patient at home who has been 'behaving oddly'. Unfortunately their medical records cannot be located in advance of the visit, so their past psychiatric history is unknown. Which of the patients below is most likely to have late onset schizophrenia?
   A. A diabetic man who reports that the police are stealing his thoughts
   B. A deaf woman who lives alone and reports that the police are trying to rob her
   C. An obese woman who lives alone and is thought disordered
   D. A blind woman who lives alone and reports seeing policemen in her living room every night
   E. A man with ischaemic heart disease who can hear talking on the police radio in all the rooms in his house

5. A 76-year-old woman who started mirtazapine for a depressive episode 4 weeks ago attends her GP. Her daughter also has depression and noticed improvement after 2 weeks of an antidepressant. She has not noticed any benefit or side-effects from mirtazapine, and is wondering if she should change treatment. What would be the best management option?
   A. Change to the antidepressant that worked for her daughter
   B. Augment mirtazapine with the antidepressant that worked for her daughter
   C. Change to a tricyclic antidepressant
   D. Continue mirtazapine for at least 8 weeks
   E. Discontinue mirtazapine and observe without antidepressant

6. A 77-year-old lady with a history of bipolar affective disorder no longer requiring medication is brought to A&E by her family. In the past 24 hours she has started behaving very oddly – getting dressed in the middle of the night, dropping to the ground and shaking her leg about, and shouting irritably at people when she is asked questions about her orientation. AMT is 2/10. What is the most likely diagnosis?
   A. Lithium toxicity
   B. Manic episode
   C. Hypomanic episode
   D. Somatization disorder
   E. Delirium

7. A GP pays a home visit to a 74-year-old man with a long history of schizophrenia. The man mentions he is more bothered by auditory hallucinations than normal. The GP notices there are little piles of olanzapine tablets on saucers in the kitchen and living room. The man admits he is struggling to keep track of whether he has taken his medication or not. What would be the best way to improve concordance?
   A. Start a depot antipsychotic
   B. Dispense medication weekly in a labelled dosette box
   C. Refer for a support worker to prompt medication
   D. Arrange daily dispensing at the local pharmacy
   E. Change the time of olanzapine so he can take it in the morning with his other medication

8. An 82-year-old widow with no past psychiatric history presents to her GP requesting a repeat prescription of temazepam. Her supply should not have run out yet, and she admits she took six extra tablets at the weekend in the hope of 'going to sleep and not waking up'. In the event she just overslept, and no harm was done. She feels foolish now and would just like to go home and stop wasting the GP's time. What is the best management option?
   A. Review by GP in a month
   B. Review by GP in a week
   C. Refer to the local lunch club
   D. Refer to psychiatic out-patients
   E. Refer for urgent, same day, psychiatric review

Chapter 27 Child and adolescent psychiatry

1. The mother of a 5-year-old boy reports that he is unable to concentrate on any task for longer than a minute, and has persistently been in trouble at school for shouting out answers and jumping on tables. At interview, he is running around the room and seems transiently interested in various toys, and the contents of his mother's bag. According to DSM-IV, the core symptoms of ADHD must have their onset before which age?
   A. 5 years old
   B. 7 years old
   C. 9 years old

   D. 13 years old
   E. 17 years old

2. The family of a 5-year-old boy raise concerns about his development. He does not like interacting with other children. His mother also notes that he seems to enjoy reading the telephone directory. Which of the following would be most useful in differentiating childhood autism from Asperger's syndrome?
   A. Acquisition of language skills
   B. Adherence to routines
   C. Making eye contact
   D. Stereotyped motor movements
   E. Lack of imaginative play

3. A 3-year-old girl has a diagnosis of a pervasive developmental disorder. Which of the following pervasive developmental disorders occurs more commonly in girls than boys?
   A. Heller's syndrome
   B. Pervasive developmental disorder, not otherwise specified
   C. Childhood autism
   D. Rett's syndrome
   E. Asperger's syndrome

4. For the past 6 months, a 12-year-old boy has repeatedly been in trouble with the police. Recently, he has been violent towards his sister and has killed her pet hamster. His mother sought help after he deliberately set the garden shed on fire. Which ONE of the following statements is TRUE regarding conduct disorder?
   A. There is an equal gender distribution
   B. It is a milder variant of oppositional defiant disorder
   C. Associated with schizoid personality disorder in later life
   D. School refusal is commonly seen
   E. There is often associated substance misuse in later life

5. For the last 4 months, a young girl who had previously achieved bladder control has been troubled by bed-wetting. What is the age criterion used to define enuresis in children?
   A. 2 years or older
   B. 3 years or older
   C. 5 years or older
   D. 7 years or older
   E. 8 years or older

6. A 10-year-old boy has a diagnosis of Gilles de la Tourette syndrome, characterized by copralalic and coprapraxic tics. Which of the following neurotransmitter systems is thought to be implicated in the aetiology of Tourette's syndrome?
   A. GABA
   B. Dopamine
   C. Glutamate
   D. Acetylcholine
   E. Serotonin

7. An 8-year-old girl presents with encopresis. During examination by the junior doctor, genital warts and vaginal trauma are noted. Which ONE of the following steps should immediately follow?
   A. The child should be sent home and seen in out-patients
   B. The parents should be confronted by the nurses
   C. The child should be directly asked what happened
   D. Police should be contacted to question the girl
   E. The duty social worker and on-call paediatrician should be alerted

Chapter 28 Intellectual disability

1. A 12-year-old boy has a profound intellectual disability. Which ONE of the following is TRUE regarding individuals with profound intellectual disabilities?
   A. They account for 10% of all people with intellectual disabilities
   B. The aetiology of their difficulties is usually unknown
   C. They will need nursing care in adulthood
   D. They are unable to benefit from behavioural therapies
   E. They cannot be diagnosed with depression

2. A 44-year-old lady with Down's syndrome is admitted to a psychiatric ward for a period of assessment. Which ONE of the following is the most commonly diagnosed psychiatric disorder in patients with Down's syndrome?
   A. Schizophrenia
   B. Alzheimer's dementia
   C. Bipolar affective disorder
   D. Borderline personality disorder
   E. Social anxiety disorder

3. A 5-year-old boy presented with symptoms similar to autism. His maternal uncle and his father had very similar symptoms. Which ONE of the following is the most likely diagnosis?
   A. Prader–Willi syndrome
   B. Velo-cardio-facial syndrome
   C. Down's syndrome
   D. Fragile X syndrome
   E. Rett's syndrome

4. A 32-year-old man has a moderate intellectual disability. Which ONE of the following is most accurate regarding individuals with moderate intellectual disabilities?
   A. They cannot sustain employment
   B. They can generally live independently
   C. They have limited language and comprehension skills
   D. They tend to require full-time nursing care
   E. They have intact self-care skills

5. A 22-year-old lady with a severe intellectual disability presents with marked behavioural disturbance, including head-banging and aggression towards carers. Which ONE of the following is TRUE regarding behavioural disturbances in people with intellectual disabilities?
   A. Behavioural disturbances are usually related to psychiatric illness
   B. Aetiology of the intellectual disability does not affect management
   C. Psychotropic medication should be prescribed in the first instance
   D. Simple psychosocial interventions usually have long-term benefits
   E. Admission to a specialist unit is almost always required

Chapter 29 Forensic psychiatry

1. A 19-year-old gentleman has been charged with a serious assault. He appears incredibly distracted and distressed, and is openly responding to auditory hallucinations. The forensic psychiatrist does not feel that he is fit to plead. Which ONE of the following is TRUE regarding the concept of being 'unfit to plead'?
   A. Commonly found in those with mental illness
   B. Is determined by the M'Naghten Rule
   C. May result in transfer to a secure hospital
   D. Is applicable if the accused cannot remember the offence
   E. Is also known as 'not guilty by reason of insanity'

2. A 32-year-old woman with a psychotic illness is arrested and charged with stalking her psychiatrist. Which ONE of the following types of delusion is most commonly seen among stalkers with psychotic disorders?
   A. Delusions of love
   B. Delusions of infidelity
   C. Delusions of reference
   D. Delusions of control
   E. Delusions of persecution

3. A 28-year-old man is charged with indecently exposing himself to a group of female university students. Which ONE of the following is most accurate regarding indecent exposure?
   A. It usually immediately precedes violent sexual assault
   B. It is a crime more commonly committed by men over 55 years old
   C. There is a high rate of re-offending in those who are convicted
   D. It is not associated with intellectual disability
   E. Exhibitionism is considered by ICD-10 to be a psychiatric disorder

4. A 24-year-old gentleman with a history of paranoid schizophrenia has been charged with attempted murder after stabbing a female lawyer in an upmarket bar. He reports that he had heard the voice of God commenting that she was the Devil, and that the Pope had been in control of his bodily movements and mood at the time of the offence. Which ONE of the following is TRUE?

A. People with psychotic disorders are twice as likely as members of the general public to acquire convictions for violent offences

B. Comorbid substance misuse is not thought to increase risk of violent offending in patients with schizophrenia

C. Command hallucinations are a specific risk factor for violence in patients with paranoid schizophrenia

D. Patients with paranoid schizophrenia are more likely to evade detection by the authorities than offenders without mental illness

E. There is a strong association between the presence of psychotic symptoms and homicide following sadistic sexual offences

5. A 36-year-old man with schizophrenia has committed a crime. He asks his lawyer if he can be considered to have had diminished responsibility. What is the only charge diminished responsibility applies to?

A. Arson

B. Rape

C. Theft

D. Grievous bodily harm

E. Murder

6. A 32-year-old man with substance misuse problems reports he is thinking of taking up mugging to fund his habit. Which ONE of the following is the best predictor of future violence?

A. Having a mental disorder

B. Using substances

C. Previous violence

D. Experiencing command hallucinations

E. Childhood abuse

Extended-matching questions (EMQs)

1. Management of antipsychotic-induced extrapryamidal side-effects

A. Intramuscular procyclidine

B. Oral procyclidine

C. Propranolol

D. Stop anticholinergics

E. Oral olanzapine

F. Intramuscular haloperidol

G. Rescuscitation

H. Baclofen

I. Dantrolene

J. Quinine

For each of the following patients, select the ONE best management option from the list above.

1. A 22-year-old woman recently commenced on an antipsychotic who is pacing her bedroom and says she feels very restless.
2. A 22-year-old woman recently commenced on an antipsychotic who is staring at the ceiling and has her jaw clenched tight.
3. A 22-year-old woman recently commenced on an antipsychotic who is collapsed in her bedroom with a fast pulse, low blood pressure, reduced consciousness level and stiff limbs.
4. A 26-year-old man who commenced antipsychotics a month ago. His face shows little expression and he does not swing his arms when he walks. He does not have a tremor and his gait is not shuffling.
5. A 34-year-old man who has been on antipsychotics and regular procyclidine for over a decade. He makes frequent darting movements with his tongue but seems unaware of this.

2. Psychodynamic psychotherapy

A. Acting out

B. Projective identification

C. Hypnosis

D. Catharsis

E. Parapraxis

F. Transference

G. Rationalization

H. Countertransference

I. Dream interpretation

J. Working through

For each of the following, select the ONE most appropriate descriptor from the list above.

1. A 32-year-old woman, who has previously been very punctual, has arrived late and slightly inebriated for the past six sessions since the therapist was on leave.
2. The therapist of a 59-year-old man realizes that he has been talking to him as if he were a father figure.
3. A 43-year-old man feels better after his first psychotherapy session, because he has 'got it off his chest'.
4. A 21-year-old says 'I'm glad we're almost finished'. She intended to say 'I'm sad we're almost finished'.
5. A 29-year-old man has been avoiding his psychotherapist for the past few weeks following what he considered to be a 'clash of personalities'. He decided to return and is keen to uncover his unconscious reasons behind this.

3. Modalities of individual psychotherapy

A. Psychoanalysis

B. Cognitive-behavioural therapy

C. Mentalization-based therapy

D. Psychodynamic psychotherapy

E. Dialectical behavioural therapy

F. Exposure and response prevention

G. Eye movement desensitization and reprocessing

H. Cognitive analytic therapy

I. Systematic desensitization

J. Mindfulness-based cognitive therapy

K. Interpersonal therapy

For the examples below, select the ONE most appropriate modality of psychotherapy from the list above.

1. A 28-year-old man has a diagnosis of borderline personality disorder. He reports that he often finds it difficult to know what others are thinking about him, and tends to expect the worst and act accordingly. He sometimes has difficulty knowing what he is thinking and feeling.
2. A 57-year-old lady has a depressive disorder of moderate severity. She attributes her symptoms to the fact that her father has recently been taken into a nursing home, that her daughter has recently left home to attend university, and that she was recently made redundant from her job in the bank.

3. A 35-year-old woman has a diagnosis of agoraphobia. She wants to start a practical sort of therapy in which she does not need to talk about her difficult past.

4. A 24-year-old ex-soldier has a diagnosis of post-traumatic stress disorder. He requests a talking therapy. In the past, he tried treatment with a therapist who 'wiggled his finger in front of my face' and found this unhelpful.

5. A 42-year-old gentleman has a diagnosis of obsessive-compulsive disorder, and is mainly troubled by having to check switches and locks in his home. He feels that a therapy that is 'more practical than talking' would be helpful.

4. Mental disorder and self-harm

A. Obsessive-compulsive disorder

B. Anorexia nervosa

C. Alcohol-dependence syndrome

D. Lesch–Nyhan syndrome

E. Mania with psychosis

F. Borderline personality disorder

G. Recurrent depressive disorder of moderate severity

H. Paranoid schizophrenia

I. Generalized anxiety disorder

J. Severe depression with psychotic features

K. Dissocial personality disorder

For each of the following patients, select the ONE most likely mental disorder from the list above.

1. A 19-year-old woman states that she is going to kill herself because 'the voices in my head are telling me to'. These started troubling her this morning after an argument with her mother. Yesterday, she felt fine with no voices. She has no symptoms of depression. She insists that 'it will be all your fault when I commit suicide' and demands admission to a psychiatric ward. She has a history of self-harm by cutting, and is well known to mental health services from previous emergency presentations.

2. A 50-year-old male bank manager is found in a remote forest clearing at 4.30 a.m. by a dog-walker, having tried to gas himself in his car. Typed letters to his wife and children (currently on holiday) were found on the passenger seat. He has no psychiatric history. He appeared intoxicated; however, he states he is not a big drinker. He described recent weight loss and wakening early in the morning. He is entirely convinced that the recent financial crisis is all his fault.

3. A 22-year-old man presents with his mother. She is concerned that he has burned his chest with cigarettes multiple times, and appears to have created the image of a crucifix. He insists that he is the second coming of Jesus Christ, and has special powers of healing that

command respect. You note that he is dishevelled, topless, talking very fast about loosely related ideas, and is very distractible. There is no history of substance misuse. He has never been to church in his life.

4. A 62-year-old lady reports that she has taken a 'handful' of her antidepressant tablets before telling her husband what she had done. She is unsure whether she wanted to die. She has been in intermittent contact with the community mental health team for much of her adult life with periods of poor motivation and alterations in her sleep pattern; however, she has also had long periods of being well and managing to work in the local supermarket. She states strong feelings of guilt, and reports recent social withdrawal. At interview, you feel that her affect is flat and she is tearful. She does not drink alcohol or use drugs.

5. A 15-year-old girl was found having tried to hang herself in the family bathroom. She left a suicide note, and was discovered by chance by the family cleaner. You notice that she looks thin. His parents report that she has been 'picky' with food over the past few months, but they have not noticed anything else because of their busy jobs as lawyers. On examination, you note that she is wearing very baggy clothes and has fine hairs over visible skin areas. She has actively resisted physical examination. She tells you that nothing is wrong at all, and that she just wants to get home to study for her forthcoming exams.

5. Methods of self-harm and suicide

A. Jumping from a high building

B. Placing head in an unlit gas oven

C. Drop hanging

D. Ingestion of razor blade

E. Suspension hanging

F. Overdose of medicinal drugs

G. Self-laceration of arms

H. Intentional motor vehicle collision

I. Self-inflicted firearm injury

J. Ingestion of methylated spirits

K. Burning with cigarette lighter

For each of the following statements, select the ONE most likely method or act from the list above.

1. The most common presentation of self-harm to hospitals in the UK

2. A method that would have been more likely to be fatal prior to the 1960s

3. The most common method of suicide in adolescent males in the USA

4. A method which, if not fatal, may result in blindness

5. The most common method of suicide in prisons

6. Immediate psychiatric management of the patient who has inflicted harm upon themselves

A. Admission to intensive psychiatric care unit

B. Admission to in-patient psychiatric ward

C. Admission to medical assessment/short stay ward

D. Discharge with immediate outreach team involvement

E. Discharge with community mental health team later in the week

F. Discharge with out-patient psychiatry clinic appointment next month

G. Discharge with appointment with alcohol addictions services

H. Discharge to police custody

I. Discharge with information on non-NHS support services

J. Discharge with prescription for antidepressant medication

K. Discharge to the care of GP

For each of the following statements, select the ONE most appropriate psychiatric management strategy from the list above.

1. A 57-year-old, unemployed, divorced man who lives alone took an overdose of a benzodiazepine. A scribbled suicide note was left, and he called emergency services before falling unconscious. He saw his keyworker from the alcohol addictions team earlier that day who provided the benzodiazepines for a community detoxification. She felt that he was in 'good humour' when she saw him. He has presented numerous times in the past with minor overdoses. At interview, he appears very drowsy and smells strongly of alcohol. He is inconsolably tearful, stating that he is 'ruined' and wants to die.

2. A 20-year-old, unemployed, single woman took an overdose of dihydrocodeine. She was found collapsed in the street, and required naloxone. Her urine drug test is positive for cannabis and cocaine. Upon wakening, she threatens to kill the nurse who has taken her cigarettes. She continues to be physically, verbally and racially aggressive to A&E staff. She has had one short admission to a psychiatric ward 2 years ago, and was discharged after assaulting a member of staff. On discharge, the consultant concluded 'no signs of mental illness'. At interview, she screams at you to supply her with more dihydrocodeine, and threatens to kill herself if you do not comply.

3. A 33-year-old, married taxi driver (male) was found by his wife in the loft, holding a nail-gun to his head. He was slightly intoxicated, and broke down in tears while agreeing to attend hospital. He has no history with psychiatric services, and – despite having taken a drink tonight – does not usually do so. He described feeling like he 'can't be bothered' since he had his pay severely cut about 2 months ago, and has since been burdened by creditors calling him. At interview, he described poor sleep, weight loss, lack of energy, and guilt about his loss of libido. While he described ongoing suicidal feelings, he described his newborn baby daughter and wife as strong protective factors, is regretful that 'things have come to this', and glad that his wife found him before he did 'something stupid'. He seems a bit more optimistic after assessment.

4. A 67-year-old, retired widow with no psychiatric history, took an overdose of four of her blood pressure tablets. She waited until after her daughter went on holiday, and was only discovered when her neighbour visited unexpectedly and saw a suicide note addressed to her daughter on the coffee table, stating that she could not go on without her recently deceased husband. She later told the psychiatrist that she was 'just a silly old lady' and denied any suicidal intent. She just wanted to go home to look at her wedding photographs.

5. A 26-year-old, single, mature student, who lives with flat-mates, presents at A&E requesting sutures for a self-inflicted laceration on her inner thigh. She has previously been involved with mental health services due to self-harming, but disengaged with them 2 years previously because she did not agree with their diagnosis of borderline personality disorder. She is on no medication. She is reluctant to talk to a psychiatrist; however, you manage to engage her and she tells you that she is not suicidal. She reports that her self-harm was previously improving, but has recently become more frequent due to academic pressures. She is keen to go home, and refuses to have any involvement in the future with mental health services.

7. Differential diagnosis of low mood

A. Mild depressive episode

B. Moderate depressive episode

C. Severe depressive episode without psychotic features

D. Severe depressive episode with psychotic features

E. Recurrent depressive episode

F. Dysthymia

G. Bipolar affective disorder

H. Schizoaffective disorder

I. Low mood secondary to a general medical condition

J. Low mood secondary to psychoactive substance use

For each of the following patients, select the ONE most likely diagnosis from the list above.

1. A 40-year-old man feels he has been depressed for 20 years. He cannot recall a lengthy period of normal mood since his early adulthood. Despite this, he is able to work as a supermarket manager, has a loving relationship with his wife and reports that he quite enjoyed his last holiday in Tenerife.

2. A 24-year-old waitress has had low mood and lethargy for 3 weeks. She finds it harder than normal to remember her customer's orders. She thinks this is because she has never been an intelligent person. She is eating normally, sleeping well and enjoyed going out to the movies last night.

3. A 71-year-old widowed woman who lives alone is brought to the surgery by her neighbour. The neighbour is shocked because the patient put a rude note through his door telling him to get his drains unblocked in order to get rid of the stench in the street. No one else has noticed a bad smell. Before her husband died the patient used to be very social and visited her neighbours frequently. On examination, she is unkempt and walks very slowly. When you ask her questions she makes poor eye contact and does not answer for a long time.

4. A 35-year-old cashier presents to his GP asking for a sick line. He feels he cannot continue at work because for the last month he has been low in mood and finds himself becoming easily tired during his shifts. He is not enjoying talking with his colleagues as much as he used to. He finds himself wakening at 5 a.m. (he normally rises at 8 a.m.) and lies in bed worrying about the day ahead. His mood is a bit better in the evenings. He has been eating poorly and lost a stone in weight over the last month.

5. A 42-year-old construction worker reports intermittent low mood. Sometimes he is so low he is unable to go to work. On closer questioning it seems it is mainly Mondays he misses, and the weekends he feels low. The problem has come on over the last year, when he has been binge drinking at the weekends after his wife left him. On weekends when he looks after his daughter he does not drink and feels fine.

8. Low mood secondary to a general medical condition

A. Huntington's disease

B. Parkinson's disease

C. Multiple sclerosis

D. Cerebral tumour

E. Cushing's disease

F. Addison's disease

G. Conn's disease

H. Thrombocytopenia

I. Hypothyroidism

J. Hyperthyroidism

K. Systemic lupus erythematosus

For each of the following patients, select the ONE key diagnosis to exclude from the list above.

1. A 52-year-old care assistant presents to her GP with a 6-month history of low mood and fatigue. She complains she has put on a lot of weight recently despite no changes in her diet or exercise. On examination she is obese, hypertensive and the blood pressure cuff leaves a bruise.

2. A 35-year-old traffic warden presents to his GP after he tripped over the curb and banged his knee. He also mentions a 3-month history of low mood. He is not sure why he tripped, but has been stumbling more often than he used to and has given up football. He does not drink. He thinks he may have a family history of depression because his father went into a psychiatric hospital in his early 40s and died there 10 years later.

3. A 46-year-old florist presents because for the last 2 months she has felt tired all the time and low in mood. She feels ugly, her hair never seems to be glossy any more and she thinks her skin is dry and flaky. On examination, her pulse is 52 regular.

4. A 26-year-old veterinary student presents with tingling in her left arm. She becomes tearful during the consultation, admitting she is finding the fourth year of her studies much more difficult than the previous years. You see she attended 3 months ago with a sore eye and blurred vision which resolved spontaneously.

9. Mental state examination in low mood

A. Poor self-care

B. Malingering

C. Reduced range of reactivity

D. Incongruous affect

E. Low mood

F. Psychomotor retardation

G. Psychomotor agitation

H. Marche à petits pas

I. Negative cognition

J. Hopelessness

K. Complete anhedonia

L. Partial anhedonia

For each of the following patients, select ONE clinical feature described from the list of options above.

1. A 76-year-old widowed retired headmistress is brought to A&E by her family who are concerned she has not been eating. She paces the cubicle, keeps buttoning and unbuttoning her coat and does not sit down when offered a chair.

2. A 44-year-old architect being treated for depression is upset because he has lost a contract after the company went bust. He says this means he will lose all his other contracts and never be asked to design another building.

3. A 22-year-old woman tells her GP she has passed a recent exam, but does not smile or appear pleased. Later

she mentions she has broken up with her partner, but does not look sad or relieved. She describes both things in a similar tone of speech.

4. A 36-year-old sales assistant attends his GP straight from work for a prescription of citalopram. He has greasy hair and stains on his shirt, and is slightly malodorous.

5. A 55-year-old lorry driver tells his GP he has lost interest in everything he used to enjoy. He no longer plays darts or watches football as he does not care who wins now. However, he did enjoy spending time with his grandson at the weekend.

10. Differential diagnosis of elevated or irritable mood

A. Hypomanic episode
B. Manic episode without psychotic features
C. Manic episode with psychotic features
D. Mixed affective episode
E. Bipolar affective disorder
F. Cyclothymia
G. Schizophrenia
H. Schizoaffective disorder
I. Elevated or irritable mood secondary to a general medical condition
J. Elevated or irritable mood secondary to psychoactive substance use
K. Delirium/dementia

For each of the following patients, select the ONE most likely diagnosis from the list above.

1. A 40-year-old lawyer attends his GP asking for a medication to reduce his sex drive because his wife is complaining. He is smartly dressed in a new suit and says he feels 'on top of the world'. He has been finding it hard to stay focused at work but so far no one has commented. Fortunately he is able to stay up late catching up on work without feeling tired the next day. He denies any drug or alcohol use.

2. A 22-year-old trainee electrician is brought to A&E by the police after he was found breaking into an electronics shop. He states he needed the parts for a new jetpack he was designing – he plans to start a new business with it which will 'revolutionize transatlantic flight'. He has resigned from his apprenticeship in order to spend more time on this venture. He is irritable with the male police officer but flirtatious towards the female police officer. He denies drug or alcohol use.

3. A 37-year-old man with a history of bipolar disorder was admitted to a psychiatric ward one day ago. The nurses tell you he has been very elated and disinhibited so far today. When you interview him he seems low and tearful, but as the interview progresses he gets very

irritable and starts to speak too quickly for you to ask him any more questions.

4. A 36-year-old secretary attends her GP because she is feeling unusually irritable at work. Sometimes she loves her job and sometimes she hates it, but forces herself to attend. Right now she is also feeling irritable with her family and neighbour. She has noticed her mood has seemed to cycle since her late teens, but it has never stopped her doing anything.

5. A 28-year-old doctor suffers from recurrent depressive disorder. He has recently started a stressful new job and his flatmates are worried because he doesn't seem to be eating or sleeping well, despite seeming quite cheerful. He paces the flat at night talking about new operative techniques he is designing. His consultant sent him home from work because he refused to scrub for theatre, stating 'I'm pristine already'.

11. Elevated or irritable mood secondary to a general medical condition or psychoactive substance use

A. Huntington's disease
B. Multiple sclerosis
C. Parkinson's disease
D. Cerebral tumour
E. Cushing's disease
F. Hypothyroidism
G. Hyperthyroidism
H. Anabolic steroids
I. Corticosteroids
J. L-dopa
K. Cocaine
L. Amfetamine

For each of the following patients, select the ONE most likely cause from the options above.

1. A 66-year-old man with a shuffling gait and reduced facial expression has recently had a medication increase. Now he is elated, spends all his time playing online poker and asked his wife where all the monkeys in the kitchen had come from.

2. A 22-year-old student is brought to A&E by his friends from a party because he tried to fly off the roof. He is adamant he is Superman. He admits to having swallowed a pill earlier. On examination he is restless with dilated pupils.

3. A 28-year-old bodybuilder has recently become convinced he will win the next world championship. He is irritable with his girlfriend whenever she queries this. He is also hypersexual and forgetful, and has been reprimanded at work.

4. A 62-year-old woman is an in-patient on an acute medical ward following a severe asthma exacerbation. The nurses notice she seems irritable and suspicious and keeps asking for a single room 'as befits someone of my status'. Her daughter says this is a complete change from normal.

5. A 45-year-old woman presents to A&E with palpitations. When not seen immediately she becomes extremely irritated and starts pacing in the waiting room. On examination she has a tremor, pupils are normal and ECG shows sinus tachycardia. She shouts at the ECG technician for not being gentle enough when she removes the electrodes.

12. Mental state examination in elevated or irritable mood

A. Pressured speech
B. Flight of ideas
C. Tangential thinking
D. Poor concentration
E. Psychomotor retardation
F. Psychomotor agitation
G. Hyperacusis
H. Visual hyperaesthesia
I. Auditory hallucination
J. Visual hallucination

For each of the following patients, select ONE clinical feature described from the list of options above.

1. There are no natural breaks in the conversation and it is impossible to interrupt the patient without speaking over them.
2. The patient comments she has never seen a blue as blue as the nurse's uniform before.
3. The patient speaks normally and initially starts to answer a question but quickly diverts onto related but unimportant topics.
4. The patient speaks rapidly and initially starts to answer a question but very rapidly diverts onto lots of other topics. It is very confusing to listen to but in retrospect there are links between the topics. Some of the links were rhyming words.
5. The patient is trying to complete serial 7s but keeps being distracted by the noise of hoovering.
6. The patient comments there is a beautiful blue bird in the corner of the room, but no one else can see it.

13. Differential diagnosis of psychosis

A. Schizophrenia
B. Schizophrenia-like psychotic disorders

C. Schizoaffective disorder
D. Delusional disorder
E. Manic episode with psychotic features
F. Depressive episode, severe, with psychotic features
G. Dementia/delirium
H. Personality disorder
I. Neurodevelopmental disorder
J. Psychosis secondary to a general medical condition
K. Psychosis secondary to psychoactive substance use

For each of the following patients, select the ONE most likely diagnosis from the list of options above.

1. The mother of a 22-year-old man asks for a home visit from their GP. For the last 6 weeks her son has barely left his room and seems to be collecting tinfoil. She is adamant that he has never used drugs. He is in second year at university having passed first year with a distinction, but 6 months ago he lost interest and stopped going to lectures. He tells the GP that a terrorist organization is trying to brainwash him into becoming a terrorist and he needs the tinfoil to make it more difficult for them to beam thoughts into him.

2. A 45-year-old man has recurrent episodes of low mood associated with third person auditory hallucinations in the form of an abusive running commentary. These symptoms do not occur separately.

3. A 52-year-old man has recurrent episodes of low mood associated with second person auditory hallucinations in the form of abusive comments. He has noticed his mood starts to dip first, and the hallucinations emerge as his mood worsens.

4. A 47-year-old teacher presents to his GP for the 25th time in 6 months convinced he has bowel cancer, despite having had a normal colonoscopy and CT abdomen/pelvis. He tells his GP he knows logically he cannot have bowel cancer but at the same time he is certain he does. His mood is normal and he is still working.

5. A 37-year-old man is brought to A&E for assessment by the police after calling them to say his neighbour is persecuting him by refusing to move his wheelie-bin. The police note multiple previous calls over the last decade about previous neighbours. The man agrees it is possible the neighbour has some other reason for not wanting to move the wheelie-bin, but thinks it is most likely because he wants to spite him. He is angry with the police for bringing him to see a doctor, stating he plans to contact his lawyer about their behaviour.

6. A woman requests a GP home visit for her 78-year-old father who has no previous psychiatric history. She is concerned that he has told her he can hear his mother and sister talking, who are both dead. She is also concerned that he seems very forgetful and does not seem to be looking after himself properly. He is quite cheerful and enjoys speaking with his relatives.

14. Psychosis secondary to a general medical condition or psychoactive substance use

A. Huntington's disease

B. Neurosyphilis

C. Cerebral tumour

D. Cushing's disease

E. Hypothyroidism

F. Hyperthyroidism

G. Vitamin B_{12} deficiency

H. Thiamine deficiency

I. Corticosteroids

J. L-dopa

K. Cocaine

L. Amfetamine

For each of the following patients, select the ONE most likely cause from the options above.

1. A 62-year-old retired navy officer is brought to his GP by his wife. She is concerned that his personality has changed over the last few months. He has been unusually cheerful and keeps mentioning that he expects to be knighted for his naval service. He has become very extravagant, wanting to sell their home and give half the proceeds to charity. He forgot their wedding anniversary. On examination he has unusually brisk reflexes.

2. A 57-year-old accountant is brought to A&E by the police after going to the supermarket in swimming trunks and flippers. He does not see what the problem is. He states he wore the flippers because he has a constant headache which worsens when he bends down to tie his shoelaces. He has no psychiatric history or previous encounters with the police.

3. A 46-year-old vegan goes to her GP because for the last 6 months she has found herself unusually clumsy, tripping over rugs and stairs in a way she never did before. She feels like everyone is watching her when she stumbles in the street, and is sure she heard a group of strangers commenting on how they planned to rob her.

4. A 42-year-old man is admitted for emergency surgery following a road traffic accident. Two days after admission he becomes agitated and asks the charge nurse why there are so many insects in the ward (there are none). He keeps rubbing his skin and saying 'get away, get away'. He has a stumbling gait and his eyes make rapid small movements to the side and back again.

15. Mental state examination in psychosis (perceptual disturbance)

A. Audible thoughts

B. Second person auditory hallucination

C. Third person auditory hallucination

D. Pseudohallucination

E. Tactile hallucination

F. Visceral hallucination

G. Kinaesthetic hallucination

H. Olfactory hallucination

I. Gustatory hallucination

J. Hypnagogic hallucination

K. Hypnopompic hallucination

L. Extracampine hallucination

For each of the following patients, select ONE clinical feature described from the list of options above.

1. I hear a man saying 'you idiot' in the corner of the room but no one's there.

2. I hear a man saying 'you idiot' inside my head.

3. I hear a man in Newcastle talking to me even though I live in Edinburgh.

4. My spleen is moving around inside me.

5. As I'm drifting off to sleep I catch a glimpse of a ginger cat beside the bed, but I have no cat.

6. I taste rotting meat all the time.

16. Mental state examination in psychosis (thought disturbance)

A. Persecutory delusion

B. Grandiose delusion

C. Delusion of reference

D. Erotomania

E. Delusion of infidelity

F. Delusion of misidentification

G. Nihilistic delusion

H. Somatic delusion

I. Delusion of control

J. Loosening of association

For each of the following patients, select ONE clinical feature described from the list above.

1. I'm sure I'm being spied on by the government, I can tell because of the amount of junk mail I get.

2. My boss definitely loves me, even though he denies it every time I remind him.

3. I can't understand why that woman has dressed up as my wife and keeps referring to me as her husband.

4. The newsreader on the radio keeps reading out my name for some reason.

5. I don't need to eat because I'm already dead.

6. Someone else's thoughts are inside my head.
7. Why should the cat indeed bend that carrot tomatoes are red.

---

17. Differential diagnosis of anxiety, fear or avoidance

A. Agoraphobia with panic disorder
B. Agoraphobia without panic disorder
C. Social phobia
D. Generalized anxiety disorder
E. Panic disorder
F. Depressive episode
G. Acute stress reaction
H. Post-traumatic stress disorder
I. Adjustment disorder
J. Personality disorder
K. Anxiety secondary to a general medical condition
L. Anxiety secondary to psychoactive substance use

For each of the following patients, select the ONE most likely diagnosis from the list above.

1. A 25-year-old librarian avoids being with others whenever possible. He does all his shopping online and always volunteers to re-shelve books rather than deal with enquiries. When he is forced to interact with people he can feel himself blushing and sweating. He feels they are scrutinizing and judging him critically, even though he knows he is not really a bad person.
2. A 43-year-old woman feels she has been on edge for 2 years. She spends most of each day worrying about many trivial topics and sometimes she feels something bad is going to happen for no reason. She lies awake at night thinking about these things. She often has a dry mouth, epigastric discomfort and a bilateral frontal headache.
3. A 28-year-old secretary presents to her GP with weight loss. Six months ago in a supermarket she suddenly felt like she was going to die. She had pain in her chest, was short of breath and her arms and lips tingled. She rushed outside and the feeling subsided, but now she does not like to go into any large shops and is eating less well. She is still going to work but now walks 5 miles each way as she does not want to be on a bus and have another attack. As long as she is in her house or with her friends she is relaxed.
4. Over the last 3 months, a 35-year-old builder has experienced several episodes of sudden onset shortness of breath, palpitations, sweatiness, nausea, feeling that the world is unreal and a feeling he is about to die. These feelings resolve spontaneously over 20 minutes. He cannot identify any triggers. In particular, they are not brought on by exercise and he can continue to do his active job. His ECG is normal.

5. A 37-year-old professional violinist finds himself unable to play concerts. He can play well when alone, but starts to sweat and shake such that he cannot play properly when in the presence of others. He has had to cancel a tour. These symptoms came on after he received a series of negative reviews. In general he is a relaxed person who enjoys socializing.
6. A 42-year-old policeman has experienced low mood, anhedonia, fatigue, early morning wakening and anorexia for the last month. He has free-floating anxiety most of the time, and has had two panic attacks. These symptoms had onset after he witnessed an armed robbery but he denies flashbacks and still buys milk in the shop where he witnessed the robbery.

---

18. Anxiety secondary to a general medical condition or psychoactive substance use

A. Cushing's disease
B. Hypoglycaemia
C. Hyperthyroidism
D. Phaeochromocytoma
E. Caffeine
F. Alcohol
G. Cannabis
H. Amfetamine
I. Fluoxetine
J. Mirtazapine
K. Trazodone

For each of the following patients, select the ONE most likely cause from the options above.

1. A 63-year-old shopkeeper with hypertension has periodic episodes of anxiety, tachycardia, sweating and pallor. She can identify no triggers but recalls her mother having a similar problem. Her random glucose is elevated.
2. A 48-year-old scientist with a past medical history of vitiligo presents with a 3 month history of anxiety, increased appetite and heat intolerance. Her hands are shaky and she has knocked over a lot of test tubes recently.
3. A 25-year-old joiner has recently been diagnosed with depression and commenced an antidepressant 4 days ago. Since then he has been very restless and agitated, and frequently called his friends for reassurance. His sleep has worsened further.
4. A 23-year-old man has started a new job as a welder. He has noticed that he gets very irritable and anxious by the end of the day, and has had to go home early a couple of times. He sweats a lot while working so is drinking a lot of his favourite soft drink, 'Go-Man'.

5. A 19-year-old man is brought to A&E by his friends. He is pacing the cubicle, is tachycardic, hyperventilating, has dilated pupils and is sweating. He jumps when his name is called. His friends saw him swallow a white tablet earlier in the evening.

5. For the last 4 months, a 27-year-old woman has experienced recurrent thoughts of herself as being fat and ugly. She feels these thoughts are her own, and are appropriate, as she believes she is fat and ugly. She has been avoiding food and exercising lots. Her periods have stopped and her BMI is 17. She still views herself as overweight.

19. Differential diagnosis of obsessions and compulsions

A. No mental illness
B. Obsessive-compulsive disorder
C. Depressive episode
D. Phobia
E. Agoraphobia with panic disorder
F. Agoraphobia without panic disorder
G. Social phobia
H. Panic disorder
I. Eating disorder
J. Personality disorder
K. Hypochondriacal disorder

For each of the following patients, select the ONE most likely diagnosis from the list above.

1. For the last year, a 27-year-old woman has experienced repetitive images of soiled hands that she acknowledges are from her own mind. Washing her hands reduces her fear that her hands are dirty, but now she spends around 2 hours a day washing and is developing contact dermatitis. She has tried to wash less but this makes her very anxious.
2. For the last year, a 27-year-old nurse has been influenced by a NHS advertising campaign featuring soiled hands spreading infection. Washing her hands reduces her fear that they are dirty. Now she washes her hands before and after every patient contact, up to 100 times a day, and is developing contact dermatitis.
3. For the last 4 months, a 27-year-old woman has experienced repetitive images of herself having sexual encounters with children. This makes her feel extremely guilty and unclean. Showering reduces her fear that she will engage in such behaviour, but she now has to spend several hours a day in the shower. She describes herself as worthless and hopeless, and admits that 6 months ago she started to feel low in mood, anhedonic and fatigued.
4. After a bad experience as a child, a 27-year-old woman has been terrified of illness. Most of the time she has no problems, but if she meets anyone who is unwell she avoids them and washes her hands thoroughly to reduce her risk of contracting their illness. If she cannot get away from the person she feels overwhelmingly anxious and may have a panic attack.

20. Differentiating types of repetitive or intrusive thoughts

A. No mental illness
B. Obsession
C. Rumination
D. Pseudohallucination
E. Hallucination
F. Over-valued idea
G. Delusion
H. Thought insertion

For each of the following descriptions, select the ONE most likely psychopathology from the options above.

1. 'I keep seeing images of germs crawling on my skin. I try to stop my mind showing them to me, but I can't'.
2. 'After I got viral gastroenteritis, I became much more careful about hygiene. I'm worried I'll get it again. Now I autoclave every utensil and piece of crockery I use. I had to give up my job at the hospital, it wasn't worth the risk'.
3. 'I lie awake at night thinking about all the ways I could have avoided getting sick. I think about it from all the different angles but never reach a conclusion'.
4. 'I keep hearing a voice inside my head saying "you're dirty". I don't know who it is but I think they're probably right'.
5. 'I keep hearing a voice outside my head saying "you're dirty". I don't know who it is but I think they're probably right'.
6. 'Someone puts ideas in my head – like thoughts of germs, and of being ill. I don't know how they get in there, but they're not my thoughts'.
7. 'When I saw a picture on TV of germs crawling on someone's skin, I knew that I was fatally ill. The doctor told me I was fine, but I know my days are numbered'.

21. Dissociative disorders

A. Stupor
B. Dissociative anaesthesia
C. Depersonalization disorder
D. Psychogenic non-epileptic seizures

E. Ganser's syndrome

F. Hysterical paralysis

G. Psychogenic amnesia

H. Fugue state

I. Hysterical blindness

J. Dissociation secondary to psychoactive substance use

K. Dissociative identity disorder

Assuming physical causes have been excluded, which ONE of the above would be the most likely diagnosis for the following?

1. A 29-year-old mother of two, with a history of depression and a family history of epilepsy, has recently started having seizures, which last for less than a minute, and do not cause tongue-biting, incontinence or post-ictal confusion. She denies alcohol or drug use, and seems indifferent to her predicament. Her husband tells you that this started when he told his wife of his new job on an oil rig. He now feels he cannot leave home for fear that she will be seriously harmed by the seizures.

2. A 46-year-old businessman from a distant city is brought to hospital by the police, after apparently trying to withdraw money from a building society and being unable to remember his name. At interview, he seems unable to recall any personal details about himself, and has no idea where he is. He is carrying a bundle of business cards for a company that was recently reported to have gone bankrupt.

3. A 21-year-old male prisoner appears to be experiencing vivid visual hallucinations, and seems drowsy. However, at interview, he is fully orientated and appears able to concentrate. He complains of lack of sensation in his right arm, anterior abdomen and left leg. When you ask him how many days are in a week, he replies 'six', and also tells you that the colour of snow is 'black'. The prison guard tells you that he has been moved to protective custody because a senior gang member has threatened to kill him.

4. An 18-year-old tells you that she feels like she is 'in a bubble', and feels that everything around her appears to be unreal and distant from her life. She has no psychiatric history, and was fine until yesterday. Her parents tell you that she returned home from a 'rave' party only a couple of hours ago.

22. Diagnosis following stressful events

A. Acute stress reaction

B. Post-traumatic stress disorder

C. Moderate depression

D. Adjustment disorder

E. Bereavement reaction

F. Acute/transient psychotic disorder

G. Alcoholic hallucinosis

H. Panic disorder

I. Conversion disorder

J. Temporal lobe epilepsy

K. Musculoskeletal injury

From the options above, which ONE of the diagnoses would be the most appropriate for the scenarios below?

1. The wife of a 35-year-old RAF pilot has been hearing the voice of her husband, who was recently killed on duty in Libya. She has been feeling very low in mood since his death.

2. An 18-year-old man complains of pains in his neck and right shoulder that seem to have developed shortly after he was driving a car that had a head-on collision with a lorry. He feels lucky to be alive, and you are unable to elicit any other psychopathology.

3. A 52-year-old deep sea diver has felt constantly 'on edge' for the last 3 months since he was involved in an incident involving loss of oxygen flow while deep under the sea. He was convinced that he was going to die. He reports vivid nightmares and has been unable to return to work.

4. A 27-year-old lady is referred from the neurosurgical unit 4 months after a fall from a first floor balcony. She reports episodes of derealization, followed by visual hallucinations, loss of memory and extreme tiredness.

23. Diagnosis of medically unexplained physical symptoms

A. Undifferentiated somatoform disorder

B. Münchausen syndrome by proxy

C. Somatoform autonomic dysfunction

D. Body dysmorphic disorder

E. Factitious disorder

F. Somatic delusional disorder

G. Schizophrenia

H. Hypochondriacal disorder

I. Somatization disorder

J. Malingering

K. Severe depression with psychotic features

For each of the following scenarios, select the ONE most appropriate diagnosis from the list above.

1. A 23-year-old quit her job as a dancer 2 years ago because she is preoccupied with the idea her breasts are misshapen. Now she barely leaves the house, wears baggy clothes and is requesting surgical augmentation. The cosmetic surgeon noted no abnormalities.

2. An 8-year-old girl is drowsy. Her mother tells you that it is sudden onset. On examination, you find subcutaneous needle marks between her toes. One of the nurses finds an insulin syringe on the bedside while her mother is at the bathroom.

3. A 21-year-old man is preoccupied by a small scar behind his ear, which he believes is where the government have implanted a microchip to insert thoughts.
4. A 65-year-old man in a surgical ward with abdominal pain believes that he is dead and rotting from the inside.
5. A 45-year-old man complains of whiplash following a road traffic accident, and asks you to complete a medical report. He tells you he has been disabled permanently and wears a neck brace. You saw him getting off the bus earlier that morning wearing no neck brace.

24. Differential diagnosis of cognitive impairment

A. Delirium
B. Dementia
C. Mild cognitive impairment
D. Subjective cognitive impairment
E. Depression ('pseudodementia')
F. Psychotic disorders
G. Mood disorders
H. Intellectual disability
I. Dissociative disorders
J. Factitious disorder and malingering
K. Amnesic syndrome

For each of the following patients, select the ONE most likely diagnosis from the list above.

1. A 62-year-old teacher presents to her GP because she feels she is not remembering the names of the children in her class as well as she used to. She is worried she has dementia like her mother. She has no difficulties in activities of daily living and her mood is normal. She scores 30/30 on MMSE. What is the most likely diagnosis?
2. A 62-year-old teacher presents to her GP because she feels she is not remembering the names of the children in her class as well as she used to. She is worried she has dementia like her mother. She has no difficulties in activities of daily living and her mood is normal. She scores 24/30 on MMSE. What is the most likely diagnosis?
3. A 62-year-old teacher presents to her GP because she feels she is not remembering the names of the children in her class as well as she used to. She is worried she has dementia like her mother. She has noticed herself getting lost in the school corridors sometimes and her husband now does all the shopping because she kept getting disorientated in the supermarket. Her mood is normal. She scores 24/30 on MMSE. What is the most likely diagnosis?
4. A 62-year-old teacher presents to her GP because she feels she is not remembering the names of the children

in her class as well as she used to. She is worried she has dementia like her mother. She has no difficulties in activities of daily living and scores 29/30 on MMSE. She admits she has been low in mood recently, is not enjoying work any more, is fatigued, has lost weight and is not sleeping well. What is the most likely diagnosis?

25. Potentially reversible causes of dementia

A. Subdural haematoma
B. Brain tumour
C. Normal pressure hydrocephalus
D. Hyperthyroidism
E. Hypothyroidism
F. Hyperparathyroidism
G. Hypoparathyroidism
H. Cushing's disease
I. Addison's disease
J. Vitamin B_{12} deficiency
K. Folate deficiency

For each of the following patients, select the ONE most likely diagnosis from the list above.

1. A 74-year-old woman presents to her GP with her husband who is concerned that over the last 8 weeks she has become increasingly forgetful and disorientated. She has burnt a couple of pans after leaving them unattended. Some days she takes afternoon naps, which is new for her. When pressed he recalls she was hit on the head by a football around 3 months ago while watching her grandson's team, but seemed fine afterwards. Past medical history includes atrial fibrillation and asthma. MMSE is 22/30 and neurological exam shows normal consciousness level and a subtle right hemiparesis.
2. A 76-year-old widower attends his GP because of urinary incontinence. As he walks into the room he has a broad based, stiff-legged gait. He is very slow to answer questions and seems not to be paying close attention to what is asked. He says he cannot remember when his incontinence started or how often it occurs. Past medical history is of a duodenal ulcer only. MMSE is 19/30 and neurological exam is normal apart from his gait.
3. A 52-year-old woman presents to her GP with memory and concentration problems. She reports feeling tired and sluggish for the last 6 months. She feels low in motivation and mood and has quit her running club because she can't be bothered to keep up any more. Past medical history is unremarkable. MMSE is 29/30. Physical examination is normal apart from dizziness when she gets off the examination couch.

4. A 43-year-old traffic warden presents to her GP with weight gain and amenorrhoea. She is surprised to be going through the menopause so soon as her mother's was in her late 50s. She is finding herself forgetful at work, checking cars on the same streets repeatedly. She has got into trouble for this and feels very low in mood. MMSE is 26/30. Physical examination shows hypertension, a plethoric complexion and central obesity.

5. A 76-year-old woman attends her GP with a 12-month history of gradually worsening memory problems and low mood. Past medical history includes renal calculi and abdominal pain for which no cause has been identified. MMSE is 24/30. Physical examination is normal.

26. Subtypes of dementia

A. Alzheimer's disease

B. Vascular dementia

C. Mixed dementia

D. Frontotemporal dementia

E. Dementia with Lewy bodies

F. Parkinson's disease with dementia

G. Progressive supranuclear palsy

H. Huntington's disease

I. Creutzfeldt–Jakob disease

J. Neurosyphilis

K. HIV-related dementia

For each of the following patients, select the ONE most likely cause from the options above.

1. A 77-year-old woman has a 9-month history of gradual onset, gradually worsening cognitive impairment. She forgets recent events and people's names. She can no longer manage her finances. Past medical history is of psoriasis and asthma. CT head showed generalized atrophy, particularly marked in the medial temporal lobes.

2. A 74-year-old man has a 10-month history of progressive cognitive impairment. His family notice he seems to worsen suddenly and then plateau before abruptly worsening again. He has marked word-finding difficulties and an abnormal gait. Past medical history is of ischaemic heart disease, hypertension and diabetes. He is a current smoker. CT head shows generalized atrophy, small vessel disease and an old lacunar infarct.

3. A 75-year-old woman has an 11-month history of gradual onset cognitive impairment. Three months ago her family noticed a sudden deterioration. Delirium was excluded. She is forgetful and gets lost easily. Past medical history is of hypertension and osteoporosis. CT head shows generalized atrophy and an old infarct in the left frontal lobe.

4. A 67-year-old retired chef has a 12-month history of gradual personality change. He was previously polite and considerate but has become very rude and tactless. He is having an affair with a waitress from his old restaurant. His wife of 40 years is thinking of leaving him but he says he does not care. CT head shows generalized atrophy, particularly marked in the frontal lobes.

5. An 81-year-old man has an 18-month history of fluctuating cognitive impairment on a background of a gradual cognitive deterioration. He has been investigated for delirium but no cause found. Sometimes he is very drowsy during the day. He is increasingly stiff and finds it hard to roll over in bed. He also finds it hard to keep his balance and has had a lot of falls recently. Sometimes he experiences visual hallucinations of cats and mice. CT head shows generalized cerebral atrophy.

6. A 71-year-old man was diagnosed with Parkinson's disease 5 years ago. He has a 1-year history of cognitive impairment causing him to forget people's names and where he has left his clothes. Sometimes he has hallucinations of former work colleagues walking around the room. CT head shows generalized cerebral atrophy.

27. Clinical features in cognitive impairment

A. Apraxia

B. Agnosia

C. Aphasia

D. Amnesia

E. Perseveration

F. Disinhibition

For each of the following patients, select ONE clinical feature described from the options above.

1. When shown a pair of scissors a woman states they are scissors but cannot work out how to cut with them. She can mimic the correct action when shown.

2. When shown a pair of scissors a woman states they are 'those things used for cutting paper' but cannot name them.

3. A woman uses scissors to cut a piece of paper into squares as asked. When asked to then cut triangles, she keeps cutting squares.

4. When shown a pair of scissors a woman is unable to name them or describe their function. When she is allowed to touch them she quickly identifies what they are. She has normal visual acuity.

5. When given a pair of scissors inside a covered box, a woman turns them around in her hands but is unable to name them. When she is allowed to look at them she quickly identifies them. She has normal sensation in her hands.

6. When asked to name a pair of scissors a woman replies 'Yes, that table smart'. She has normal hearing.

28. Substances of abuse

A. MDMA
B. Cannabis
C. Alcohol
D. Heroin
E. Amfetamine
F. Diazepam
G. Cocaine
H. Ketamine
I. Mephedrone
J. Buprenorphine
K. LSD

For each of the following statements, select the ONE most appropriate answer from the options above.

1. Chronic usage can degrade the septum nasi.
2. Causes a dissociative anaesthetic effect.
3. Follows zero-order eliminatory pharmacokinetics.
4. The most widely used illegal drug in the UK.
5. A partial opioid agonist.

29. 'Street' names, or slang terms for drugs

A. 'Skag'
B. 'Trips'
C. 'Poppers'
D. 'Charlie'
E. 'Weed'
F. 'Pills'
G. 'Roofies'
H. 'Miaow'
I. 'Mushies'
J. 'Base'
K. 'Special K'

Pair the following drug names with the ONE most appropriate 'street' name from the list above.

1. Lysergic acid diethylamide.
2. Tetrahydrocannabinol.
3. Cocaine hydrochloride.
4. 3,4-methylenedioxy-N-methylamphetamine.
5. Diacetylmorphine.

30. Diagnosis of personality disorder

A. Paranoid personality disorder
B. Schizoid personality disorder
C. Schizotypal personality disorder
D. Borderline personality disorder
E. Antisocial personality disorder
F. Narcissistic personality disorder
G. Histrionic personality disorder
H. Dependent personality disorder
I. Avoidant (anxious) personality disorder
J. Anankastic personality disorder

For the following, select the ONE most appropriate personality disorder from the list above. Assume absence of axis I psychiatric disorder, and that diagnosis of a personality disorder is appropriate.

1. A 24-year-old accountant wears inappropriate clothes to work. Her colleagues feel that she is always flirtatious, and always seeks to be the centre of attention. When this does not happen, she tends to become very upset, and dramatically displays emotion.
2. A 47-year-old housewife refuses to leave her abusive partner, despite having recently been hospitalized after he assaulted her. She feels that she could never manage without him.
3. A 26-year-old unemployed man is constantly preoccupied by the mischief of local youths, and is concerned that he is a 'marked man'. He cannot hold down a job as he always becomes concerned that colleagues are talking about him behind his back. His last girlfriend left him 3 years ago after he accused her of cheating on him.
4. A 49-year-old successful entrepreneur feels that others have trouble getting on with him. His fourth marriage has recently ended because of his affairs. He has always been incredibly confident and able to succeed.
5. A 35-year-old website designer has difficulty making friends because of his fear of others criticizing, rejecting or disliking him. Instead, he socializes mainly using social networking sites, and will not physically meet others until he is sure they will like and accept him.

31. Traits of personality disorder

A. Callous unconcern for the feelings of others
B. Excessive sensitivity to setbacks and rebuffs
C. Consistent preference for solitary activities
D. Perfectionism that interferes with task completion

E. Over-concern with physical attractiveness

F. Frantic efforts to avoid real or imagined abandonment

G. Allowing others to make most of one's important life decisions

H. Excessive preoccupation with being rejected in social situations

For the personality disorders listed below, pick ONE trait from the above examples.

1. Histrionic personality disorder.
2. Schizoid personality disorder.
3. Obsessive-compulsive personality disorder.
4. Paranoid personality disorder.
5. Dependent personality disorder.

32. Psychiatric causes of low weight

A. Chronic schizophrenia

B. Anorexia nervosa, restrictive type

C. Specific phobia

D. Depression, severe without psychosis

E. Bulimia nervosa

F. Alcohol dependence syndrome

G. Alzheimer's disease

H. Acute paranoid psychosis

I. Anorexia nervosa, purging type

J. Obsessive-compulsive disorder

For the case vignettes below, pick the ONE most appropriate psychiatric cause from the list above.

1. A 42-year-old man was discharged to his own flat from a long-stay psychiatric rehabilitation ward 2 months ago. He has a BMI of 17, with evidence of rapid weight loss. He denies any problems with body image. He seems cheerful, and there are no acute psychotic symptoms.
2. A 19-year-old male student was admitted to a general medical ward after collapsing in the street. He denies any problems and tells you it was 'probably just a funny turn'. His BMI is 22, serum potassium is 2.1 mmol/L, there are U waves on his ECG, and you notice that his parotid glands appear swollen.
3. A 16-year-old girl has lost 15 kilos in the last 3 months, giving her a BMI of 16. She denies any body image concerns, but tells you that she is only able to eat food prepared in a specific manner. She knows this is irrational; however, the prospect of contamination with food-borne pathogens causes her to have unpleasant panic attacks.
4. A 62-year-old ex-model has recently begun to lose weight, and her BMI is 18. She has a past history of anorexia nervosa. She described that she could not bring herself to eat because of intense worry that she would

vomit. Any time that she has tried to eat, she has suffered a panic attack and has ended up vomiting. She suffered from a severe case of norovirus about 6 weeks ago.

5. A 21-year-old plumber has recently lost 12 kilos, causing his BMI to fall to 15. He appears incredibly frightened, and tells you that the owners of all the food shops in his locality are poisoning his food on behalf of government agents, who want him dead because of his involvement in the London terrorist bomb attacks in 2005.

33. Physical consequences of eating disorders

A. Lanugo

B. Caries

C. Xerosis

D. Russell's sign

E. Onychorrhexis

F. Alopecia areata

G. Cheilitis

H. Acrocyanosis

I. Perimylolysis

J. Striae distensae

For the statements below, select the ONE most appropriate descriptive term from the list above.

1. The fine, downy hair often seen on the body of sufferers of anorexia nervosa.
2. Erosion of dental enamel caused by repeated vomiting.
3. Dry nails, often associated with anorexia nervosa.
4. Stretch marks on the abdomen, associated with rapid changes in body weight.
5. A callus on the knuckle that may develop as a result of self-induced vomiting.

34. Treatment setting for depression

A. Admit to psychiatric hospital

B. Admit to general medical hospital

C. Manage in primary care

D. Refer to psychiatric out-patients routinely

E. Refer to psychiatric out-patients urgently

F. Refer to crisis team

For each of the following patients, select the ONE best management option from the list above.

1. A 55-year-old man with a severe depressive episode who has sent goodbye emails to his family. A dog walker

alerted the police after he found him in isolated woodland tying a noose to a tree.

2. A 55-year-old man with a moderate depressive episode which has not responded to adequate trials of two antidepressants. He denies suicidal ideas and maintains an oral intake.
3. A 55-year-old man with a severe depressive episode who reports derogatory second person auditory hallucinations. He denies suicidal ideas and maintains an oral intake.
4. A 55-year-old man with a severe depressive episode who has lost 3 stone in weight over 3 months and has refused food and fluids for the last 2 days.
5. A 55-year-old man with a mild depressive episode who has not benefited from self-help CBT.

35. First line antidepressants

A. SSRI
B. Venlafaxine
C. Duloxetine
D. Mirtazapine
E. Amitriptyline
F. Lofepramine
G. Phenelzine
H. Moclobemide
I. Lithium

For each of the following patients with moderate to severe depression, select the ONE best first line antidepressant from the options above.

1. A 49-year-old stunt man on long-term ibuprofen for back pain.
2. A 23-year-old shop assistant with no past medical history.
3. A 32-year-old teacher whose chief complaint is insomnia.
4. A 45-year-old butcher who says he will stop any antidepressant that affects his sexual function.
5. A 64-year-old librarian with stress incontinence.

36. Antipsychotic choice in schizophrenia

A. Chlorpromazine
B. Haloperidol
C. Flupentixol depot
D. Clozapine
E. Quetiapine
F. Aripiprazole
G. No antipsychotic indicated

For each of the following patients, select the ONE best management option from the options above.

1. A 47-year-old woman with schizophrenia. She remembers a good response to haloperidol in her 20s and would like to try it again.
2. A 28-year-old model experiencing a first episode of psychosis. She is very keen to avoid weight gain.
3. A 33-year-old man experiencing his second episode of psychosis. He recalls very unpleasant tremor and rigidity with the antipsychotic he used previously, and would like to avoid these symptoms.
4. A 36-year-old man with schizophrenia who has had multiple relapses after forgetting to take oral medication.
5. A 26-year-old woman who has tried 3 months of olanzapine and 3 months of risperidone at optimum doses but remains troubled by distressing psychotic experiences associated with functional impairment.

37. Presentations of antipsychotic side-effects

A. Photosensitivity
B. Postural hypotension
C. Hypersalivation
D. Dry mouth
E. Agranulocytosis
F. Parkinsonism
G. Akathisia
H. Dystonia
I. Somnolence
J. Hyperprolactinaemia

Select the ONE term used to describe the following side-effects from the list of options above.

1. A 27-year-old man wakes up each morning drooling onto a wet pillow.
2. A 57-year-old woman describes feeling dizzy. On examination, she has an erect blood pressure of 140 systolic and a supine of 100 systolic.
3. A 22-year-old woman has noticed milk coming from her nipples bilaterally, but is not pregnant or breast feeding.
4. A 43-year-old man collapses with a severe pneumonia. He has an undetectable neutrophil count.
5. A 30-year-old woman keeps crossing and uncrossing her legs during an interview. She also keeps smoothing her hair and handbag. She says she feels like she is 'crawling out of my own skin'.

38. Management of post-traumatic stress disorder

A. Self-help
B. Watchful waiting

247

C. CBT with exposure response prevention

D. Eye movement desensitization and reprocessing therapy

E. Applied relaxation

F. SSRI

G. TCA

H. Benzodiazepine

I. Venlafaxine

J. Pregabalin

K. Mirtazapine

For each of the following patients, select the ONE best first line management option from the list above.

1. A 23-year-old woman has symptoms of PTSD following being raped 2 weeks ago. She is no longer attending classes at university as she avoids leaving her house.

2. A 23-year-old woman has symptoms of PTSD following being raped 2 weeks ago. She is still able to attend classes at university.

3. A 23-year-old woman has symptoms of PTSD following being raped 2 months ago. She is still able to attend classes at university.

4. A 47-year-old former soldier has tried trauma-focused CBT for PTSD but continues to have symptoms which markedly affect his functioning. He would like to try a medication, but is keen to avoid sexual dysfunction as a side-effect.

5. A 35-year-old survivor of an airplane crash has tried talking therapies and two first line drug therapies for severe PTSD symptoms. She would like to try a further medication.

39. Management of generalized anxiety disorder and panic disorder

A. Self-help

B. Watchful waiting

C. CBT

D. Eye movement desensitization and reprocessing therapy

E. Applied relaxation

F. SSRI

G. MAOI

H. Benzodiazepine

I. Pregabalin

For each of the following patients, select the ONE best first line management option from the choices above.

1. A 27-year-old female grocer has panic disorder. She has had to leave her shop on several occasions in the last month because of panic attacks.

2. A 27-year-old female grocer has panic disorder but does not feel it stops her from doing anything.

3. A 44-year-old zoo keeper has generalized anxiety disorder and is unable to work. He has tried CBT in the past and would now like to try a different talking therapy.

4. A 44-year-old zoo keeper has generalized anxiety disorder and is unable to work. He has tried CBT in the past and would now like to try a medication.

5. A 44-year-old zoo-keeper has generalized anxiety disorder and is unable to work. He has tried CBT and an SSRI in the past and would now like to try a different class of medication.

40. Pharmacological management of opiate dependence

A. Naloxone

B. Dihydrocodeine

C. Levacetylmethadyl

D. Buprenorphine

E. Lofexidine

F. Naltrexone

G. Loperamide

H. Methadone

I. Paracetamol

J. Diazepam

For the following questions, select the ONE most appropriate drug from the list above.

1. A 37-year-old man is admitted to A&E via emergency ambulance. He is GCS 5/15, with pinpoint pupils and a respiratory rate of six per minute. He has syringes and hypodermic needles in his pocket.

2. A 22-year-old man wants to become entirely abstinent from opiates. He is not interested in substitution therapy; however, he asks if he can be prescribed something to 'take the edge off' the withdrawal state.

3. A 30-year-old woman is motivated to stop injecting heroin; however she feels that she needs to be prescribed a substitute for the long term. She was previously spending £100 per day on heroin.

4. A 27-year-old man is undergoing a detoxification from dihydrocodeine but he is troubled by profuse diarrhoea.

5. A 38-year-old lady who intermittently abuses opiates asks to be prescribed a drug to reduce the associated 'high', as she feels this will discourage her from using.

41. Prochaska and DiClemente Transtheoretical Model of Change

A. Pre-contemplative

B. Relapse

C. Preparation

D. Action

E. Contemplative

F. Maintenance

G. Termination

H. Recycling

For the following questions, select the ONE most appropriate term from the list above.

1. A 31-year-old nurse has set a 'quit date' to stop smoking.
2. A 62-year-old salesman has been abstinent from alcohol for 30 years, and is no longer even tempted by the thought of drinking.
3. A 22-year-old female student does not consider her heavy cannabis use to be a problem.
4. A 29-year-old banker is considering stopping his cocaine use; however, he is worried about what his friends will say.
5. A 33-year-old unemployed man has been using heroin on a daily basis for the last 2 weeks since his partner left him. He had previously been clean for 3 years.

42. Treatment of alcohol dependence

A. Alcoholics anonymous

B. Lorazepam

C. Psychoeducational group

D. Disulfiram

E. Thiamine

F. Chlordiazepoxide

G. Naltrexone

H. Cognitive-behavioural therapy

I. Acamprosate

J. Motivational interviewing

K. Diazepam

For the questions below, select the ONE most appropriate treatment option from the list above.

1. A 55-year-old man, currently drinking 70 units of alcohol per day, requires a benzodiazepine during an in-patient detoxification. He suffers from severe chronic liver failure.
2. A 45-year-old woman drinker is uncharacteristically confused, walking with an ataxic gait, and has nystagmus on examination of the eyes. She does not smell of alcohol.
3. A 57-year-old woman with a history of alcohol dependence is currently abstinent; however, she wants help to 'avoid temptation'. She does not want drugs, and is frightened by the prospect of group therapy.
4. A 36-year-old man is currently abstinent from alcohol but has experienced a couple of 'slips' that he attributed to powerful cravings. He is also prescribed tramadol for knee pain.

5. A 44-year-old man has recently stopped drinking and wants to remain abstinent for life. He considers alcohol to be a 'disease', and does not really want to be involved with health services. He is socially isolated and feels that he would benefit from meeting like-minded individuals.

43. Management of patients with personality disorders

A. Weekly dispensing of medication

B. Detention under mental health legislation

C. Informal, time-limited admission to psychiatric ward

D. Removal to police custody

E. Referral for mentalization-based therapy

F. Encouragement to engage with existing care-plan

G. Referral to social work

H. Trial of antipsychotic medication

I. Advice regarding lifestyle choices

J. Day-hospital referral

K. Urgent multi-agency meeting

For the vignettes below, choose the ONE most appropriate intervention from the list above.

1. A 36-year-old lady with dependent personality disorder arrives at A&E demanding admission to the hospital because she feels that she is not coping at home. She has missed her last two appointments with the occupational therapist.
2. A 22-year-old lady with borderline personality disorder was brought to hospital by police after being restrained to prevent her from jumping from a railway viaduct. She is covered in bruises and reports that her partner assaulted her and threw her out of the house. She is inconsolably upset, extremely pessimistic and voicing ongoing suicidal intent and plans.
3. A 43-year-old man has paranoid personality disorder. He is socially isolated, and has longstanding worries that he will be targeted by local youth gangs. He does not trust doctors; however, he has recently acknowledged that his concerns are perhaps unfounded.
4. A 19-year-old lady has a diagnosis of borderline personality disorder, and an extensive history of self-harm. She has recently developed a comorbid depressive illness that her GP feels would benefit from treatment with an antidepressant. However, the GP is reluctant to prescribe because of previous overdoses.
5. A 39-year-old man with a diagnosis of anxious personality disorder reports recent initial insomnia. He attributed this to worries about his future. Since he was made homeless, he has been spending his days drinking complimentary coffee in the support centre. When he cannot sleep at night, he lies in bed and smokes cigarettes.

44. Treatment strategies for patients with eating disorders

A. Nutritional advice from GP

B. High-dose fluoxetine

C. Voluntary sector referral

D. Motivational interviewing

E. Cognitive-behavioural therapy

F. Interpersonal therapy

G. Family therapy

H. Community mental health team involvement

I. Intensive home treatment by specialist eating disorder service

J. Informal admission to general psychiatric ward

K. Forced, involuntary nasogastric feeding under mental health legislation

For the scenarios below, select the ONE most appropriate management strategy from the list above.

1. A 23-year-old pole-dancer has a diagnosis of anorexia nervosa. Her weight has recently stabilized and is slowly increasing. She has previously appeared fairly bubbly and cheerful. However, she reports a 3-week history of tearfulness, loss of interest in all hobbies, early morning wakening and strong suicidal thoughts. When questioned directly, she tearfully discloses that she bought a rope and posted final letters earlier today, and intends to hang herself this evening when her flatmate goes out to work. She says she is amenable to whatever management is suggested.

2. A 19-year-old male medical student has a diagnosis of bulimia nervosa. He is motivated to change, has engaged well with his cognitive-behavioural therapist, and has found himself worrying a lot less about his shape and weight recently. However, despite his best efforts, he is still troubled by compulsive binge/purge behaviours.

3. A 16-year-old schoolgirl has a diagnosis of anorexia nervosa. She has been under the care of the specialist intensive team, but has continued to lose weight. Her BMI is currently 11.7. On examination, it is noted that she has incredible difficulty concentrating. She is hypotensive and bradycardic. Blood tests show profound hypoglycaemia and hypokalaemia. There are U waves on ECG. She vehemently refuses to eat, refutes that she has a problem, and categorically declines hospital admission. She just wants to be left alone to study for her A levels.

4. A 28-year-old lawyer has a diagnosis of anorexia nervosa. She is motivated to engage with treatment. She feels that a number of her past difficulties, including the death of her mother, starting work in her current firm, and not being able to stand up to dominant male partners, have played a role in the development of her illness. She is keen to explore these.

5. A 14-year-old schoolboy was recently diagnosed with anorexia nervosa. It is noted that his parents consistently correct him when he is trying to tell his story. Mum is a consultant surgeon, and dad is a barrister, and both subsequently spend a lot of time at work. They have persistently told him that they want him to be a doctor when he grows up and have set high standards for him. However, when interviewed alone, he stated that he aspired to attend art college and hoped for a career in photojournalism.

45. Management of mental illness in the puerperium

A. Lithium

B. Interpersonal therapy

C. Sertraline

D. Maternal skills teaching

E. Doxepin

F. Reassurance and check-up in 1 week

G. Olanzapine

H. Sodium valproate

I. Cognitive-behavioural therapy

J. Mother and baby groups

K. Electroconvulsive therapy

For the situations below, select the ONE most appropriate management strategy from the list above.

1. A 17-year-old mother of a 3-month-old baby reports that she is finding motherhood to be a burden, and is worried that she is not 'doing it properly'.

2. A 26-year-old lady appears weepy and reports feeling 'down' 3 days after the birth of her son.

3. A 24-year-old lady with a history of bipolar affective disorder is 1 week postpartum, and presents with auditory hallucinations and ideas that the father of the child is Jesus Christ.

4. A 33-year-old lady with a history of depression is 4 weeks postpartum. She has marked psychomotor retardation. Her husband reports that she has not been eating or drinking for the past week.

5. A 29-year-old mother of a 2-month-old girl is tearful and reports feeling low in mood. She appears to be ruminating about being a bad mother because, despite her best efforts, she has been physically unable to feed the baby purely by breast as she 'should' be doing.

46. Psychotropic medication in pregnancy

A. Paroxetine

B. Haloperidol

C. Olanzapine

D. Diazepam

E. Lamotrigine

F. Imipramine

G. Lithium carbonate

H. Carbamazepine

I. Fluoxetine

J. Chlorpromazine

K. Sodium valproate

From the list above, select ONE medication applicable to each of the statements below.

1. Should be prescribed with extreme caution to women of childbearing age, due to the high risk of neural tube defects.
2. Associated with increased risk of gestational diabetes.
3. Discontinuation in pregnancy is strongly advised due to increased risk of fetal heart defects and pulmonary hypertension.
4. May be continued in pregnancy if risks of discontinuation are high, but should be balanced against the risk of increased risk of fetal heart defects.
5. May be continued in pregnancy if benefits outweigh risks, but associated with an increased risk of pulmonary hypertension in the neonate.

DISCLAIMER: Information on the effects and complications of the use of psychotropic medication during pregnancy and breast feeding is continuously evolving. Seeking up-to-date information from the National Institute for Health and Clinical Excellence (NICE), the British National Formulary (BNF) and the Maudsley Prescribing guidelines is always advised.

47. Management of dementia

A. Donepezil

B. Rivastigmine

C. Galantamine

D. Memantine

E. Citalopram

F. Methylphenidate

G. Quetiapine

H. Trazodone

I. No treatment recommended by current guidelines

For each of the following patients, select the ONE best treatment for maintaining cognition from the options above.

1. A woman with a diagnosis of Alzheimer's dementia and MMSE of 20.
2. A woman with a diagnosis of Alzheimer's dementia and MMSE of 8.

3. A woman with a diagnosis of Alzheimer's dementia and MMSE of 20 with sick sinus syndrome, COPD and an active peptic ulcer.
4. Parkinson's disease with dementia.
5. Frontotemporal dementia.

48. Adverse drug reactions in older adults receiving psychotropic medication

A. Lithium

B. Sodium valproate

C. Diazepam

D. Lorazepam

E. Trazodone

F. Mirtazapine

G. Amitriptyline

H. Fluoxetine

I. Olanzapine

J. Haloperidol

For each of the following patients, select the ONE medication most likely to be implicated in their presentation from the options above.

1. A 67-year-old woman complains of insomnia, anxiety and anorexia. She has tinnitus and keeps mistaking her oxygen tubing for a snake. She was admitted 10 days ago with a myocardial infarction and her sleeping tablet was stopped.
2. A 72-year-old man receiving treatment for depression presents with general malaise. His serum sodium is 126 mmol/L.
3. A 69-year-old man receiving treatment for bipolar affective disorder presents with vomiting and diarrhoea. His serum sodium is 151 mmol/L.
4. A 74-year-old man collapses. His ECG shows torsade de pointes. He was admitted 5 days ago with delirium requiring pharmacological management.
5. An 81-year-old woman has delirium. She has recently been started on analgesia for trigeminal neuralgia.

49. Pharmacotherapy in child and adolescent psychiatry

A. Paroxetine

B. Methylphenidate

C. Haloperidol

D. Venlafaxine

E. Sodium valproate

F. Sertraline

G. Olanzapine

H. Imipramine

I. Risperidone

J. Atomoxetine

K. Dexamphetamine

L. Fluoxetine

For each of the questions below, select the ONE most appropriate option from the list above.

1. A 15-year-old girl has moderate symptoms of depression. She has recently been referred for cognitive-behavioural therapy, but found it difficult to concentrate.

2. An 8-year-old boy has ADHD, which is causing significant problems with his schoolwork. He has never been on medication for this before.

3. A 7-year-old girl suffers from nocturnal enuresis. Behavioural strategies and psychosocial interventions have been unsuccessful.

4. A 13-year-old boy has Tourette's syndrome. There is no suggestion of ADHD or OCD. His symptoms are troublesome and he has not responded to psychosocial interventions.

5. An 11-year-old girl has ADHD. Her symptoms responded well to methylphenidate; however, she developed tics.

2. The father of a 6-year-old girl is concerned that she has recently started wetting the bed, and also wetting her clothes during the day. Her mother committed suicide 3 months ago.

3. A 6-year-old boy is referred by educational psychology, due to his behaviour at school. He seems to be unable to concentrate on his schoolwork, and has been running around the classroom distracting fellow pupils from completing their work, often by jumping on tables and throwing chairs around. On one occasion, he flooded the play area when he broke a water pipe. His parents are very surprised, because he is entirely normal at home.

4. A 12-year-old boy has been incredibly disobedient, both at school and within the home. He has been dancing in front of the TV when his father has been watching the football. He has also been using curse words in the house, and – on two occasions in the last week – has run away from home after being confined to his room. His parents are surprised that he has not been bullying others, or in trouble with the police.

5. An 11-year-old girl has stereotyped hand-flapping and appears obsessed with trains. She does not appear interested in playing or interacting with others. Her parents report that her development was entirely normal until just after she was 2 years old, after which she seemed to deteriorate.

50. Diagnosis of psychiatric disorders with onset in childhood or adolescence

A. Rett's syndrome

B. Asperger's syndrome

C. Age-appropriate behaviour

D. Conduct disorder

E. Secondary enuresis

F. Heller's syndrome

G. Childhood autism

H. Attention deficit hyperactivity disorder

I. Oppositional defiant disorder

J. Academic setting inappropriate to ability

K. Primary enuresis

For the following examples, select the ONE most likely diagnosis from the list above.

1. The mother of a 7-year-old boy raises concerns about his behaviour. He becomes distressed when they drive a different route to school, and the family have been unable to go on holiday because of this. He spends much of his spare time looking at road maps, and seems very interested about the UK motorway network. There have been no concerns about his speech and language development.

51. Functional estimation of IQ in intellectual disability

A. 100 > (above average intelligence)

B. 86–100 (below average intelligence)

C. 71–85 (borderline intellectual disability)

D. 50–69 (mild intellectual disability)

E. 35–49 (moderate intellectual disability)

F. 20–34 (severe intellectual disability)

G. <20 (profound intellectual disability)

For each of the scenarios below, select the ONE most appropriate estimation of IQ and level of disability from the list above.

1. A 24-year-old woman lives alone and works in a bakery. She cannot serve customers as she finds it very difficult to use the cash register or give the correct change. She needed extra help at school with reading and writing, and did not achieve any qualifications.

2. A 19-year-old man lives alone, does not see his family and is unemployed. He has no support at home, and spends much of his time writing programmes on his computer and reading about the mathematics of quantum mechanics. He has always found social interactions to be difficult, and strongly dislikes socializing with others. There were no problems with language development.

3. A 14-year-old boy is wheelchair-bound and incontinent. He lives with his mother, who is his main carer. He is unable to undertake any activities of daily living, and his mother has to feed him.
4. A 35-year-old woman lives in sheltered accommodation, and requires support to cook meals, to keep her flat tidy and to do laundry. She has a job at a local toy factory, where she works on a production line and is closely supervised by a trained support worker.
5. A 22-year-old man lives with his family, who are his main carers. He requires some assistance getting dressed and tending to his personal hygiene; however, he can do this by himself on good days. He can feed himself, and spends his days watching children's television programmes and playing with Lego.

52. Genetic disorders in intellectual disability

A. Down's syndrome
B. Lesch–Nyhan syndrome
C. Prader–Willi syndrome
D. Turner's syndrome
E. Fragile X syndrome
F. Cri-du-chat syndrome
G. Angelman's syndrome
H. Edward syndrome
I. Rett's syndrome
J. Patau syndrome

For each of the scenarios below, select the ONE most likely genetic syndrome from the list above.

1. A 6-year-old girl with a mild intellectual disability is short in height and obese. Her parents report that she seems to have an excessive appetite, and never seems to stop eating.
2. A 2-year-old boy recently started biting his fingers and banging his head off walls.
3. A 7-year-old girl initially met developmental milestones, but then seemed to regress. She has a severe intellectual disability, and stereotyped tortuous 'hand washing' movements are noted.
4. A 14-year-old girl with a mild intellectual disability remains pre-pubertal. Her verbal IQ is greater than her performance IQ.
5. A 4-year-old boy has a severe intellectual disability. He appears hypotonic, with microcephaly, low set ears, and single palmar crease. His mother reported that he used to make odd crying noises as an infant, but has stopped now.

53. Diagnosis of mental disorder in offenders

A. Othello syndrome
B. Paranoid schizophrenia
C. Dissocial personality disorder
D. Mania with psychotic symptoms
E. Severe depression with psychotic symptoms
F. Borderline personality disorder
G. De Clerambault syndrome
H. Delirium tremens
I. Obsessive-compulsive disorder
J. Mild intellectual disability
K. Drug-induced psychosis

For each of the following scenarios, select the ONE most appropriate diagnosis from the list above.

1. A 35-year-old man was arrested after he assaulted a bus driver. He believed that the driver was trying to procure the services of his wife, who he is convinced is working as a prostitute. He has dismissed extensive reassurances from his wife and his own siblings. He reports that he has a sword in the back of his car, and intended to 'get the truth out of her'. He has a history of alcohol abuse.
2. A 50-year-old man with no psychiatric history was arrested after committing a public order offence on a train home from a music festival. He assaulted three police officers and required restraint. At interview, he appears distressed and is clearly responding to auditory hallucinations. He is convinced that the police are Nazis who plan to use his brain for experimentation.
3. A 21-year-old woman has been charged with fraud. She has applied for several credit cards and bank loans in the last fortnight, and has used a number of different names to do so. She says that she is a pop star and needs money to fund a world tour. She was recently discharged from hospital following a depressive episode.
4. A 44-year-old man is arrested and charged with murdering a sandwich shop clerk, who was on his way home from work. He has an extensive forensic history and is a well-known member of an organized criminal gang. He denies any psychiatric history, and admits killing the man because he got his order wrong. He appears cold and emotionless.
5. A 30-year-old man is arrested and charged with setting his neighbour's caravan on fire. He appears to be from a distant town; however, he reports that he used to have contact with psychiatric services as a youngster. He thought his actions would please people in his neighbourhood because the flames were 'pretty'.

BOF answers

Chapter 2 Pharmacological therapy and electroconvulsive therapy

1. B – Looking at his drug kardex. Although the two syndromes have features in common they can nearly always be easily distinguished by medication history (see Fig. 2.11).
2. E – Assess ABC. This man is likely to be experiencing neuroleptic malignant syndrome. After ABC has been addressed all antipsychotics should also be discontinued. The other answers are all possible treatment options, but none are first line. Before they are considered he needs initial resuscitation and then is likely to need transfer to a general hospital for investigation and monitoring. See Fig. 2.11.
3. C – Weekly FBC. Without monitoring, just under 3% of patients treated with clozapine develop neutropenia (low neutrophil count) and just under 1% develop agranulocytosis (negligible neutrophil count). This is most likely to occur early in treatment. Therefore weekly FBC are advised initially. As with all antipsychotics, she will also require regular checks of blood pressure, liver function, lipid profile and glucose. These parameters should be checked 1–3 monthly initially, then annually.
4. E – Egg mayonnaise toastie is the only safe option given the dietary restrictions required for irreversible monoamine oxidase inhibitors such as phenelzine. See Fig. 2.5. They should also avoid drinking Chianti wine with lunch.
5. E – 1.8 mmol/L. Her symptoms are consistent with lithium toxicity in the 1.5–2.0 mmol/L range. However, symptoms of toxicity can manifest at lower levels, particularly in older adults. Toxicity is likely to have been precipitated by the recent course of nonsteroidals. See Fig. 2.6.
6. B – Discontinue lamotrigine. This woman has erythema multiforme with mucosal involvement: Stevens–Johnson syndrome. This can be fatal. It is often drug-induced, and lamotrigine is a candidate cause. Wegener's granulomatosis and HIV can cause erythema multiforme but no reason to suspect them is given in the question so screening is not a priority. Oral aciclovir can be used for recurrent erythema multiforme.

Chapter 3 Psychological therapy

1. C – This man is suffering from a prolonged grief reaction. In the first instance, it would be helpful to refer him to bereavement counselling, which most commonly takes the form of person-centred counselling. In the UK, Cruse are a large voluntary sector run service offering bereavement counselling. Psychodynamic therapy, cognitive-behavioural therapy and mindfulness-based cognitive therapy have little evidence to support their use in this instance. Exposure and response prevention is a behavioural therapy used in the treatment of obsessive-compulsive disorder.
2. B – A comprehensive review of psychotherapy research showed that common factors (operable in any model of therapy) account for 85% of the therapeutic effect, whereas theoretical orientation only accounts for 15%. Common therapeutic factors include client factors (personal strengths, social supports), therapist–client relationship factors (empathy, acceptance, warmth), and the client's expectancy of change. Therefore, the use of a modality with which the patient can identify and work may be more important than the theoretical basis of the therapy itself.
3. C – Transference is the theoretical process by which the patient transfers feelings or attitudes experienced in an earlier significant relationship onto the therapist. Counter-transference refers to the feelings that are evoked in the *therapist* during the course of therapy. The therapist pays attention to noticing these feelings, as these may be representative of what the patient is feeling, and so helps the therapist to empathize with the patient. Often the therapist has undergone therapy themselves as part of their training: this helps the therapist to separate out what feelings belong to them, and what feelings to the patient.
4. A – Assertiveness training is not associated with graded exposure.
5. E – This cognitive distortion is an example of magnification (also known as 'catastrophization'), where things get 'blown out of proportion'. An example of emotional reasoning in this context would be 'I feel so miserable, so I must have failed my exam'. An example of fortune telling would be

'I failed my exam, so in the future no one will employ me'. An example of personalization would be 'it is all my fault: I failed my exams'. An example of labelling would be 'I am stupid'. Note that more than one type of cognitive distortion can exist in the same patient in the same circumstances.

6. B – There is a strong evidence base to support the use of interpersonal therapy in the treatment of mild to moderate depression.

Chapter 4 Mental health and the law

1. E – Patient A lacks capacity as he will not be able to communicate his decisions. Patient B is likely to lack capacity for any decisions requiring more consideration than is available in working memory as he will not be able to retain information for long enough to weigh it up. Patient C lacks capacity for the decision about surgery as she does not believe the information because of a delusion. However, she is likely to have capacity for decisions about which she does not have delusions. Patient D is very likely to lack capacity for this decision as she is unlikely to be able to understand the risks and benefits of contraception. However, she may have capacity for simpler decisions and patients with less severe intellectual disabilities may be able to decide about contraception. Patient E should be assumed to have capacity to make a decision about a statin, unless his psychotic symptoms relate to cholesterol.

2. D – She needs to notify the DVLA of her diagnosis. They will then ask for a doctor's report and potentially a driving assessment, and are likely to arrange more frequent review of the licence than otherwise (e.g. annually). It is the DVLA's decision as to whether she is fit to drive or not. Many patients with mild dementia are found fit to continue to drive. Patient and partner reports of driving can be unreliable as patients can have poor insight and partners may not want to act in a way they perceive as harming the patient, or themselves. It is the patient's responsibility to notify the DVLA although doctors may need to do so if patients ignore this advice and present a significant risk to others through driving.

Chapter 5 Mental health service provision

1. A – The other options demonstrate treatment resistance, bipolar disorder, significant risk to self

and diagnostic uncertainty, all of which means referral to secondary care should be considered.

2. B – Early intervention in psychosis team. This man may be experiencing prodromal psychosis. He does not currently appear to be at high enough risk to require home treatment or admission. As he does not have an established diagnosis of mental illness, an assertive outreach team is not appropriate. A community mental health team could manage him, but early intervention teams are expert at identifying early psychosis so are best placed to monitor him.

Chapter 6 The patient with thoughts of suicide or self-harm

1. D – While all of these symptoms are common in those with depression, suicide is more common in those with insomnia, psychomotor agitation, feelings of worthlessness and psychotic symptoms.

2. A – By far the most common reason given in a large recent study was to 'escape from a terrible state of mind'. This could similarly be described as 'releasing tension'. The other reasons were far less common.

3. C – Measuring serum paracetamol levels (plus INR, liver function, etc.) to determine the requirement for potentially life-saving treatment is the priority in this case. This can be measured from 4 hours post-ingestion although levels become harder to interpret after 15 hours. Psychiatric evaluation and risk assessment can be initiated after this.

4. E – Veterinary surgeons have a very high rate of completed suicide. This may relate to their easy access to lethal medications. There is also a high rate of burnout and stress associated with the job.

5. D – While researching methods is also worrying, acts of closure (such as making a will, organizing finances, writing suicide notes) are the most worrying signs, and may suggest strong suicidal intent. Contacting voluntary support agencies (such as the Samaritans) suggests emotional distress, but also a degree of ambivalence. Telling his wife of his plans may be a way of communicating his feelings to her, but is not necessarily a final act.

6. C – Suspension hanging is the most common method of completed suicide in England and Wales, and many other countries. Means are widely available, and lethality is high. Self-inflicted firearm wounds are most common in the USA. Paracetamol is the most common drug of overdose in the UK;

however, advances in medical treatment and public health measures have reduced mortality associated with this. Jumping from height is a fairly 'public' method of suicide, and is thus often reported in the news (although media coverage of all suicides has reduced in recent years due to campaigns to reduce 'advertising' suitable locations). Carbon monoxide poisoning used to be fairly common; however, catalytic converters on modern motor vehicles has reduced fatality of this method.

Chapter 7 The patient with low mood

1. E – Prednisolone is the only medication listed commonly associated with depression.
2. B – The midline neck swelling may represent a goitre. Given the patient's symptoms are mild, there is time to check her thyroid function. If she is hypothyroid this should be treated first, which may normalize her mood without need for an antidepressant.
3. D – The patient reports a nihilistic delusion. This is mood-congruent. Therefore the most likely diagnosis is depression with psychotic features. Schizoaffective disorder, schizophrenia and bipolar disorder are unlikely to have onset at his age.
4. D – Suicidal ideation should be checked at every appointment.
5. D – This patient is in a situational crisis. It is likely that her symptoms will resolve spontaneously. She needs reassurance and to be offered a follow-up appointment to check on her progress. She cannot be diagnosed with depression as her symptoms are present for less than 2 weeks. However, she may still be at risk of self-harm and should be screened for this.

Chapter 8 The patient with elevated or irritable mood

1. E – Irritability is the commonest mood state in mania, not euphoria. Often patients fluctuate. Delusional mood is seen in the prodrome to schizophrenia (see p. 68).
2. A – Thought disorder due to mania. Dysarthria or Broca's asphasia would not lead to rapid incoherent speech, but to slow, halting speech. A partial seizure would not cause incoherent speech, although confusion may be present postictally. Substance use would be important to exclude.
3. B – Bipolar affective disorder. An episode of depression is not necessary to meet criteria for bipolar affective disorder. Recurrent mania and hypomania are not diagnoses. No first rank symptoms are mentioned, making schizoaffective disorder unlikely.
4. D – Urine drug screen. This will demonstrate recent use of common recreational drugs (although not newer drugs such as 'legal highs'). The main differentials in a healthy young man are a manic episode or mania secondary to psychoactive substance use. FBC should be performed to check for evidence of infection, but is likely to be normal. TFT should be checked to exclude hyperthyroidism but is also likely to be normal. EEG and CT head should only be requested if there are neurological abnormalities.
5. D – Emotionally unstable personality disorder. This woman describes a persistent pattern of maladaptive behaviour present since childhood associated with social and occupational dysfunction. This is a personality disorder. The mood swings are faster than would occur within bipolar affective disorder and she has never had a period of normality, required for a diagnosis of a mental illness. The symptoms cause marked functional impairment, excluding cyclothymia. Dysthymia is prolonged low mood, not mood swings. Although multiple sclerosis can present with emotional lability it would not have onset in childhood.

Chapter 9 The psychotic patient

1. B – Charles Bonnet syndrome. On the basis of the information given here, Charles Bonnet syndrome (see p. 67) is the most likely diagnosis. However, it is crucial to exclude delirium with a physical examination and cognitive assessment.
2. E – Ischaemic heart disease. This man has risk factors for ischaemic heart disease (age, male, smoker) and gives a description of exercise-induced chest pain with a classic 'weight on chest' description typical of cardiac ischaemia. People with schizophrenia may be at increased risk of cardiovascular disease. Although this symptom could also be a tactile hallucination it is important to exclude a physical origin before making this attribution.
3. D – Over-valued idea. Delusional jealousy is the key differential here, but the belief his wife is having an affair appears to be based on logical grounds, so he cannot be said to be delusional. The belief is not described as recurrent or intrusive so is not an obsession. However, the impact of the belief on this man's life is substantial as he has become

preoccupied with it to an unreasonable extent. This is an over-valued idea (see p. 68).

4. E – Psychosis secondary to psychoactive substance use (a drug induced psychosis). This is the most likely diagnosis; however, a definite diagnosis requires a longitudinal assessment. The diagnosis would be confirmed if he stops using substances and his symptoms resolve. However, chronic cannabis use is a risk factor for schizophrenia and if his symptoms persist despite abstaining from substances this may emerge as the diagnosis. At present he has not had the symptoms long enough to meet criteria for schizophrenia in any case.

5. E – Hebephrenic. This boy shows prominent thought disorder, incongruous affect and negative symptoms. Hebephrenic schizophrenia has an early onset and a poor prognosis.

Chapter 10 The patient with anxiety, fear or avoidance

1. D – Panic attack. This is the most likely diagnosis based on the history. However, it is important to take a full medical history (e.g. asthma, congenital heart disease) and family history (e.g. sudden death in young relatives) and to exclude other causes such as hyperthyroidism and hypoglycaemia, particularly given her repeat attendances. It would also be useful to know whether the attacks appear to have triggers (e.g. substance use/withdrawal/going to the library).

2. C – Blood–injection–injury phobia. This is suggested by his situational paroxysmal anxiety and avoidance.

3. B – Observations. The first step in management is ABC. She is speaking to you so her airway is maintained independently. The next step is to ascertain her breathing and circulation status. Although the differential includes a panic attack, she could also be experiencing a wide range of acute medical problems requiring urgent management.

4. E – Check blood sugar. Someone with type 1 diabetes will be receiving insulin. The description sounds very much like hypoglycaemia. If hypoglycaemia is confirmed it is important to treat the episode by consuming carbohydrate, and then examine his insulin/food/activity regime to reduce further episodes.

5. D – Alcohol withdrawal. This man is drinking at least 60 units/week. He is experiencing physiological withdrawal symptoms after a few hours without alcohol, and the symptoms are relieved by further alcohol. Although anxiety in the morning may be part of diurnal variation in a depressive disorder, this man's mood is generally good.

Chapter 11 The patient with obsessions and compulsions

1. A – No mental illness. Lay people often use 'obsession' loosely. Her thoughts of the show are not obsessional as they are ego-syntonic, pleasurable and not resisted. She describes no compulsions. Calling in sick represents unethical behaviour rather than a mental illness.

2. C – Depressive episode. This man reports obsessions, but they are concurrent with the change in his mood, meeting the criteria for a depressive episode of moderate severity (five depressive symptoms). The obsessions are mood-congruent. Depression rather than obsessive-compulsive disorder is the primary diagnosis.

3. D – Obsessive-compulsive disorder with comorbid depressive episode. This man describes obsessions and compulsions associated with functional impairment of greater than 2 weeks duration, giving him a diagnosis of OCD. Superimposed on this he has developed a depressive episode, mild severity (four symptoms).

4. B – Obsessive-compulsive (anankastic) personality disorder. This is suggested by her lifelong history of unusual conscientiousness and perfectionism which has caused some functional impairment (reduction of leisure time and being made redundant). Her thoughts of perfection are ego-syntonic and not resisted, meaning they are not true obsessions. Staying late to check is not a compulsion as it is not an unreasonable way to achieve her goal (assuming she does not check an excessive number of times).

5. B – Pseudohallucination. She reports a perception in the absence of a stimulus from within internal space. A hallucination would occur in external space. An obsession would be attributed to herself. A thought insertion would be attributed to an external agency. See Fig. 11.4.

Chapter 12 The patient with a reaction to a stressful event or bereavement

1. D – It is vital to aggressively exclude physical aetiology prior to attributing symptoms to psychological causes. In this case, excluding intracranial haemorrhage secondary to head injury should take priority. This should include a history of the

mechanism of assault (with corroboration from a witness if possible), full neurological examination, and appropriate investigations (which may include a CT brain).

2. C – This describes symptoms of fairly marked psychomotor retardation, which would be suggestive that a depressive illness has developed from the bereavement reaction. The other symptoms (wanting to be dead, poor concentration, intense guilt, hallucinations involving the deceased) are typical of normal bereavement.

3. B – This woman is suffering from an adjustment disorder, characterized by difficulty coping with a significant change in circumstances. Feelings of inability to cope are fairly typical of difficult adjustment. Note the duration of onset of symptoms, and the fact that she has been signed off work, suggesting disruption to occupational functioning (which suggests that a diagnosis is appropriate, as opposed to 'no mental illness'). Also, she does not appear to be suffering from other symptoms that would suggest an affective or anxiety disorder.

4. B – While traumatic stressors can exacerbate pre-existing (or precipitate initial onset of) major psychotic illnesses such as schizophrenia, developing these as a sole result of trauma is unusual. Acute and transient psychotic illnesses are more common. Note this gentleman is 34 years old. The fact that he has been employed as a soldier is suggestive that he has no pre-existing schizophrenia. Psychotic SYMPTOMS, on the other hand, are very common in those with PTSD as part of the disorder itself, associated with alcohol (alcoholic hallucinosis, withdrawal state), or associated with comorbid depression.

5. A – This case is fairly typical of dissociative amnesia. She has no memory of a circumscribed period of her life, with intact memory for her past and the more recent present. While head trauma is naturally a concern, she appears to have been able to make her way to the UK and apply for asylum, which would suggest that cognitive impairment has not been global, and she has been able to function at a reasonable level. She has no symptoms suggestive of PTSD at this time, and the memory loss is more prolonged than would be expected in this disorder. In terms of stressful events, while she is unable to recall anything, she is seeking asylum from an area in which human rights violations are widely reported. The fact that she was pregnant with no recollection of conception or termination may suggest that she has been the victim of rape (which would be a traumatic stressor).

6. B – According to ICD-10, symptoms must occur within 1 month of the original stressor. This is extended to 3 months when DSM-IV criteria are applied. There is no indication of severity of the actual stressor, and instead it is the subjective experience of the stressor that is important. Suicidal ideation is common in adjustment disorder; however, this is not a criterion. Alcohol consumption may increase, but this is not a criterion. Also, if a patient meets criteria for another psychiatric disorder, this is the diagnosis, not an adjustment disorder.

Chapter 13 The patient with medically unexplained physical symptoms

1. A – These situations are commonly encountered by GPs. The patient may well be developing multiple sclerosis; however, his symptoms are minimal and insufficient to make any diagnosis. Overzealous attempts to take his problems seriously by a well-intentioned doctor (such as referral to neurology, advanced investigations or arranging urgent follow-up) may reinforce his belief that something is wrong. However, dismissal by telling him it is 'all in his head' (or – at this stage – even empathic suggestion of psychiatric illness) is likely to cause him to seek a second opinion, and in any case is irresponsible given the inconclusive evidence. In the first instance, empathic acknowledgement and explanation, and inviting the patient to re-attend if further symptoms arise (watchful waiting) is the most balanced option of the above.

2. D – This lady describes classic symptoms of body dysmorphic disorder, which some consider to be a subtype of hypochondriacal disorder. However, the psychopathology would suggest that she is concerned with her appearance as opposed to an underlying disease. If she did hold the over-valued idea with delusional intensity, somatic delusional disorder should be considered. Note that some patients may exaggerate (or even feign) psychological sequelae of imagined or minor flaws in their appearance in order to receive cosmetic surgery paid for by the state, which would be malingering.

3. E – Irritable bowel syndrome (IBS) is an example of somatoform autonomic dysfunction. Note the absence of other symptoms, the presence of clinical signs, and the fact the gut is largely under autonomic control.

4. D – ICD-10 criteria state that symptoms need to have been present for at least 2 years. If this is not the case but the symptoms are suggestive of

somatoform illness, the diagnosis of 'undifferentiated somatoform disorder' should be considered.

5. D – This history is highly suggestive of factitious disorder (female, healthcare professional, symptoms without signs, great knowledge, specific demands, far from home). It is imperative to contact previous hospitals to get more information; however, asking the patient for such contact details may yield vague answers (in some cases, requesting such details will result in the patient discharging themselves). Details of such patients are often shared between local A&E departments.

6. B – Onset of such symptoms in older people with no significant medical or psychiatric history is more likely to be indicative of insidious organic disease. Prior to attribution of symptoms to a psychological origin, physical disease needs to be aggressively excluded. In this case, physical investigations have been inappropriate to exclude likely physical illnesses.

7. C – This presentation is classic somatization disorder (Briquet's syndrome). Note the multiple and changing symptoms, refusal to accept the absence of physical cause, and duration of more than 2 years.

Chapter 14 The patient with impairment of consciousness, memory or cognition

1. D – Delirium. This is suggested by her acute onset objective cognitive impairment associated with sleep–wake cycle disturbance. Suspicion and visual hallucinations are common in delirium. Although Lewy body dementia is commonly associated with visual hallucinations it is excluded by the acute onset. Similarly Alzheimer's is excluded by the acute onset. Late onset schizophrenia remains a possibility but is far less likely than delirium. Charles Bonnet syndrome would not account for all the features here, e.g. persecutory beliefs, sleep–wake cycle disturbance, cognitive impairment.

2. A – Amnesic syndrome. This man has an isolated long-term anterograde and retrograde memory impairment with intact working memory and other cognitive function. He is confabulating. A history of alcohol excess raises the possibility of Korsakoff's syndrome as the cause. He does not have dementia because the impairment is not global or progressive.

3. D – This gentleman has a likely diagnosis of dementia. NICE (2010) recommends the blood tests this man

has already received, vitamin B_{12} and folate level and structural neuroimaging as a minimum assessment for reversible causes of dementia. However, there is some clinical judgement involved. There is no reason to think this man needs syphilis and HIV serology but for other patients it may be appropriate. Practice varies locally and some centres would not request a CT head unless there are neurological signs. See Fig. 14.13.

4. A – Delirium. This woman has recently been extremely unwell. Even though her UTI has been successfully treated the brain can often lag behind the rest of the body when recovering from a serious illness. The fluctuation in her mental state may reflect a resolving or a new delirium. It would be wise to reassess for other causes that may have been missed initially or occurred since admission, e.g. a hospital acquired pneumonia. It may be that she does not regain her premorbid cognitive functioning and in due course is diagnosed with dementia, but it is too early to make this diagnosis.

5. E – Anticholinergic medication. This man has a delirium. Amitriptyline is sometimes used to reduce insomnia, although this is extremely inadvisable in an older adult, so this may be the precipitant. The other options are all causes of delirium but have been excluded by his normal investigations.

Chapter 15 The patient with alcohol or substance use problems

1. E – The Edwards and Gross criteria do not include 'increased use of other substances'.

2. D – This is classic alcoholic hallucinosis. Note the absence of memory or attentional problems. Late onset schizophrenia should be in the differential diagnosis, but is unlikely in this case.

3. D – This man's presentation is highly suggestive of delirium, and the history of heavy alcohol use is likely to be of aetiological significance. Note the 'lilliputian hallucinations' – visual hallucinations of small figures (in his case, a horse). Any surgical intervention should be delayed pending clinical improvement. Also note that it is very difficult to exclude Wernicke–Korsakoff syndrome in delirious patients, and therefore this should be empirically treated with parenteral thiamine.

4. C – Prior to any substitute prescribing, it is vital to establish that the drug being substituted is actually being used, making urine drug testing the first step.

5. B – To calculate alcohol units, take the %ABV and multiply by volume (in litres): e.g. $40 \times 0.350 = 14$ units; 350 mL of a 40% ABV spirit contains

14 units. Six pints (3.408 L) of continental lager (5.3%ABV) contains 18 units; two bottles (1.5 L) of red wine (12.5%ABV) contains 18.75 units; 3 L of strong white cider (8.4%ABV) contains 25.2 units; and six bottles (1.980 L) of alco-pops (4.9% ABV) contains 9.7 units. It should be recommended that she takes no more than 2–3 units per sitting, and has at least two alcohol-free days per week.

6. E – Hypotension is not generally associated with cocaine intoxication. More commonly, blood pressure is significantly increased during intoxication with cocaine. Hypotension may be observed as a result of cardiac arrhythmia associated with cocaine use/toxicity, which would suggest imminent circulatory collapse ('peri-arrest'), necessitating emergency treatment with antiarrhythmics, cardioversion and intensive specialist in-patient care.

Chapter 16 The patient with personality problems

1. A – Chronic feelings of emptiness is the only criterion listed here for borderline personality disorder. According to DSM-IV, diagnosis of borderline personality disorder requires a pervasive pattern of instability of interpersonal relationships, self-image and affects, as well as marked impulsivity, beginning by early adulthood and present in a variety of contexts.

2. D – This man is likely to have schizoid personality disorder, as suggested by his stable and pervasive traits of social isolation and indifference to the opinions of others, with no evidence of an axis 1 mental disorder.

3. C – This man is likely to have antisocial personality disorder. Antisocial personality disorder is very prevalent within prisons.

4. C – The difficulties associated with personality disorders start in adolescence or early adulthood. Also, the enduring pattern of psychological experience should be longstanding and relatively stable over time – not only when stressed. It should manifest in at least two domains (cognition, affect, interpersonal functioning, impulse control), and should appear inflexible and pervasive across a wide range of situations, leading to clinically significant distress or impairment in important areas of functioning. The pattern must not be better accounted for as a manifestation of another mental disorder, or to the direct physiological effects of a substance (e.g. drug or medication) or a general medical condition (e.g. head trauma).

5. E – In this case, there is too little information to make or exclude any diagnosis. The man is in a state of emotional distress following a significant life event (breakdown of a relationship, potential homelessness), which is compounded with acute intoxication. Initial management should focus on physical care, alleviating distress, ensuring his (and her) safety, and achieving sobriety. Further psychiatric assessment (including collateral history) at a later time is needed to establish a diagnosis, or absence of mental illness.

6. D – Obsessive thoughts are not ego-dystonic ('against the mind') or distressing in obsessive compulsive personality disorder. Instead, they are ego-syntonic ('with the mind'). This is one of the main features that distinguishes the psychopathology of obsessive-compulsive personality disorder from obsessive-compulsive disorder. The rest of the answers are true.

7. A – From this man's difficulties, it is likely that he has borderline personality disorder. Note the link between childhood sexual abuse and borderline personality disorder.

Chapter 17 The patient with eating or weight problems

1. A – A body weight of at least 15% below expected for height is suggestive of anorexia nervosa. Patients with bulimia nervosa are often of normal or increased weight. Preoccupation with being thin, as well as a dread of fatness and a distorted perception of being too fat are associated with both anorexia and bulimia nervosa. Again, use of medication and exercise as means of controlling weight can occur in both disorders.

2. C – While patients with eating disorders often deny their symptoms, it is very important to exclude insidious physical illness as a cause of weight loss before attributing to psychiatric disorder. Physical causes can include malignancy, inflammatory disorders, infection and endocrine abnormalities. In this case, assessment of weight loss by a paediatrician would be helpful.

3. E – The use of alcohol or substances, along with resultant self-neglect, can cause significant weight loss. Prior to diagnosing an affective, anxiety or eating disorder, a thorough drug and alcohol history should be taken to exclude this as a cause. Bear in mind that drug or alcohol misuse can also be a comorbidity of many other psychiatric disorders.

4. C – Patients with anorexia nervosa usually have high serum cholesterol (hypercholesterolaemia). All

other abnormalities occur frequently in starvation states.

5. D – This lady has anorexia nervosa. She is dangerously underweight. While all of the above mental illnesses can cause weight loss, they are differentiated from specific eating disorders by the presence of dread of fatness, distortion of body image and subsequent restriction of her dietary intake. Although it is not sure whether she is vomiting or not, the diagnosis of bulimia is unlikely given her restrictive pattern of eating and her low BMI (if she was vomiting, this could be described as 'anorexia nervosa, purging type' rather than 'restrictive type').

Chapter 18 The mood (affective) disorders

1. E – Treatment-resistant depression is an indication for ECT but if the patient has capacity and does not wish it, it is not given. No information is given to suggest she lacks capacity, which is presumed to be present in adults unless proven otherwise. Life-threatening reduction in oral intake, psychotic depression and previous good response to ECT are all other indications for ECT.

2. C – Admission under mental health legislation. This man is experiencing a manic episode with psychotic features. His psychotic beliefs place him at high risk of injury or death and are impairing his ability to make decisions regarding management of his mental health. It is not safe to let him go home and police custody is not appropriate given his behaviour is driven by illness. He may be persuadable to be admitted informally but if not he would meet criteria for detention under mental health legislation (see Ch. 4).

3. D – Citalopram and quetiapine. This man has a severe depressive episode with psychotic features. A combination of an antidepressant and an antipsychotic is indicated. Citalopram is normally tried before amitriptyline as it has fewer side-effects. Also, amitriptyline is more toxic than citalopram in overdose. Given his suicidal ideation it is best to choose the less toxic medication. Quetiapine or any other second generation antipsychotic would be reasonable to treat his psychosis.

4. A – Her family history suggests she has may have genes that increase her susceptibility to depression. All the other options are risk factors for depression too, but no information is given in the question to suggest them.

5. B – Olanzapine. Olanzapine, lithium or valproate are the antimanic agents recommended by NICE (2006). Lithium should not be started in the acute situation in someone with a history of non-concordance. Valproate should be avoided where possible in a woman of childbearing age. Lamotrigine is not recommended during acute mania. Citalopram, or any other antidepressant, should be discontinued in a manic patient. This woman is likely also to need rapid tranquillization with a benzodiazepine (see p. 146).

6. C – Individual cognitive-behavioural therapy. Self-help CBT and structured group physical activity are recommended by NICE for mild depression (2011). Dialectical behaviour therapy is a psychological therapy for borderline personality disorder. Graded exposure therapy is used to treat obsessive-compulsive disease and phobias.

Chapter 19 The psychotic disorders: schizophrenia

1. B – If one parent has schizophrenia, the probability of their offspring having schizophrenia is 13%. The population lifetime risk is 1%. See Fig. 19.1.

2. E – If both parents have schizophrenia, the probability of their offspring having schizophrenia is 50%. The population lifetime risk is 1%. See Fig. 19.1.

3. C – This is a difficult question as there is little solid evidence about the optimum period of treatment for a first episode of psychosis. Without prophylactic antipsychotics following a first episode of schizophrenia, over half of patients will relapse within a year. The current recommendation is to continue antipsychotics for 1–2 years after a first episode. However, many patients wish to stop sooner. In this case, a gradual reduction over a few weeks reduces the risk of relapse. Alternatively, this man may prefer to switch to an antipsychotic less associated with weight gain.

4. D – Cognitive-behavioural therapy. The other modalities are not recommended in schizophrenia. Family therapy is also recommended if the patient lives with or is in close contact with their family.

5. D – Temperature, pulse, blood pressure and respiratory rate should be checked every 5–10 minutes following any parenteral administration of rapid tranquillization. Observations should be every 5–10 minutes for 1 hour, then every half hour until the patient is able to walk. If the patient refuses or remains too behaviourally disturbed to allow observations, they should be regularly observed for

respiratory effort, airway and consciousness level. If the patient has received haloperidol or is at high risk of arrhythmia for other reasons, ECG monitoring is also advised. See Fig. 19.3.

6. E – Hypoglycaemia. Hypoglycaemia is unlikely – hyperglycaemia secondary to stress would be expected. She is at increased risk of all the other options: benzodiazepines can cause respiratory depression, over-sedation by any means can cause loss of airway, antipsychotics and hyperarousal increase the risk of arrhythmia and benzodiazepines and antipsychotics can both cause hypotension. Further complications of antipsychotic use include seizures and dystonias. All these complications can occur with oral formulations also, but are more likely when large doses are given via a fast acting method.

Chapter 20 The anxiety and somatoform disorders

1. D – Social phobia and OCD have roughly equal prevalence in men and women. All other anxiety disorders, and depression, are more common in women.

2. E – Around half of patients with post-traumatic stress disorder will recover fully within 3 months. Around half of patients with panic disorder will recover fully within 3 years. The other anxiety disorders are more likely to have a chronic course.

3. E – Specific phobia. SSRI is the first line pharmacological option for moderate to severe forms of all other anxiety disorders (for PTSD, mirtazapine is an alternative first line treatment). This man has a severe disorder in view of the impact of his symptoms on his ability to work.

4. B – Seeing patients with anxiety about their physical health on a regular basis can help contain their anxieties and reduce the total number and number of urgent appointments they need. However, this does not mean they should not be allowed access to urgent appointment slots – they will experience physical health problems along with somatization. Similarly, investigations should be carefully considered and avoided if possible, but some are likely to still be required to safely exclude other disorders. Benzodiazepines are not indicated for somatization disorder, but may be indicated for some other reason. The nature of somatization disorder should be explained to patients, but it should not be done in a confrontational manner. Phrases such as 'all in the mind' should be avoided as patients are genuinely experiencing symptoms. See Fig. 20.4.

5. B – Cognitive-behavioural therapy with desensitization is recommended for phobias with mild to severe functional impairment. Trauma-focused CBT is for post-traumatic stress disorder. PRN diazepam would not be advisable given she is likely to come into contact with bodily fluids on a daily basis. SSRIs are not recommended for specific phobias.

6. C – An SSRI is the first line drug therapy for obsessive-compulsive disorder. Clomipramine is a second line drug therapy. Mirtazapine and pregabalin are not recommended by current guidelines. Self-help is recommended for mild symptoms but this woman's symptoms are associated with marked functional impairment. Talking therapies are first line for moderate to severe OCD and she should be encouraged to reconsider a talking therapy if a SSRI is ineffective.

Chapter 21 Alcohol and substance-related disorders

1. B – This man is currently contemplating changing his behaviour. He recognizes the need for change (he wants to give up), but is ambivalent about it (worrying he will lose all his friends). Motivational interviewing may be helpful to allow him to progress to the next stage of preparation for change.

2. E – Prior to prescribing methadone, it is essential to confirm the use of opiates. A urine drug test can be used to do this. Admission to psychiatric hospital is not necessary, although dose titration should be undertaken in a controlled clinical environment with facilities to measure physiological response to opiates, and with emergency treatment for opiate toxicity (i.e. naloxone) close to hand. Viral serology testing and physical examination is important screening for health complications from intravenous drug use, but is not necessary for a methadone prescription. Forcing a patient to identify a confidant for the purposes of corroboration can lead to problems, either placing false security in a possibly inaccurate historian, or causing disengagement with services.

3. D – Methylphenidate (Ritalin) is frequently (legitimately) prescribed. However, unlawful possession (i.e. without a prescription) or unauthorized supply (i.e. someone who is prescribed the drug selling/giving it to someone without a prescription) is an offence. Methylphenidate is considered to be a Class B

drug under the Act, therefore supplying/dealing can result in a maximum of 14 years custodial sentence, or an unlimited fine, or both. Heroin (diamorphine) used to be prescribed as an analgesic but is generally avoided now.

4. C – Naltrexone is an opioid receptor antagonist. This may control cravings, and reduces the pleasurable effects of drinking alcohol, reducing 'reward' and – by operant conditioning – can 'extinguish' the desire to drink (the 'Sinclair method'). Disulfiram causes an unpleasant reaction when taken with alcohol. Acamprosate may be helpful in controlling cravings. Long-term antidepressants or benzodiazepines are not recommended for the sole purpose of maintaining abstinence; however, antidepressants may be helpful for treating comorbid depression.

5. A – A needle exchange service, where users can obtain clean syringes, hypodermics and preparation equipment, has the role of reducing the risks of injecting (not the risks of the drug itself). Therefore this is an example of a 'harm reduction service.

6. C – Buprenorphine (Subutex) is a partial opioid agonist, and can be used for substitution therapy. The other drugs can be used in treating various stages of opiate dependence; however, none are true 'substitutes'.

Chapter 22 The personality disorders

1. D – Patients with borderline personality disorder require far longer durations of treatment than those with depression, and therefore are far costlier to treat. The prevalence of comorbid substance misuse is incredibly high in patients with borderline personality disorder, and the lifetime risk of completing suicide is also very high (1 in 10 sufferers of borderline personality disorder will complete suicide). Borderline personality disorder patients also tend to be more difficult to engage in psychotherapy, and are usually far less responsive to treatment with antidepressants than patients with depression.

2. D – In the treatment of patients with antisocial personality disorder, a history of violence towards others is a predictor of a negative treatment outcome. Other factors associated with a negative response include: history of arrest and conviction for a crime; a history of repeated lying, confidence tricks or the use of aliases; unresolved legal situations on admission; hospitalization as an alternative to imprisonment; and the presence of an organic brain disorder. Predictors of a positive response to therapy include the presence of anxiety, diagnosis of depression and diagnosis of psychosis (other than organic conditions).

3. E – The Cochrane Collaboration systematic review included 27 randomized controlled trials. As well as showing that flupentixol decanoate (depot) reduced suicidal behaviour, it concluded that current evidence from RCTs suggested that drug treatment – especially mood stabilizers (topiramate, lamotrigine, valproate semisodium) and the second generation antipsychotics olanzapine and aripiprazole – may be effective in treating a number of core symptoms and associated psychopathology of borderline personality disorder. However, it acknowledged that the clinical evidence did not currently support effectiveness for any drug treatment in reducing the overall severity of borderline personality disorder, and recommended that pharmacotherapy should be targeted at specific symptoms.

4. C – Psychodynamic psychotherapy is intentionally unstructured, and agendas are never set by the therapist. This is to allow exploration of what is (unconsciously) important to the patient without interference.

5. E – Consideration should be given to the 'weekly dispensing' of any prescribed medication, to avoid the patient having immediate access to large quantities of potentially harmful drugs which they may impulsively take in overdose. Psychological therapies can be helpful, even during periods of acute illness. Care plans may need to be changed to allow for increased support during periods of depression. Benzodiazepines should be avoided if possible, due to the risk of dependence or misuse. Admission to a psychiatric ward may be necessary to manage risk or to treat severe illness; however, this can prove counterproductive and other measures should be considered in the first instance.

6. C – Given the significant risk to another person, confidentiality needs to be broken in this case. The psychiatrist has a duty to immediately warn the police. Also, the specific and detailed content of the threat necessitates that the intended victim be warned (see the Tarasoff case for further details). The responsibility for this falls on the doctor; however, in practice the police will usually be happy to facilitate this. Detention under mental health legislation would not be appropriate, as the threat should be addressed by law enforcement agencies in the first instance. Meticulous notes would need to be kept. It is likely that he would be held criminally responsible for his actions.

Chapter 23 Eating disorders

1. D − Around 5% (1 in 20) of the female population have eating habits that give cause for concern. Most of these women are between the ages of 14 and 25 years. Anorexia nervosa, and indeed eating disorders in general, are about 10 times more common in females than males. About 0.5–1% have a diagnosis of bulimia nervosa. Anorexia nervosa used to be considered to be more common in higher socioeconomic classes; however, the evidence for this is variable and continues to be debated (both anorexia nervosa and bulimia nervosa are thought probably to have an equal prevalence across socioeconomic classes). Eating disorders are more common in gymnasts, ballet dancers and athletes.

2. B − Bulimia nervosa is commonly associated with a long history of exposure to dieting behaviour. There is subsequently often a history of childhood obesity, parental obesity and early menarche. Genetic factors are thought to play a significant role in the aetiology of bulimia nervosa although individual genes have not yet been identified. Family enmeshment (over-involvement between parent and child) is more commonly associated with anorexia nervosa, and sufferers of bulimia nervosa often have conflict-ridden family dynamics. Substance misuse is a common comorbidity in bulimia nervosa. Previously, a history of childhood sexual abuse was thought to be common in individuals with bulimia nervosa; however, recent studies have shown that rates of this are about the same as for other mental illnesses, suggesting that it is a general risk factor for all mental illnesses rather than just bulimia nervosa.

3. A − Personality traits commonly seen in individuals with anorexia nervosa include perfectionism, harm-avoidance, inhibition and obsessionality. Novelty-seeking personality traits are associated with impulsivity and often recklessness, and are more frequently seen in patients with addictions.

4. E − Motivational interviewing would probably be the most useful in the first instance. He does not feel that there is a problem; however, the fact that he is agreeable to meeting a therapist is suggestive that he may have some ambivalence. Motivational interviewing uses Prochaska and DiClemente's Transtheoretical Model of Change, and focuses on helping patients consider the need to change behaviour. All the other modalities may be useful in treating the illness, and should be considered once he feels that he is ready to change his behaviour.

5. C − The presence of binge–purge symptoms are associated with a poorer prognosis in sufferers of anorexia nervosa, as is late age of onset, very low weight (not rapid weight loss), long duration of illness, personality difficulties, difficult family relationships and poor social adjustment. The presence of a family history of anorexia is not necessarily indicative of poor prognosis, neither is the rate of engagement with psychotherapy.

Chapter 24 Disorders relating to the menstrual cycle, pregnancy and the puerperium

1. C − While 'mood swings' are thought to be a common symptom of the premenstrual syndrome, elevated mood is not. If a woman presents with elevated mood and a cyclical pattern of symptoms, diagnoses such as bipolar affective disorder, cyclothymia or substance use should be considered.

2. E − While the woman in the case description attributes her symptoms to the menopause, the duration of the symptoms accompanied by the presence of suicidal thoughts are more suggestive of a depressive illness. Around the menopausal years, there can be an increase in psychosocial stressors (children leaving home, 'facing up' to growing older, changes in personal relationships, etc.), which may increase the risk of developing depression independently of the hormonal changes that arise during the menopause. Thus, psychological therapies and social supports may be helpful. Hormone replacement therapy can be useful in certain circumstances; however, it does not suit everyone, and should not be used as a substitute for a recognized antidepressant in the management of major depression. The use of omega-3 fish oils as treatment for depression during the menopause is currently being studied, but at the time of writing there is insufficient evidence to support this. Dietary and lifestyle advice (avoiding alcohol, tobacco, eating a balanced diet, exercising) should be given to all patients who report low mood.

3. B − Lithium is thought to be teratogenic, and is probably associated with the development of Ebstein's anomaly (a congenital heart defect). While the relative risk is increased, the absolute risk still remains fairly low. This needs to be balanced with the individual risk of relapse on stopping lithium (as acute mental illness and associated risk-taking behaviours or acute phase drug treatment are likely to have a profound effect on the fetus). Discussion of risks and

benefits of stopping vs not stopping the lithium can help women make informed choices. Ultimately, the doctor is responsible for prescribing the drug, but this should be in the best interests of the patient, and therefore the decision should be made jointly. If lithium is continued, the dose will need carefully monitored (as changes in body water during pregnancy can affect levels). Sodium valproate carries a much higher risk of teratogenicity, and should be avoided during pregnancy. This woman is at high risk of relapse should she become pregnant and should be referred to perinatal psychiatry services prior to conception.

4. E – Reassurance that she will not become unwell cannot be given. This lady has a history of postnatal depression and is at greatly increased risk of suffering a further episode. She should be referred to the perinatal mental health team. Given this history, and also her good response to medications in the past, commencing antidepressant treatment later in pregnancy or in the early postpartum may be beneficial. The perinatal mental health team would explore the risks vs benefits of this option. When choosing an agent, consideration should be given to previously effective drugs, and the mother's choice to breast feed.

5. D – A troubled relationship is not thought to be a major risk factor for puerperal psychosis; however, it is a risk factor for postnatal depression. The rest of the list above are considered to be risk factors for the development of puerperal psychosis.

Chapter 25 Dementia and delirium

1. A – Aromatherapy. This woman has a behavioural and psychological symptom of dementia. Non-pharmacological options are recommended as first line by NICE (2010), unless there is immediate risk of harm or severe distress. Referral to speech and language therapy is unlikely to be of benefit given her severe dementia.

2. C – Vascular and Alzheimer's dementia. Vascular risk factors are important for both these dementias.

3. A – Antipsychotics. Antipsychotics can cause irreversible severe parkinsonian reactions in patients with Lewy body dementia. The other options may all potentially be of benefit – if his delusion is due to concurrent infection (antibiotics), depression (antidepressants) or worsening dementia – cholinesterase inhibitors can improve behavioural and psychological symptoms of dementia. Nutritional supplements

may be of benefit whatever the cause if he is losing weight.

4. C – Co-codamol. This contains both codeine and paracetamol. Opiates are very common causes of delirium in older adults. Opiates are often started during acute admissions for pain or surgery.

5. D – Acute medical ward. This lady is delirious. This is a medical emergency. She needs to be fully physically investigated. Her acute onset psychotic symptoms are almost certainly due to her delirium, not a psychiatric disorder.

Chapter 26 Older adult psychiatry

1. A – Antidepressant. The key issue here is the diagnosis. She presents with a common triad in older adults: depressive symptoms, cognitive impairment and functional impairment. It is often difficult to tease out whether someone is experiencing a pseudodementia (depression manifesting as dementia) or an early dementia leading to comorbid depression. Ideally depression is treated first, then cognition reassessed once mood is euthymic. An antidepressant would be preferable to counselling for treating depression in this lady as her cognitive impairment is likely to limit the benefit of psychological therapies.

2. C – Depressive episode. It is common for depression to manifest with prominent features of anxiety, psychomotor agitation and hypochondriacal ideas in older adults. Mild cognitive impairment is the next most likely differential – although her MMSE of 28/30 is reassuring, a more sensitive test such as the ACE-R may still show an objective impairment. Generalized anxiety disorder or hypochondriacal disorder are unlikely to have onset so late in life, and diagnosis would require a longer duration of symptoms. There are no psychotic features to suggest schizophrenia.

3. A – ECT. All of the suggested management strategies are reasonable but ECT is preferable because of this man's potentially life-threatening poor oral intake and poor concordance. Depot medication would get round the concordance problem but is not as effective as ECT and would take longer to work. ECT is the quickest and most effective treatment for depression known and seems to work particularly well in older adults.

4. B – All of these patients could potentially have late onset schizophrenia. However, symptoms of late onset schizophrenia are predominantly delusional, rather than bizarre or negative symptoms (as in patients A and C). Patient D is more likely to have Charles Bonnet syndrome (see p. 67). Late onset

schizophrenia is far more common in women than men, and social deprivation and hearing impairment are also risk factors.

5. D – Continue mirtazapine for at least 8 weeks. Older adults can take longer to show response to antidepressants, so an adequate trial is at least 8 weeks. Augmentation is not necessary at this stage and increases the risk of drug interactions. Tricyclics are best avoided in older adults because of dangerous side-effects.

6. E – Delirium. This lady has acute onset cognitive impairment: delirium until proven otherwise. The history is concerningly suggestive of a focal seizure. She needs admitted to a medical ward for investigation. A manic or hypomanic episode would be highly unlikely to have such a rapid onset. Were she on lithium, it would be crucial to check a random lithium level as her presentation could also be due to lithium toxicity.

7. B – This is the simplest and easiest of the options. If concordance remains poor despite this, prompting by a carer could be considered. A depot could be useful if the patient wishes it, or his insight reduces and he requires compulsory treatment. Daily dispensing is normally reserved for methadone or for those at high risk of overdose. In general, simplifying medication regimes to once daily is a good idea, but unfortunately olanzapine is likely to be too sedating to allow use in the mornings. Potentially his other once daily medication could be changed to the evening.

8. E – Refer for urgent psychiatric review. This lady has recently attempted to commit suicide. Older adults are at high risk of completed suicide. She may perceive taking extra benzodiazepines as far more harmful than they actually are, as she may have memories of barbiturates – highly toxic sleeping tablets which were fatal in minor overdose. Her ongoing intent is unclear from the vignette. She may require admission or urgent community support from mental health services.

Chapter 27 Child and adolescent psychiatry

1. B – According to DSM-IV, some of the core symptoms need to be present before the age of 7 years to make the diagnosis of ADHD. This is not to say that ADHD cannot be diagnosed in children older than 7 years: often, it is not diagnosed until their behaviour causes problems in school or other situations.

2. A – In Asperger's syndrome, there are no significant abnormalities in language acquisition and ability,

or in cognitive development and intelligence. Indeed, IQ and language may be superior in some cases.

3. D – Rett's syndrome is an X-linked dominant disorder, and so it occurs almost exclusively in girls. All other pervasive developmental disorders are more common in boys.

4. E – Conduct disorder is associated with the development of antisocial personality disorder, criminality and substance misuse in later life. It is approximately four times as common in boys than girls. Oppositional defiant disorder is often considered to be a 'milder' variant of conduct disorder, where defiant behaviour is characteristic, but this tends not to involve criminality or violating the rights of others. Truancy, as opposed to school refusal, is commonly seen.

5. C – Normally, the age criterion used to define enuresis in children is 5 years old, in children whose chronological age corresponds with their development. It is thought that, by this stage, children should have established consistent bladder control.

6. B – Given the effectiveness of first generation antipsychotics (dopamine antagonists) in reducing tics, functional excess of dopamine is thought to be implicated in the aetiology of tic disorders.

7. E – Vaginal trauma and genital warts are not normal in an 8-year-old girl, and the findings should immediately raise suspicions of sexual abuse. The safety of the child is paramount, and steps should be taken to maintain this. While protocols vary slightly between areas, child protection procedures usually advise contacting the duty social worker and/or the local paediatrician on-call for child protection. If in any doubt about a possible child protection concern, either of these parties will usually be more than happy to offer guidance. The child should not be directly asked about what happened at this stage: a formal interview needs to be arranged involving police, social work and paediatric staff. Police will not question the girl just now. Parents should never be 'confronted' by medical staff; however, it is obviously courteous (if possible) to let them know what is going on and what will happen next. The child should not be allowed home until all relevant agencies are involved and safety at home can be ensured. This may not be possible, and an alternative place of safety may have to be sought. Should the parent remove the child from safety, it would be appropriate to contact the police given the magnitude of the concerns.

Chapter 28 Intellectual disability

1. C – Profound intellectual disabilities are diagnosed when IQ is estimated to be less than 20. These people comprise about 1–2% of all people with intellectual disabilities. They are severely limited in their abilities, often have severe motor impairment, and invariably need nursing care in adulthood – usually in a residential setting. However, they can be diagnosed with depression, can benefit from behavioural therapies and aetiology is (more often than not) known.

2. B – From the list given, Alzheimer's disease is the most commonly diagnosed mental disorder in patients with Down's syndrome. This is thought to be because of the triplication of chromosome 21, and the subsequent over-expression of the amyloid precursor protein which is located on chromosome 21.

3. D – Fragile X syndrome is the most common single-gene cause of autism, and the most common inherited cause of intellectual disability. It is caused by the expansion of the CGG trinucleotide repeat affecting the Fragile X mental retardation 1 (or FMR1) gene on the X chromosome. Because men have only one X chromosome they are more severely affected by the mutation. It results in a spectrum of intellectual disability ranging from mild to severe, as well as physical characteristics such as an elongated face, large or protruding ears, and larger testes (macroorchidism), behavioural characteristics such as stereotypical movements (e.g. hand-flapping), and social anxiety.

4. C – Individuals with moderate intellectual disabilities have limited (but not absent) language and comprehension skills. Some can sustain employment if well supported: usually simple practical work. They tend to require some assistance with self-care and supported living but do not tend to need full-time nursing care.

5. D – Simple psychosocial and environmental interventions often have long-term benefits. When a behavioural disturbance occurs in an individual with intellectual disability, it is important to consider what may have changed in their life. This may include changes to accommodation or carers, changes to routine or social circumstances, changes in the family (e.g. divorce, bereavement), physical illness (e.g. toothache, constipation). Behavioural disturbances can be associated with the onset of comorbid mental illness, but this is less common. The aetiology of the intellectual disability can help guide management. Psychotropic medication can be helpful, but should be given in conjunction with appropriate psychosocial supports. Admission to a specialist unit may be required in extreme cases; however, the individual should continue to be supported in their own (familiar) environment if possible.

Chapter 29 Forensic psychiatry

1. C – An individual being considered unfit to plead through mental illness is relatively uncommon. In England and Wales, fitness to plead is determined by the Pritchard criteria (the M'Naghten Rule applies to mens rea, and being not guilty by reason of insanity at the time of the alleged offence, which is a different concept). Amnesia for the offence does not mean that the accused cannot stand trial (although someone who is unfit to plead might also have amnesia for the offence). While not always the case, the court will usually recommend that the accused is transferred to a secure psychiatric hospital for assessment and/or treatment.

2. A – Among stalkers with psychotic disorders, delusions of love are most commonly present. This is known as erotomania or De Clerambault syndrome, and is characterized by the abnormal belief that the subject of the stalking is in love with the perpetrator. Approximately one in three members of the Royal College of Psychiatrists have experienced stalking behaviours that met the legal definition of harassment.

3. E – Exhibitionism is considered as a psychiatric disorder by ICD-10, under the classification of paraphilia. It rarely immediately precedes violent sexual assault. Individuals with intellectual disability are over-represented in the statistics, although this may reflect the fact that the perpetrator is often known to the victim and therefore the rate of detection is high. Recidivism (re-offending) rates are fairly low, although those who do are more likely to commit more serious sexual crimes in the future.

4. C – Command hallucinations are associated with an increased risk of violence in patients with schizophrenia. People with psychotic disorders are approximately eight times more likely than members of the general public to acquire convictions for violent offences. There is no strong association between sexual offending and active psychotic symptoms. Comorbid substance misuse significantly increases the risk of violent offending in patients with psychotic disorder. There are far

higher arrest rates among psychiatrically ill patients than offenders without mental illness.

5. E – Murder is the only charge for which diminished responsibility may apply. If the accused is found to have diminished responsibility, the conviction is reduced to manslaughter (or culpab Scotland). This was particularly import historically when murder carried the deat

6. C – The best predictor of future violence is pa violence.

le homicide in
ant
h penalty.
st

EMQ answers

1.

1. C – Propranolol. This woman is probably experiencing akathisia. This is hard to treat but propranolol or benzodiazepines can help. See Fig. 2.10. Ideally the dose of antipsychotic is reduced. Quinine can be used for restless leg syndrome when in bed. The differential includes agitation secondary to psychosis.

2. F – Intramuscular procyclidine. This woman is experiencing a dystonia with an oculogyric crisis and trismus. Her clenched jaw means oral procyclidine is not possible. Baclofen and dantrolene are for chronic spasticity.

3. G – Rescuscitation. This woman is acutely unwell. She needs ABC and probably a peri-arrest call/999 ambulance. She may have neuroleptic malignant syndrome, or a range of other differentials (e.g. meningitis, substance intoxication). Dantrolene is not an emergency treatment and is not indicated until the diagnosis is clearer.

4. B – Oral procyclidine. This man has drug-induced parkinsonism. In the early stages the features are different to idiopathic parkinsonism. Anticholinergics can help but ideally the dose of antipsychotic would be reduced or an alternative antipsychotic trialled.

5. D – Stop anticholinergics. This man has tardive dyskinesia. This is hard to treat but stopping anticholinergics (in this case procyclidine) and reducing or withdrawing antipsychotics if possible can help.

2.

1. A – This is an example of acting out: behaving in a certain way in order to express thoughts or feelings that the person feels otherwise incapable of expressing.

2. H – Countertransference is the process whereby the therapist unconsciously interacts with the patient as if they were a significant figure from the patient's past.

3. D – Catharsis is a Greek word meaning 'cleansing' or 'purging'. It is often used to describe a feeling of relief after an outpouring of emotive material.

4. E – Parapraxis is a term used to describe an error of memory, speech, writing, reading or action that may be due to the interference of repressed thoughts and unconscious features of the individual's personality. It is referred to in common culture as a 'slip of the tongue' or a 'Freudian slip'.

5. J – Working through describes the concept of working over one's emotional difficulties from the past. In psychotherapy, it usually follows an 'impasse', which can be thought of as a therapeutic stalemate.

3.

1. C – Mentalization is the process by which we implicitly and explicitly interpret the actions of ourselves and others as meaningful on the basis of intentional mental states. Mentalization-based therapy is a treatment intended to improve the capacity to mentalize, which is often a specific difficulty in those with borderline personality disorder. This is thought to improve emotional regulation and interpersonal relationships.

2. K – Interpersonal therapy is based on the assumptions that problems with interpersonal relationships and social functioning contribute significantly to mental illness. Main areas of focus include role disputes, role transitions, interpersonal deficits and grief.

3. I – Systematic desensitization is a type of behavioural therapy that can be useful in the treatment of phobias. It involves compilation of a hierarchy of phobic stimuli (e.g. standing at the front door, going into the garden, going to the end of the street, going to the supermarket) and – with support from the therapist and the use of appropriate relaxation techniques – working through the hierarchy in order to face increasingly anxiety-provoking scenarios.

4. B – Cognitive-behavioural therapy can be useful in the treatment of post-traumatic stress disorder. The 'wiggly finger' type of therapy that the gentleman in the scenario describes is eye movement desensitization and reprocessing, which can also be helpful for some; however, evidently not in this case.

5. F – Exposure and response prevention is a type of behavioural therapy in which the patient is encouraged not to respond to the obsessional thought with a compulsive act. Relaxation techniques are used instead to overcome the anxiety associated with not carrying out the compulsion.

4.

1. F – Borderline personality disorder. She is a young woman with a long history of self-harm, difficulties with interpersonal relationships and auditory pseudohallucinations at times of stress. Of note, she has no symptoms suggestive of a depressive illness.

2. J – Severe depression with psychotic features. This man has made a serious suicide attempt. Note that he went to some effort to prevent discovery (remote location, unsocial hour) and made acts of closure (typed letters implies that some thought had gone into these). He has biological and psychotic symptoms of depression. He may have intoxicated himself to reduce his inhibitions prior to the act and is not necessarily alcohol dependent.

3. E – Mania with psychosis. This young man's self-inflicted injuries are in keeping with his grandiose beliefs (of a religious nature), of which he is entirely convinced. He is disinhibited and feels that he has special powers. He also exhibits flight of ideas on mental state examination. Important differential diagnoses in this case would be a drug-induced state, or an organic illness.

4. G – Recurrent depressive disorder of moderate severity would be the most fitting of the listed diagnoses. Note the pattern of previous periods of illness, punctuated by periods of relatively good functioning. There is no mention of psychotic symptoms, and drugs or alcohol are not thought to be implicated.

5. B – Anorexia nervosa. Although a full history and physical examination would be required to definitively establish this diagnosis, the patient's history and presentation is fairly typical of a serious eating disorder. Note the baggy clothes and the 'lanugo' hair. Anorexia nervosa is much more common in females, but males also suffer from it.

5.

1. F – Overdoses of medicinal drugs account for 80–90% of self-harm presentations to hospitals in the UK.

2. B – This was previously a relatively common method of suicide, as domestic gas was derived from coal. This had a high concentration of carbon monoxide, which meant it was regularly fatal. Since the 1960s, 'natural' gas has been used, which is non-toxic. However, because an oven is a very enclosed space, the presence of any gas is likely to displace oxygen and therefore there is a risk of asphyxia.

3. I – Self-inflicted firearm injuries are the most common method of suicide in males in the USA. In the UK, suicide by firearm is much more common in farmers, who often have (legitimate) access to them.

4. J – Ingestion of as little as 10 mL of methyl alcohol (methylated spirits) can result in blindness by destruction of the optic nerve.

5. E – Suspension hanging is a method in which a ligature is secured in a 'noose', placed around the neck, and the other end attached to a fixed point. Upon the application of weight, the noose tightens around the neck, occluding the jugular veins, carotid arteries, and (if heavy enough) the trachea. This results in death by strangulation, as opposed to 'drop hanging', where the goal is typically to cause traumatic (usually fatal) spinal cord injury. In prisons, the ligature used is usually fashioned from bed-sheets, and attached to the cell bars or a door handle. Note that full suspension (i.e. entire body weight) is not required to be fatal, and that it is often used in the sitting or kneeling position, and can even be effective when supine.

6.

1. C – An admission to a medical/short stay ward is necessary, with a psychiatric evaluation when he sobers up. He is currently too intoxicated (with drugs and alcohol) to undertake an adequate mental state examination and risk assessment. Discharging a patient in this state is unacceptable, as he is at risk of not only committing further acts of self-harm, but of medical complications from his intoxication. He is also possibly unable to look after himself and could be vulnerable from exploitation or accidents.

2. H – This lady should be discharged to police custody. Her overdose does not appear to have been with strong suicidal intent (she was found in the street), and she is exhibiting drug-seeking and manipulative behaviour. While many patients like this do not require police involvement, she has committed physical, verbal, and racial assaults on healthcare workers, and needs to face consequences for these actions. Admission to a psychiatric ward is unlikely to be beneficial, and may even prove detrimental by reinforcing the suggestion that behaviour of this nature is driven by mental illness.

3. E – This gentleman should be referred for semi-urgent (later in the week) input from the community mental health team. He is likely to be suffering from a depressive illness, probably precipitated by financial and employment difficulties. While he is clearly remorseful about his suicidal behaviour, he appears to be struggling with his current situation and could well benefit from input by the community mental health team. He has a concerned and

supportive wife and a relatively stable domestic situation, which is why immediate outreach team involvement is not necessary at present.

4. **B** – This lady most likely requires admission to a psychiatric ward for further assessment and management of her mental state and risk. Should she refuse, use of mental health legislation may need to be considered. Despite the overdose being relatively small, this is likely due to lack of knowledge and there appears to have been clear suicidal intent. First presentations of self-harm in older adults should be considered to be with suicidal intent unless there is clear evidence to the contrary. Intensive outreach support in this case would be inappropriate given the very high risk of imminent further acts, despite her pleas that she will be fine.

5. **I** – Discharge with information on non-NHS support services. Despite her history and diagnosis, this woman appears to be functioning at a relatively high level (studying, not self-harming until recent stressors). She has made it clear that she is not wishing mental health service input; however, it could be that she would benefit greatly from non-NHS resources. Information on local student support agencies or voluntary support services for people who self-harm should be offered. Most of these agencies accept self-referrals, and distribute leaflets to local mental health bases.

7.

1. **F** – Dysthymia. This man describes subsyndromal symptoms of depression which emerged in adulthood and do not significantly interfere with his functioning. The lack of discrete episodes excludes recurrent depressive disorder.

2. **A** – Mild depressive episode. This woman has two out of three of the core symptoms of depression, poor concentration and poor self-esteem. There are no biological symptoms mentioned. She has four symptoms of depression in total and is able to continue her normal activities, meeting criteria for mild depression.

3. **D** – Severe depression with psychotic features. This woman has a clear change in functioning from her baseline, psychomotor retardation and what may be olfactory hallucinations of foul smells leading to the secondary delusional belief that her neighbour's drains are clogged. Although her mood is not reported, she is at risk of depression following a bereavement and these hallucinations are typical of severe depression.

4. **B** – Moderate depression. This man has the three core symptoms of depression and two further symptoms (disturbed sleep and appetite). This

gives him five symptoms of depression in total, and he is having great difficulty continuing his normal activities, meeting criteria for moderate depression.

5. **J** – Low mood secondary to psychoactive substance use. This would normally be diagnosed as harmful use of alcohol (see Ch. 15). This man gives a clear history of low mood following alcohol excess. This is impacting upon his mental health and occupational functioning. He is easily able to abstain from drink, indicating he is not dependent.

8.

1. **E** – Cushing's disease is an excess of cortisol. It can present with depression or psychosis. Clinical features include obesity, hypertension and easy bruising.

2. **A** – Huntington's disease is an autosomal dominant neurodegenerative disorder beginning in the basal ganglia. Depression is often an early symptom. Increased clumsiness and poor coordination can be subtle early features of the movement disorder which progresses to marked ataxia with choreiform movements (see p. 108). Huntington's disease is not always talked about in families and the description of the patient's father is more typical of the course of Huntington's than of depression.

3. **I** – Hypothyroidism is suggested by this woman's fatigue, low mood, dry, thin hair, dry skin and bradycardia.

4. **C** – Multiple sclerosis would be an important differential. This is suggested by her two neurological symptoms separated in time and place. Depression is common in multiple sclerosis.

9.

1. **G** – Psychomotor agitation. This is a common feature of depression in older adults.

2. **I** – Negative cognition. When considering the loss of the contract this man has demonstrated Beck's cognitive triad: negative views of himself, the world and the future.

3. **C** – Reduced range of reactivity (blunted affect). This woman's affect does not vary as would be appropriate when discussing content of different types.

4. **A** – Poor self-care. This is particularly concerning as personal appearance is important to this man's job.

5. **L** – Partial anhedonia. This man reports a markedly reduced interest in all activities with loss of the ability to derive pleasure from most, but not all, activities he previously enjoyed.

10.

1. A – Hypomanic episode. This man describes elated mood with a decreased need for sleep, poor concentration, increased energy, increased recent expenditure and increased libido. It is interfering with his social and occupational functioning but these activities are not completely disrupted. We are not given information on past mood abnormalities so the diagnosis of bipolar affective disorder is not appropriate.

2. C – Manic episode with psychotic features. This man has irritable mood, sexual disinhibition and grandiose delusions which have led him to commit an offence and quit his career. Schizophrenia is made less likely by the presence of mood symptoms and disinhibition. It would be important to check a urine drug screen to exclude mania secondary to psychoactive substance use. We are not given information on past mood abnormalities so the diagnosis of bipolar affective disorder is not appropriate.

3. D – Mixed affective state. This man shows rapid changes between an elated, low and irritable mood within 24 hours.

4. F – Cyclothymia. This woman describes alternating periods of mild elation and mild depression since early adulthood which do not impact on her functioning.

5. E – Bipolar affective disorder – manic episode with psychotic features. This man has a history of depression and now presents with reduced sleep, reduced appetite, psychomotor agitation and a grandiose delusion which has resulted in marked disruption to his occupational function.

11.

1. J – L-dopa. This man probably has Parkinson's disease and is likely to be treated with dopaminergic agents such as L-dopa, a precursor to dopamine. Excess dopamine is associated with euphoria, psychosis and a reduction in impulse control. Note it is the treatment rather than Parkinson's disease itself which is associated with these symptoms.

2. L – Amfetamine. Amfetamine intoxication can be associated with an acute psychosis. It is a sympathomimetic and so associated with dilated pupils. Cocaine can have similar effects but is normally smoked or snorted.

3. H – Anabolic steroids. These are commonly used by bodybuilders to increase muscle bulk, but can be associated with changes in mood, arousal and cognition.

4. I – Corticosteroids. High dose corticosteroids are often prescribed for severe acute asthma. Mood changes and psychosis are common psychiatric complications of steroid use.

5. G – Hyperthyroidism. This is suggested by tremor, tachycardia and irritability. Substance use is an important differential although her normal pupils make use of a stimulant less likely.

12.

1. A – Pressured speech.
2. H – Visual hyperaesthesia. This is an increased intensity of perception.
3. C – Tangential thinking.
4. B – Flight of ideas.
5. D – Poor concentration (or distractibility).
6. J – Visual hallucination. A perception in the absence of a stimulus.

13.

1. A – Schizophrenia. This man describes the symptom of thought insertion for greater than 1 month. The diagnosis is supported by his age and functional decline prior to the onset of symptoms. Although his mother does not think he misuses substances it would be important to exclude this by asking the man himself and performing a urine drug screen.

2. C – Schizoaffective disorder. This man has concurrent mood symptoms and first rank symptoms of schizophrenia. His mood and psychotic symptoms are equally prominent, making a recurrent psychotic depression unlikely.

3. F – Depressive episode, severe, with psychotic features. This man has mood symptoms and psychotic symptoms which are not typical of schizophrenia (because they are second rather than third person). The mood symptoms appear to be more prominent than the psychotic symptoms, making schizoaffective disorder unlikely.

4. D – Delusional disorder. This man has a longstanding unshakeable belief arrived at through faulty reasoning: a delusion. He has insight into this. Schizophrenia is unlikely because the delusion is non-bizarre and functioning is intact.

5. H – Personality disorder (although a fuller personal history would be required to confirm this diagnosis). This man is not delusional as his belief is not fixed. He is suspicious and litigious. The history from the police of multiple previous calls suggests his difficulties are longstanding. This would be consistent with a paranoid personality disorder. However, a fuller background history would be required to make a definite diagnosis.

6. G – Dementia/delirium. This man has cognitive impairment, functional decline and auditory hallucinations. It is crucial to exclude delirium by clarifying the onset of these symptoms (acute or chronic), by assessing his consciousness level and by completing a full physical examination and basic investigations. Dementia can also be associated with hallucinations. A mood disorder is made less likely by the description of him as 'cheerful', but otherwise a severe depressive episode could also account for his symptoms. Schizophrenia is unlikely to have such late onset.

14.

1. B – Neurosyphilis. This is now a rare diagnosis in the UK, but should always be considered in those with work or travel histories that may have placed them at risk of contracting syphilis. Neurosyphilis is a type of tertiary syphilis that emerges several years after initial infection. Clinical features are diverse but can include personality change, grandiose behaviour and dementia, along with upper motor neurone abnormalities such as brisk reflexes and extensor plantars.

2. C – Cerebral tumour. This man is socially disinhibited with a headache suggestive of raised intracranial pressure. The presence of focal neurological signs would further support the diagnosis.

3. G – Vitamin B_{12} deficiency. As a vegan, this woman is at risk of vitamin B_{12} deficiency (which is present only in meat and dairy products). She describes ataxia and paranoia, both of which can be features of vitamin B_{12} deficiency.

4. H – Thiamine deficiency. This man is likely experiencing Wernicke's encephalopathy. He is experiencing visual hallucinations and possibly tactile hallucinations of insects beneath the skin (formication). He is ataxic and has nystagmus. Thus he has the classic triad for Wernicke's: confusion, ataxia and ophthalmoplegia. Although this man's alcohol history is unknown, the time course of these symptoms is consistent with the onset of alcohol withdrawal and alcohol use may have predisposed him to being in a road traffic accident.

15.

1. B – Second-person auditory hallucination.
2. D – Pseudohallucination.
3. L – Extracampine hallucination.
4. F – Visceral hallucination.
5. J – Hypnagogic hallucination.
6. I – Gustatory hallucination.

See page 66–67 for explanations.

16.

1. A – Persecutory delusion.
2. D – Erotomania.
3. F – Delusion of misidentification (Capgras syndrome).
4. C – Delusion of reference.
5. G – Nihilistic delusion.
6. I – Delusion of control.
7. J – Loosening of associations.

See EMQ questions for explanation.

17.

1. C – Social phobia. This man has a generalized social phobia shown by his avoidance of social situations, and marked anxiety and distress when in them.

2. D – Generalized anxiety disorder. This lady has experienced continuous anxiety and apprehension about minor matters associated with autonomic overactivity and muscle tension for over 6 months.

3. A – Agoraphobia with panic disorder. This lady had a panic attack in a supermarket and has now become increasingly avoidant of crowding and confinement. Her symptoms are restricted to these situations. The weight loss may well be explained by her reduced dietary intake and increased exercise, but other disorders should be screened for, for example, hyperthyroidism.

4. E – Panic disorder. This man reports repeated non-situational panic attacks including a sensation of derealization. His symptoms could be due to cardiac problems but his young age, lack of exercise-induced symptoms and normal ECG are reassuring.

5. C – Social phobia (specific to playing a musical instrument in concert). This man has a social phobia as shown by his situation-specific anxiety and avoidance. This is not a generalized social phobia but is limited to one specific situation. DSM-IV codes for generalized and specific social phobias whereas ICD-10 does not differentiate.

6. F – Depressive episode. This man has the three core symptoms of depression and two further biological symptoms. His anxiety symptoms are concurrent with his depression so the primary diagnosis is of a depressive disorder rather than an anxiety disorder. Although his symptoms had onset following a traumatic event, they are too prolonged to be an acute stress reaction, too severe to be an adjustment disorder, and he denies two of the three key symptoms of post-traumatic stress disorder (flashbacks, avoidance and hyperarousal).

18.

1. D – Phaeochromocytoma. Although, because of its rarity, this remains an unlikely diagnosis for the scenario, it is the most likely from the options given. The features suggestive of phaeochromocytoma are the family history (not always present), hypertension, hyperglycaemia and intermittent episodes of increased catecholamine release. The history alone is not diagnostic: urinary or serum catecholamine assays and imaging of the adrenals would be required.

2. C – Hyperthyroidism. This lady already suffers from one autoimmune disorder (vitiligo) which increases her risk of another (Grave's disease). Tremor, heat intolerance, anxiety and increased appetite are classic symptoms of hyperthyroidism.

3. I – Fluoxetine. Selective serotonin reuptake inhibitors can initially be alerting and agitating, particularly in young people. This can increase the risk of suicide in the severely depressed. Use of an alternative antidepressant should be considered.

4. E – Caffeine. Caffeine has anxiogenic effects. Many soft drinks contain large amounts of caffeine.

5. H – Amfetamine. This drug increases concentrations of dopamine and noradrenaline (norepinephrine), leading to increased sympathetic nervous system activation. Cocaine intoxication would give a similar presentation.

19.

1. B – Obsessive-compulsive disorder. This woman has a greater than 2-week history of both obsessions and compulsions associated with functional impairment.

2. A – No mental illness. This woman is not experiencing obsessions or compulsions. She is responding to external influences and her handwashing may realistically reduce the feared outcome of infection transmission.

3. C – Depressive disorder. This woman has the three core symptoms of depression and two further symptoms. Her obsessions and compulsions are concurrent with her depression so the primary diagnosis is of a depressive disorder rather than obsessive-compulsive disorder.

4. D – Phobia. This woman has situation-specific anxiety with avoidance and panic attacks. She does not have obsessional thoughts, rather her anxiety is brought on by external stimuli. Although she washes her hands to reduce her anxiety, it is not a purposeless or excessive action, meaning it is not a compulsion. She is not hypochondriacal as she does not believe she is ill.

5. I – Eating disorder. This woman's low body weight, self-induced weight loss, body image disturbance and amenorrhoea mean she meets criteria for anorexia nervosa. She is not experiencing obsessions as she describes ego-syntonic thoughts which she does not resist. Rather they are over-valued ideas as they are plausible beliefs which have come to dominate her life.

20.

1. B – Obsession. The patient knows the images originate from their mind and is trying to resist.

2. F – Over-valued idea. The fear of infection is logical but held with undue importance. It is not an obsession as it is not viewed as abnormal or resisted.

3. C – Rumination.

4. D – Pseudohallucination.

5. E – Hallucination.

6. H – Thought insertion.

7. G – Delusion (strictly, a delusional perception). This belief is fixed, was arrived at illogically, and is not amenable to reason. The patient experienced a normal perception but interpreted it with delusional meaning, termed a 'delusional perception'. This is a first rank symptom of schizophrenia.

See Figure 11.4.

21.

1. D – This lady appears to be suffering from psychogenic, non-epileptic seizures. This is suggested by the chronological association with a significant stressor (being told that she will be left alone when her husband starts work). These are often more common in those with a family or personal history of epilepsy.

2. H – This is a classic presentation of a dissociative fugue, or 'fugue state'. The man is unable to recount any personal details, and appears to have travelled from a distant city. Note the possible severe stressor of being involved with a company that has recently been bankrupted.

3. E – Ganser's syndrome is an incredibly rare disorder, characterized by near-miss answers (implying that the patient has understood the question). It is often accompanied by florid hallucinations and conversion symptoms. It was initially studied in prison inmates, and was previously considered a factitious disorder.

4. J – Dissociation secondary to psychoactive substance use. Given the history of onset, and the fact that she was at a party the previous evening, initial consideration should be given to substance-induced dissociation. Common substances associated with

this include ketamine and tranquillizers; however, it can also occur following ingestion of less common substances such as mescalin or peyote.

22.
1. E – Bereavement reaction – note the chronological proximity to his death, and that the psychotic content features her husband.
2. K – Musculoskeletal injury. Note the distribution of injuries, and given the fact he was a driver (in the UK, the driver's seatbelt crosses the right shoulder) this is likely to be a whiplash/seatbelt-related injury. There is no suggestion of psychogenic origin in this case.
3. B – PTSD is the likely diagnosis in this case. Note the hyperarousal, avoidance and nightmares. Also note the persistent duration of the symptoms.
4. J – These symptoms are fairly typical of temporal lobe epilepsy. Note the history of likely head injury (implied by the fact she was referred from the neurosurgical unit). She should be referred for EEG.

23.
1. D – Body dysmorphic disorder.
2. B – This is highly suggestive of Münchausen syndrome by proxy. The safety of the child should be the immediate concern.
3. G – This is a first rank symptom of schizophrenia.
4. K – Psychotic depression (Cotard's syndrome).
5. J – While more information would ideally be required, this scenario is suggestive of malingering.

24.
1. D – Subjective cognitive impairment. This woman presents with concerns about her memory but has a normal score on standardized cognitive assessment. This may reflect her high educational level. It would be important to clarify how old her mother was when she was diagnosed with dementia, to guide frequency of follow-up (above 65 suggests the teacher has a 3-fold increased risk, under 65 suggests the possibility of a stronger genetic risk).
2. C – Mild cognitive impairment. This woman has a below normal score on standardized cognitive assessment but no impairment in activities of daily living. This low score is quite concerning in view of her young age and high educational attainment and she should be referred to a young onset memory clinic for comprehensive investigation.
3. B – Dementia (early onset). This woman has a below normal score on standardized cognitive assessment and impairment in activities of daily living. She should be referred to a young onset

memory clinic for comprehensive investigation. In view of her family history, genetic testing and counselling of any children may be considered.
4. E – Depression. This woman has symptoms of a depressive episode of moderate severity. This is likely to account for her cognitive symptoms and loss of one mark on the MMSE.

25.
1. A – Subdural haematoma. This woman has atrial fibrillation and so is likely to be on warfarin. There should therefore be a low threshold for suspecting an intracranial bleed after minor or no injury. A chronic subdural haematoma as opposed to neurodegenerative cause of dementia is suggested by her relatively quick cognitive deterioration, possible fluctuating consciousness level (uncharacteristic afternoon naps), neurological signs and history of head injury. It is not uncommon for there to be a latent period of days to weeks between injury and symptoms. The next step should be brain imaging.
2. C – Normal pressure hydrocephalus. This is suggested by this man's incontinence, ataxia and cognitive impairment, the classic triad of 'wet, wobbly, wacky'. Often this disorder is idiopathic. The next step should be brain imaging.
3. I – Addison's disease. This often presents insidiously with fatigue, loss of stamina, weight loss, apathy and memory problems. Postural hypotension is common and is suggested by her dizziness on rising. Hyperpigmentation of the palmar creases and buccal mucosa is often present but easy to miss. Addison's disease is rare, so this woman is most likely to be suffering from depression, but it would be important to check U&Es (hyponatraemia, hyperkalaemia) and glucose (hypoglycaemia) and consider a short synacthen test (diagnostic test).
4. H – Cushing's syndrome. This is suggested by the central obesity, amenorrhoea, hypertension, plethoric face and characteristic psychiatric symptoms of low mood and forgetfulness. Glucose is likely to be elevated. The next step would be to refer for a dexamethasone suppression test to confirm the diagnosis.
5. F – Hyperparathyroidism. Hyperparathyroidism causes hypercalcaemia. Mild hypercalcaemia (<3.0 mmol/L) is common in older women and often asymptomatic. Symptoms when present include low mood, abdominal pain, bone pain and renal calculi. Mild memory problems often occur, progressing to a delirium if calcium levels are very high (>3.8 mmol/L). The next step should be to check serum calcium and phosphate.

26.

1. A – Alzheimer's disease. Medial temporal atrophy is an early change in Alzheimer's.
2. B – Vascular dementia. Note this man's multiple vascular risk factors and evidence of cerebrovascular disease on imaging.
3. C – Mixed dementia. This woman's history sounds like Alzheimer's disease with a further insult to her cognition from a cerebrovascular accident 3 months ago. Hypertension is a risk factor for both Alzheimer's and vascular dementia.
4. D – Frontotemporal dementia. This is particularly common in younger adults.
5. E – Dementia with Lewy bodies.
6. F – Parkinson's disease with dementia. Parkinson's disease is associated with an increased risk of dementia.

See Fig. 14.7.

27.

1. A – Apraxia (intact motor ability shown by her ability to mimic).
2. C – Aphasia (expressive nominal aphasia).
3. E – Perseveration (receptive aphasia is less likely as she understood the initial instructions).
4. B – Agnosia (visual).
5. B – Agnosia (tactile, also called astereognosia).
6. C – Aphasia (receptive aphasia). This woman has not understood the question. Grammatical errors are common in those with receptive aphasia, perhaps because it is difficult to monitor what is being said.

See Fig. 14.2.

28.

1. G – Chronic insufflation ('snorting') of cocaine can cause damage to the nasal septum.
2. H – Ketamine is a potent glutaminergic (NMDA) antagonist, and is a potent short-acting dissociative anaesthetic. It is legitimately used in veterinary surgery as an anaesthetic agent. It can also be used as an anaesthetic analgesic agent in human medicine.
3. C – Alcohol follows zero-order eliminatory pharmacokinetics.
4. B – Cannabis is the most widely used illegal drug in the UK, with over half of 16–29-year-olds admitting to having tried it at least once.
5. J – Buprenorphine is a partial opioid agonist.

29.

1. B – 'Trips' is a common slang name for lysergic acid diethylamide (LSD). The name 'trips' may reflect the hallucinogenic effects of LSD.

2. E – 'Weed' is a common slang name for cannabis, usually of the herbal variety (as opposed to the resin or plant oil varieties). The main psychoactive ingredient of cannabis is thought to be tetrahydrocannabinol.
3. D – 'Charlie' is one of many street terms used to describe cocaine hydrochloride, the alkaloid salt derived from the coca plant. It is a widely abused substance.
4. F – While the term 'pills' could be thought to colloquially refer to any drug in a tablet or capsule form, it is generally used in the context of illicit drugs to refer to 3,4-methylenedioxy-N-methylamphetamine. Other street terms for this drug include MDMA, or Ecstasy.
5. A – 'Skag' is one of many slang terms for diacetylmorphine, or heroin. The term 'skag' may originate from Scotland, and achieved wider usage following the book/movie *Trainspotting* by Edinburgh author Irvine Welsh.

30.

1. G – Histrionic personality disorder.
2. H – Dependent personality disorder.
3. A – Paranoid personality disorder.
4. F – Narcissistic personality disorder.
5. I – Avoidant (anxious) personality disorder.

31.

1. E – Over-concern with physical attractiveness.
2. C – Consistent preference for solitary activities. This differs from avoidant (anxious) personality disorder in that the latter tend to avoid social activities for fear of rejection or criticism, while the former appear to lack any real desire for social activities.
3. D – Perfectionism that interferes with task completion.
4. B – Excessive sensitivity to setbacks and rebuffs.
5. G – Allowing others to make most of one's important life decisions. Note that 'Frantic efforts to avoid real or imagined abandonment' is a trait of borderline personality disorder. A trait of dependent personality disorder is the preoccupation with being abandoned rather than the frantic attempts to avoid it. Although be aware that the disorders commonly overlap or exist together.

32.

1. A – Given the history (recently discharged from 'a long-stay psychiatric rehabilitation ward'), it is likely this man suffers from a severe and enduring mental illness. Having been in hospital for a long

period of time, there is a very real risk that he may not know how to care for himself, which could be the reason for his rapid weight loss on discharge. It would be important to exclude depression, alcohol or drug misuse, or residual psychotic symptoms as cause for his weight loss.

2. E – Even though he has told you that he is fine, it is likely that he is suffering from bulimia nervosa. Both hypokalaemia and swollen parotid glands can be caused by excessive vomiting. The hypokalaemia is probably responsible for the U waves on the ECG.

3. J – This girl describes classical obsessive-compulsive symptoms: obsession (fear of infection); compulsion (having to prepare food in a specific manner), with awareness that it is irrational, but severe anxiety if the compulsion is not used to 'cancel out' the obsession.

4. C – Despite this lady's past history of anorexia nervosa, her current presentation is not majorly suggestive of relapse. She appears to have developed a specific phobia (with panic attacks) of vomiting, which has probably resulted from her recent physical illness (norovirus, the 'winter vomiting bug'). The link between the two could be understood as an example of psychological 'conditioning'.

5. H – The cause of weight loss in this case does not suggest any concern with body shape. Instead, this man appears not to be eating food because of a delusional belief that the food would be poisoned. He is suffering from an acute paranoid psychosis.

33.
1. A – Lanugo.
2. I – Perimylolysis.
3. E – Onychorrhexis.
4. J – Striae distensae.
5. D – Russell's sign.

34.
1. A – Admission to psychiatric hospital. This man is at high risk of suicide because of his age, sex, violent method of planned suicide, final acts and mental disorder. The extremely high suicidal intent indicated by the circumstances of his presentation means hospital admission is the only safe management option.

2. D – Refer to psychiatric out-patients routinely. A psychiatric referral is advisable given his treatment-resistant depression. There is no suggestion of acute risk to necessitate an urgent referral.

3. F – Refer to crisis team. Even without evidence of risk to self or others, psychotic features are suggestive of a very severe depression that could worsen rapidly.

4. A – Admit to psychiatric hospital. This man has depression with poor oral intake. This is not manageable in the community. He needs an urgent physical exam and bloods. If his renal function is acutely impaired he may need transfer to a general hospital for intravenous fluids. If this man is in a general hospital at the time of mental health assessment he should be physically assessed prior to transfer.

5. C – Manage in primary care. The next step for this man is to consider a higher intensity psychological intervention or an antidepressant.

35.
1. D – Mirtazapine. SSRIs increase risk of bleeding when co-prescribed with nonsteroidals and anticoagulants. Mirtazapine is suggested as an alternative first line antidepressant by NICE (2009).

2. A – SSRI. NICE (2009) recommends SSRIs as first line antidepressants if there are no cautions.

3. A – SSRI. NICE (2009) recommends SSRIs as first line antidepressants. Sleep disturbance often resolves as depression improves. A more sedating antidepressant such as mirtazapine would be a good second line option.

4. D – Mirtazapine. Although first line, SSRIs often cause sexual dysfunction. If avoidance of this side-effect is very important to patients, an alternative such as mirtazapine can be considered.

5. C – Duloxetine. Duloxetine is licensed for both stress incontinence and depression. It is a joint serotonin and noradrenaline (norepinephrine) reuptake inhibitor. This action in the spinal cord leads to increased tone in the urethral sphincter.

36.
1. B – Haloperidol. Although haloperidol is not first line for schizophrenia, patient preference is important in the choice of antipsychotic. She should have an ECG before recommencing as haloperidol can prolong the QTc.

2. F – Aripiprazole. This is the antipsychotic least likely to be associated with weight gain and the metabolic syndrome. First generation antipsychotics would be the next best choice.

3. E – Quetiapine. From the options given, haloperidol and chlorpromazine are most likely to be associated with extrapyramidal side-effects. Aripiprazole is less associated with extrapyramidal side-effects, but quetiapine has an even lower likelihood. Flupentixol is a depot medication and the majority of patients prefer oral. Clozapine is not indicated as the patient is not treatment-resistant.

4. C – Flupentixol depot formulation. Long-acting intramuscular injections (depot formulations)

administered 1–4 weekly are a good option for patients with poor concordance.

5. D – Clozapine. This woman has treatment-resistant schizophrenia as she has had two trials of antipsychotic at adequate doses for adequate durations, including at least one second generation drug.

37.

1. C – Hypersalivation. This is most commonly seen with clozapine. Most antipsychotics cause a dry mouth.
2. B – Postural hypotension. This is a side-effect of most antipsychotics, secondary to adrenergic receptor blockade.
3. J – Hyperprolactinaemia, causing galactorrhoea. This is a side-effect of most but not all antipsychotics, secondary to D_2 receptor blockade in the tuberoinfundibular pathway.
4. E – Agranulocytosis. Without monitoring, this is seen in just under 1% of patients taking clozapine.
5. G – Akathisia. This is frequent purposeless movement associated with a subjective inner restlessness. It is very unpleasant for patients, and a risk factor for suicide. It is a side-effect of most antipsychotics and some other psychotropics also. High doses are a risk factor.

38

1. D – Eye movement desensitization and reprocessing therapy. This or trauma-focused CBT are recommended for moderate to severe post-traumatic stress disorder even if the trauma occurred less than 4 weeks ago.
2. B – Watchful waiting. This is recommended for symptoms of mild post-traumatic stress disorder within 4 weeks of the trauma.
3. D – Eye movement desensitization and reprocessing therapy. This or trauma-focused CBT are recommended for all severities of post-traumatic stress disorder where the trauma occurred more than 4 weeks ago.
4. K – Mirtazapine. Mirtazapine or paroxetine are recommended as first line medications for post-traumatic stress disorder. Mirtazapine is less likely to be associated with sexual dysfunction than a SSRI. Paroxetine is the only SSRI licensed for post-traumatic stress disorder, although it is likely to be a class effect.
5. G – TCA. Amitriptyline (a tricyclic antidepressant) or phenelzine (MAOI) are second line drug therapies for post-traumatic stress disorder.

39.

1. C – CBT. First line therapy for moderate-severe panic disorder is cognitive-behavioural therapy.

2. A – Self-help. First line therapy for mild panic disorder is self-help materials.
3. E – Applied relaxation. This or CBT are the two psychological therapies recommended for moderate to severe generalized anxiety disorder.
4. F – SSRI. First line drug therapy for moderate to severe generalized anxiety disorder is an SSRI.
5. I – Pregabalin. This is a second line drug therapy for moderate to severe generalized anxiety disorder.

40.

1. A – This man has likely overdosed on intravenous opiates, leading to respiratory depression and a reduced consciousness level. Naloxone is an opioid antagonist, and needs to be given to reverse toxicity. Naltrexone is also an opiate antagonist but it needs to be given orally so is not suitable for someone with a reduced GCS (risk of aspiration).
2. E – Lofexidine can be helpful in reducing the unpleasant symptoms of opiate withdrawal. It would not be advisable to prescribe benzodiazepines to someone who already has a substance dependence.
3. H – While methadone, buprenorphine and dihydrocodeine are used as 'substitution therapy', this lady's heavy use of heroin means that she is likely to have severe withdrawal symptoms. As a partial opioid agonist, buprenorphine is likely to precipitate a withdrawal state given the magnitude of her usage. There is some evidence to suggest that dihydrocodeine can be as effective as methadone; however, its use is not widespread as – being in tablet form – it is easier to divert onto the black market.
4. G – This man could benefit from loperamide.
5. F – Naltrexone is an opioid receptor antagonist that can be used to reduce the euphoric effects of opiates. Naloxone would also have this effect but it needs to be given parenterally and is short-acting, so naltrexone is preferred.

41.

1. C – Preparation.
2. G – Termination.
3. A – Pre-contemplative.
4. E – Contemplative.
5. B – Relapse.

42.

1. B – Lorazepam. Given that benzodiazepines are metabolized in the liver, and that impaired liver function can delay metabolism and excretion, drugs with long half-lives can accumulate and

increase the risk of toxicity. From the three benzodiazepines listed, lorazepam has the shortest half-life, and is therefore safest to use for detoxification in this case.

2. E − Thiamine. From the history given, this lady is not intoxicated. She appears to be suffering from the triad of symptoms associated with Wernicke's encephalopathy, and needs urgent treatment with parenteral thiamine.

3. H − Cognitive-behavioural therapy, focusing on identifying cues and preventing relapse, could be very helpful for this lady. Motivational interviewing, with a focus on 'promoting change', may not be so useful as she is already abstinent. Psychoeducation tends to happen in groups, and because she is not keen on this there is a risk of early disengagement.

4. I − Acamprosate may be helpful in reducing cravings. Naltrexone is also thought to reduce cravings, but would be likely to reduce the efficacy of the tramadol.

5. A − Alcoholics Anonymous is a 12-step programme that could be useful for this man. It is not run by health services, and tends to consist of self-funded groups. Their ethos is one of complete abstinence, and their system of peer support (or 'sponsorship') can be very beneficial for some.

43.

1. F − Patients with dependent personality disorder can quickly become institutionalized, and alternatives to admission should be preferred. In this case, the lady should be empathically reassured, and encouraged to engage with her existing care plan.

2. C − While some practitioners would argue that this patient does not have a mental illness, she is clearly distressed and − in the short term − at incredibly high risk of completing suicide or otherwise harming herself. It would also appear that there is no safe place to which she could be discharged. A short 'crisis' admission to a psychiatric ward, of agreed duration and with clear goals and boundaries, would allow for her distress and short-term risk to be managed, and longer term support organized. Discharging her to police custody is not appropriate.

3. H − It may be worth offering this gentleman a trial of antipsychotic medication. While psychotherapeutic measures would be more likely to be effective in the long term, he appears to be untrusting of services, and it would be unlikely that he would engage with this. A small dose of an antipsychotic may be enough to reduce his paranoia to the extent that he may engage with a psychotherapist, and may also provide a reason

for ongoing contact with doctors such that trust and rapport can be established.

4. A − Depression arising in patients with personality disorders can be amenable to drug treatment; however, the benefits of this need to be balanced with the risk of overdosing on potentially harmful drugs. Antidepressants dispensed on a weekly/twice-weekly/three times weekly/daily basis can, to some degree, modify this risk.

5. I − This gentleman could benefit from lifestyle advice. His situation has recently changed, which may explain his increased anxiety. However, it is likely that his caffeine consumption is contributing to his insomnia, and that smoking cigarettes all night is perpetuating the problem. Advice regarding caffeine, nicotine, diet and exercise should be given in the first instance.

44.

1. J − It would appear that this lady has developed a comorbid depressive illness. Her eating appears to have been improving. Therapeutic priority should be given to managing her depressive symptoms and her high risk of completing suicide. From the options listed, the most appropriate would be an informal admission to a general psychiatric ward. Out-patient or home treatment may be considered; however, given the levels of risk involved, admission to hospital would probably be more appropriate.

2. B − There is some evidence to suggest that brain serotonin function is abnormal in patients with bulimia nervosa. There is also evidence to suggest that antidepressants (specifically high-dose fluoxetine) can be very useful in treating binge/purge behaviours. In this case, prescribing fluoxetine would be appropriate.

3. K − This girl is incredibly unwell, and her current physical condition poses a threat to her life. By virtue of her mental illness, and probably also her state of malnutrition, she clearly lacks capacity to make decisions regarding her healthcare. Immediate hospital treatment is required, and she should be transferred urgently under mental health legislation. Also, given her persistent refusal to eat, and her lack of capacity and insight, it is likely that involuntary nasogastric feeding will be required to save her life. This is both a clinically and medico-legally difficult situation, and should be managed by a specialist.

4. F − Interpersonal therapy, or IPT, is a type of psychotherapy that aims to change the person's interpersonal behaviour by fostering adaptation to current interpersonal roles and situations. The four areas of focus are grief, role dispute, role transition and interpersonal deficits. This lady has clearly stated that she wishes to address her

problems with grief (the death of her mother), role transition (and possibly role dispute) (starting work at her new firm), and interpersonal deficits (standing up to dominant male partners). In doing this, issues which have predisposed, precipitated, and perpetuated her illness can be addressed.

5. G – This boy lives in a family in which both parents are high-achievers, and subsequently feels pressured to live up to their expectations. Family therapy would be likely to be incredibly useful in this case, assuming that all parties involved are willing to engage.

45.

1. D – This lady may benefit from maternal skills teaching. The health visitor can be an invaluable resource for providing this.

2. F – This lady appears to be suffering from the 'baby blues'. Simple reassurance should be given. This will likely pass after 10 days or so, but follow-up is important to ensure that she is not developing postnatal depression.

3. G – This lady appears to be developing a puerperal psychosis. Given her symptoms, the use of an antipsychotic medication is indicated. Olanzapine is widely used for puerperal psychosis. ECT may be required if she does not respond to pharmacological treatment.

4. K – This lady is likely to have a severe postnatal depressive illness. Given her presentation and her poor oral intake, her illness should be considered to be potentially life-threatening. Electroconvulsive therapy should be considered.

5. I – This lady is tearful and low in mood. It is not clear whether she meets criteria for diagnosis of a depressive illness; however, she appears to be incredibly troubled by not meeting her (fairly high) personal expectations regarding pure breast feeding. Cognitive-behavioural therapy would allow her to explore this with the aim of allowing her to view the situation from a more balanced perspective.

46.

1. K – Sodium valproate is strongly associated with the development of neural tube defects. It is preferable not to prescribe sodium valproate to women of childbearing age, and less teratogenic alternatives should be considered. If it is considered necessary, risk counselling and reliable contraception are necessary.

2. C – Olanzapine is associated with an increased risk of gestational diabetes. It should be prescribed with caution in all pregnant women, and alternatives should be used in women who are already at increased risk of gestational diabetes (e.g. obesity, gestational diabetes during previous pregnancy, strong family history of diabetes). In any case, blood and/or urinary glucose should be regularly monitored.

3. A – The use of paroxetine during pregnancy (particularly during the first trimester) has been associated with an increased risk in heart defects (particularly atrial and ventricular septal defects). Use in later pregnancy has been associated with neonatal pulmonary hypertension. Lithium has also been associated with heart defects; however, there is no strong association with pulmonary hypertension in the neonate. It should also be noted that it may be safer to prescribe an alternative antidepressant to paroxetine (if required) during pregnancy. However, swapping to a different medication is associated with a risk of relapse.

4. G – The use of lithium during pregnancy has been associated with an increased risk of fetal heart defects, specifically Ebstein's anomaly (displacement of the opening of the tricuspid valve). The absolute risk may be as low as 0.1%, but this is still 20 times greater than the general population. This risk needs to be balanced against the risk of relapse of illness associated with discontinuation of lithium, as untreated affective/psychotic illness can place the fetus at greatly increased risk.

5. I – Fluoxetine is one of the better studied antidepressants in pregnancy. Some studies have suggested that *in utero* exposure to fluoxetine can cause pulmonary hypertension and low birth weight in the neonate. As with all drugs taken during pregnancy, risk vs benefit needs to be considered on an individual basis.

47.

1. A – Donepezil. This woman has mild to moderate dementia for which cholinesterase inhibitors are recommended. Donepezil is first line.

2. D – Memantine. This woman has severe dementia (MMSE <10) for which memantine is recommended.

3. D – Memantine. This woman has mild to moderate dementia for which cholinesterase inhibitors are recommended. However, she has a number of relative contraindications to cholinesterase inhbitor use – their cholinergic effects can induce bradycardia, which may be particularly problematic in those with conduction deficits. Similarly cholinergic drugs can cause bronchoconstriction, which may be problematic in COPD and asthma, and increase gastric acid secretions, which could worsen peptic ulceration. Overall, it would probably be better to try memantine first for this woman.

4. B – Rivastigmine. This is the cholinesterase inhibitor with the best evidence for maintaining cognition in Parkinson's disease with dementia, although it is likely a class effect.

5. I – No treatment recommended by current guidelines. Unfortunately no medications have yet been found to slow the progression of frontotemporal dementia.

48.

1. C – Diazepam. Abruptly discontinuing benzodiazepines can result in withdrawal symptoms. These can have onset within a day of stopping a short-acting benzodiazepine (e.g. lorazepam) or up to 3 weeks for a longer acting drug (e.g. diazepam). Symptoms include insomnia, anxiety, anorexia, tremor, perspiration, tinnitus and perceptual disturbances – such as this woman's visual illusion.

2. H – Fluoxetine. All antidepressants, but particualrly SSRIs, can be associated with the syndrome of inappropriate secretion of antidiuretic hormone, leading to hyponatraemia. This is particularly likely in older adults.

3. A – Lithium. Lithium can induce nephrogenic diabetes insipidus, leading to hypernatraemia if fluid intake cannot be maintained, e.g. due to diarrhoea and vomiting. Dehydration increases the risk of lithium toxicity (which is renally excreted) so a random lithium level should also be urgently checked for this man.

4. J – Haloperidol. This man is likely to have received haloperidol to manage his delirium. Haloperidol can cause prolongation of the QT interval. In extreme cases this can lead to torsade de pointes. Olanzapine is less likely to have this side-effect.

5. G – Amitriptyline. Anticholinergic medication is a big risk factor for delirium. Amitriptyline is often prescribed for neuropathic pain.

49.

1. L – Fluoxetine has the best evidence for the treatment of depression in children and adolescents. It should be noted that it is only recommended in the treatment of moderate to severe depression. At the time of going to press, fluoxetine does not have a marketing licence in the UK, and use in under 18s should be considered to be 'off label'.

2. B – While dexamfetamine and atomoxetine are also indicated for the pharmacological management of ADHD, methylphenidate is recommended as a first line treatment in cases where drugs are indicated. Be aware that there are various preparations of methylphenidate, each with its own pharmacokinetic profile (Concerta XL®, Ritalin®, Equasym XL®), and therefore the drug should be prescribed by brand name.

3. H – Imipramine is a tricyclic antidepressant. By virtue of its anticholinergic effects, it has been shown to be effective in the management of enuresis.

It should be used only when behavioural modification strategies have been ineffective.

4. C – Haloperidol is licensed for the treatment of tics, and can be effective.

5. J – Atomoxetine is a noradrenaline (norepinephrine) reuptake inhibitor, that can be very effective in the management of ADHD. It is not recommended for use as a first line agent; however, it does not appear to be associated with tics, and may be a more appropriate agent for this girl.

50.

1. B – Given the degree of impairment to both him and his family, this boy is likely to have an autistic spectrum disorder. The absence of the delay of language development is suggestive of Asperger's syndrome rather than childhood autism.

2. E – This history is suggestive of secondary enuresis. While it would be important to exclude physical causes (urinary infection, epilepsy, diabetes), there is a clear psychological stressor that seemed to precede the problem. While not explicitly stated in the case, it is suggested that she had initially gained bladder control ('... recently started wetting'), which differentiates this from primary enuresis.

3. J – While many of the behaviours are suggestive of the core symptoms of ADHD, note that they appear to be limited to the academic setting (he appears fine at home). ADHD is pervasive rather than situational, and this case is suggestive that the boy may be having difficulties with schoolwork (either because it is too difficult or too easy).

4. I – Oppositional defiant disorder is similar to conduct disorder in that behaviour is negativistic, rebellious, defiant and disruptive. However, unlike conduct disorder, the behaviour associated with oppositional defiant disorder does not violate the rights of others and troubles with the law are less common.

5. F – Heller's syndrome – also known as childhood disintegrative disorder – is characterized by normal development until around the age of 2 years, followed by a loss of previously acquired skills (language, social and adaptive skills, play, bowel and bladder control and motor skills) before age 10. It is also associated with an autism-like impairment of social interaction as well as repetitive, stereotyped interests and mannerisms. Thus, after the deterioration, these children may resemble autistic children. It is more common in boys, but can occur in girls (as opposed to Rett's syndrome, which occurs almost exclusively in girls). It is different from Rett's in that development tends to be further advanced prior to deterioration.

51.

1. D – This lady has a mild intellectual disability, and will have an estimated IQ of 50–69. Individuals in this group comprise the majority (85%) of all people with intellectual disabilities.

2. A – From the information given, this gentleman manages to live alone without support. His symptoms suggest that he suffers from a pervasive developmental disorder, likely Asperger's syndrome (which is not an intellectual disability). His interests would suggest that he has above-average intelligence (IQ 100>).

3. G – This boy has a profound intellectual disability (IQ <20). He is unable to care for himself and fully dependent on the support of others.

4. E – This woman has a moderate intellectual disability (IQ 35–49). Note that she is able to live on her own, albeit in a supported housing complex with a great deal of support.

5. F – This gentleman has a severe intellectual disability (IQ 20–34). He lives with his family, who are his main carers, and is able to perform simple tasks under supervision. His self-care skills are limited, but he seems to be able to sometimes contribute to these.

52.

1. C – Prader–Willi syndrome is characterized by low muscle tone, short stature, incomplete sexual development, cognitive disabilities, problem behaviours and a chronic feeling of hunger that can lead to excessive eating and life-threatening obesity.

2. B – Behavioural disturbances in Lesch–Nyhan syndrome emerge between 2 and 3 years of age. Persistent self-injurious behaviour is a hallmark of the syndrome.

3. I – Rett's syndrome. Apparently normal or near-normal early development is followed by partial or complete loss of acquired cognitive and motor skills. Stereotyped tortuous wringing of the hands is a distinctive feature.

4. D – Turner's syndrome occurs exclusively in girls. It is very occasionally associated with mild intellectual disability, with specific deficits in visuospatial tasks, visual memory and arithmetic, although most patients have normal IQ. Physical features usually include gonadal failure, which results in primary amenorrhoea and failure to develop secondary sexual characteristics.

5. F – Cri-du-chat syndrome is so called due to the distinctive kitten-like crying sounds that these individuals often make (due to problems with the larynx and nervous system). About 30% lose the cry by the age of 2.

53.

1. A – This man has morbid jealousy. He is convinced that his partner is being unfaithful, despite extensive reassurances and evidence to the contrary. The name 'Othello syndrome' is derived from the play *Othello* by William Shakespeare, in which the protagonist murders his wife (Desdemona – which means 'the unfortunate' in Greek). Othello syndrome is associated with alcohol misuse and violence. Treatment includes antipsychotic medication and psychotherapy; however, given the very poor prognosis, it is often said that the most effective treatment is 'geographical' (i.e. relocation of the spouse to a distant area).

2. K – The symptoms present in this man (delusions, hallucinations) are suggestive of a paranoid psychotic state. Given his age, the implied rapid onset of symptoms and the fact that he has no psychiatric history, this is unlikely to be a first presentation of paranoid schizophrenia. The fact that he has been at a music festival should be a pointer that substances may be implicated in his presentation. His symptoms are not typical of an alcohol withdrawal delirium; however, this is an important differential.

3. D – This lady is likely to be suffering from a manic illness. She has grandiose delusions (that she is a pop star). Note that she has recently been hospitalized with a depressive illness: her mania may be associated with drug treatment or may signify the presence of a bipolar illness. Crimes related to mania include financial offences and occasionally aggression.

4. C – The nature of this crime (killing a man in retribution for a mistake in making a sandwich) is alarming. The fact this man has an extensive forensic history, is actively involved with organized crime and appears cold and emotionless in the face of a crime of such magnitude is strongly suggestive of antisocial personality disorder. It could be that the man also meets ICD-10 criteria for dissocial personality disorder, and may also score highly on the PCL-R (the 'gold standard' for assessing psychopathy). Further assessment would be required to confirm this diagnosis.

5. J – There is an association between fire-setting and mild intellectual disability. This should be differentiated from arson (deliberate fire-raising for secondary gain, e.g. insurance money), pyromania (compulsion to set fires, followed by a 'release of tension'), wilful destruction of property (e.g. in antisocial personality disorder), or fire-setting driven by other mental disorders.

Glossary

Affect Affect refers to the transient ebb and flow of emotion in response to particular stimuli, e.g. smiling at a joke or crying at a sad memory. It is assessed by observing the patient's posture, facial expression, emotional reactivity and speech. The two components that should be assessed are the appropriateness of the affect and its range. See pages 6 and 50.

Anxiety Anxiety is a mood state. It can be defined as a response to an unknown, internal or vague threat. This is distinct from fear, which is defined below. The experience of anxiety consists of both apprehensive or nervous thoughts and the awareness of a physical reaction to anxiety. See page 77.

Attempted suicide An episode of deliberate self-harm, which did not end in death but was driven by suicidal intent. This is in contrast with episodes of non-fatal deliberate self-harm driven by other motivations. See page 45.

Capacity Capacity is the ability of an individual to make their own decisions. See page 38.

Circumstantiality Circumstantiality describes over-inclusive speech that is delayed in reaching its final goal. This is because of excessive detail and diversion. However, the final goal will be reached, which distinguishes it from flight of ideas. Circumstantiality can be found in the normal population but is increased in anxiety disorders and hypomania. See page 59 and 70.

Compulsions Compulsions can be defined as repetitive mental operations (such as counting) or physical acts (such as checking) that a patient feels compelled to perform in response to their own obsessions. The motivation for compulsions is the reduction of anxiety generated by an obsession. The compulsion may be either unrelated to the preceding obsession (e.g. counting) or an unnecessarily excessive response to the obsession (e.g. handwashing). See page 86.

Delusion A delusion is the most severe form of an abnormal idea. It is a fixed belief arrived at illogically and is not amenable to reason. It is not accepted in the patient's cultural background. The presence of a delusion signifies a psychotic disorder. See page 67.

Delusional perception Experiencing a normal perception but interpreting it with delusional meaning. For example, 'I heard the clock chime and I knew that meant the aliens were planning to kill me'. This is a first rank symptom of schizophrenia. See page 68.

Depersonalization Depersonalization is feeling yourself to be strange or unreal.

Derealization Derealization is feeling that external reality is strange or unreal.

Depression A depressed mood is when a patient describes feeling depressed, sad, dejected, despondent or low. A depressive disorder is a specific psychiatric condition where the mood change is sufficiently severe, chronic and occurring with other symptoms.

Dissociation Dissociation is an altered state of consciousness in which normally integrated experiences or processes are disrupted. For example, walking to work on 'autopilot' and not noticing a new shop front – the sensory information has not been integrated with the conscious experience. Depersonalization or derealization are dissociative symptoms (see above). Extreme dissociative states can be associated with disorders including non-epileptic convulsions and fugue. See page 93.

Dysphasia Dysphasia is an impairment of language abilities despite intact sensory and motor function. See page 105.

Dyspraxia Dyspraxia is an impairment of the ability to carry out skilled motor movements despite intact motor function. See page 105.

Dysgnosia Dysgnosia is an impairment in the ability to interpret sensory information despite intact sensory organ function. See page 105.

Echolalia Echolalia is when a patient senselessly repeats words or phrases that have been spoken near them. It can be viewed as a form of disorganized thinking or as an abnormality of speech. It occurs in a range of psychiatric conditions such as schizophrenic catatonia, autism and brain injury.

Fear Fear, similar to anxiety, is an alerting signal in response to a potential threat. It differs from anxiety in that it is a response to a known, external or definite object. Anxiety and fear are discussed on page 77.

First rank symptoms First rank symptoms were described by Schneider who suggested that the presence of one or more first rank symptoms, in the absence of organic disease, was sufficient to diagnose schizophrenia. These symptoms still feature strongly in modern diagnostic criteria for schizophrenia. See page 72.

Flight of ideas Flight of ideas can be described as either a disorder of thought form or an abnormality of speech. It describes thinking that is markedly accelerated and results in a stream of loosely connected concepts. The link between concepts can be normal, tenuous or through puns and clanging. It differs from circumstantiality in that the links between concepts are more tenuous and the final goal is less likely to be reached. In its extreme form, speech can become unintelligible or approach the incoherent thought disorder of schizophrenia. See page 59 and 70.

Functional symptoms Functional symptoms are physical symptoms without identifiable structural cause. See page 97.

Hallucination Hallucinations are perceptions that occur in the absence of external stimuli and are indistinguishable from normal sensation. See page 66.

Illusion Illusions are misperceptions of real external stimuli. For example, spots on the carpet are perceived as insects. Illusions can occur in healthy people particularly when tired, not concentrating, experiencing strong emotions or intoxicated with substances.

Insight Insight describes a patient's understanding of the nature and degree of his or her mental illness and the recognition of the need for treatment. An assessment of insight is an integral part of the mental state examination. See page 7.

Mood Mood is sustained emotion over a period of time. This differs from a 'feeling', which is a short-lived experience, and 'affect', which is the external expression of transient emotion.

Neologism Neologism is an example of disorganized thinking. It is a new word created by the patient, often combining syllables rather than words. It is classically associated with schizophrenia and can also occur in organic brain disorder.

Obsession An obsession is an involuntary thought, image or impulse, which is recurrent, intrusive, unpleasant and enters the mind against conscious resistance. Patients recognize that the thoughts are a product of their own mind even though they are involuntary and repugnant. See page 85.

Over-valued idea An over-valued idea is an incorrect belief that is not impossible (in contrast to some schizophrenic delusions), is held with marked emotional investment but not with unshakable conviction. See page 68.

Perseveration Perseveration is when a patient inappropriately repeats an initially correct action. For example, unnecessarily repeating a word or phrase, or applying the rules of one task to a second task.

Pseudohallucinations Pseudohallucinations are perceptions that occur in the absence of external stimuli but are experienced in the internal world rather than the external world. For example, hearing a voice 'inside my head'. See page 66.

Psychosis Psychosis is the presence of hallucinations, delusions or thought disorder.

Psychotherapy Psychotherapy is an umbrella term for psychological or talking therapy. There is a large number of psychological therapies; the most common ones include supportive therapy, cognitive-behavioural therapy, psychodynamic psychotherapy, family therapy and group therapy.

Psychotropic medication Psychotropic medication influences cognition, mood or behaviour. All medications used to treat psychiatric disorders are psychotropic.

Rumination Repeatedly thinking about the causes and experience of previous distress and difficulties. Voluntary thinking which is not resisted.

Self-harm Self-harm is a blanket term used to mean any intentional act done in the knowledge that it was potentially harmful. It can take the form of self-poisoning (overdosing) or self-injury (cutting, slashing, burning, etc.). See page 45.

Suicide Suicide is the act of intentionally ending one's own life.

Note: Page numbers followed by
b indicate boxes and *f* indicate figures.

A

Abbreviated Mental Test 113*f*
abnormal beliefs 59, 67–68
acamprosate (Campral) 24, 155
accommodation 43
activities of daily living (ADL) 107
acute stress reaction 92
Addenbrooke's Cognitive Examination-
    Revised 113*f*
adjustment disorder 92
adolescents *see* child/adolescent
    psychiatry
Adults with Incapacity (Scotland) Act
    (2000) 38
Advance Decisions/Directives 38
adverse drug reactions 252
    see also specific drugs
adverse life events 46
aetiology 8–10
affect 6, 50
age-related physiological changes 183,
    183*f*
ageing *see* older adults, mental illness in
agitation 50–51
agnosia 105*f*
agoraphobia 79
akathisia 6*b*, 21*f*
alcohol abuse 4, 116–120, 153–156
    aetiology 153–154
        psychological factors 153–154
        social and environmental factors
            154
    assessment 121–122
    cognitive disorders 119–120
    complications 118*f*
    course and prognosis 155–156, 156*f*
    and crime 198*f*
    epidemiology 153
    genetics 153
    harmful use 116–117
    intoxication 117
    management 24, 154–155
        pharmacological therapy 155
        psychotherapy 155
    questions 222–223, 226, 249, 260,
        263
    safe daily limits 117*f*

suicide risk 47*f*
    see also substance abuse
alcohol dependence 117, 118*f*
alcohol withdrawal 117–119, 119*f*,
    154–155, 155*f*
all-or-nothing thinking 29*f*
Alzheimer's disease 109*f*, 114*f*,
    173–174
    environmental factors 174, 174*f*
    genetic factors 173–174
    neuropathology 175*f*
    see also dementia
amisulpride 19*f*
amitriptyline 14*f*, 15*f*
amnesia 51, 105, 105*f*
    dissociative 93*f*
amnesic syndrome 112, 112*f*
anaesthesia, dissociative 93*f*
anorexia nervosa 127, 128*f*, 163–166
    aetiology 163
    epidemiology 163, 164*f*
    management 164–165, 165*f*
    prognosis 165*f*, 166
    refeeding syndrome 165*f*
    symptoms 128
    see also eating disorders
antidepressants 10, 13–17, 135–136
    choice of 136*f*
    history 13
    indications 13–15
    mechanism of action 13, 14*f*
    questions 247
    side-effects and contraindications
        15–17
    see also individual drugs
antipsychotics 19–21, 19*f*
    contraindications 19–21, 20*f*, 21*f*
    history and classification 19
    indications 21
        schizophrenia 143
    mechanism of action 19–21
    in pregnancy 168*f*
    questions 233, 247, 248
    side-effects 19–21, 20*f*, 21*f*, 144*f*
    see also individual drugs
antisocial personality disorder 125*f*, 160*f*
anxiety disorders 6–7, 77–84, 147–151
    aetiology 147–148
    alcohol-related 120
    assessment 82
    course and prognosis 150–151

definitions and clinical features 77–78
diagnosis 80*f*
differential diagnosis 78–81, 79*f*
epidemiology 147, 148*f*
generalized 77, 79*f*, 80
genetics 147–148
management 148–150, 149*f*
    drugs 150
    psychotherapy 150
medical conditions and substance
    abuse 81
non-situational 80–81
paroxysmal 78, 79*f*, 81
physical signs 78*f*
psychiatric problems associated with
    81, 81*f*
questions 219, 225–226, 240, 258,
    263
see also specific disorders
anxiolytics/hypnotics 22–24
    classification 22, 23*f*
    history 22
    indications 23
    mechanism of action 22–23
    in pregnancy 168*f*
    side-effects 23
    see also individual drugs
apathy 105*f*
aphasia 105*f*, 109*f*
apolipoprotein E 173–174
appearance 5
appetite, loss of 50
Approved Clinician (AC) 34*f*
Approved Mental Health Practitioner
    (AMHP) 34, 34*f*
apraxia 105*f*, 109*f*
aripiprazole, side-effects 144*f*
Asperger's syndrome 188, 188*f*
assertive outreach teams 42
assessment 1–12, 2*f*
    interview 1–2
    see also specific conditions
atomoxetine (Strattera) 189
attempted suicide 45
    management 48
attention deficit/hyperactivity disorder
    188–189
    diagnosis and clinical features
        188–189
    epidemiology/aetiology 189
    management and prognosis 189

AUDIT questionnaire 122
auditory hallucinations 66–67
autism 187–188, 188*f*
  diagnosis and clinical features 187
  epidemiology/aetiology 187
  management and prognosis 188
Autism Diagnostic Observation
    Schedule (ADOS) 185
autochthonous delusions 68
automatic thoughts 28–29
automatism 200
avoidance 77–84
  questions 219, 240, 258
avoidant (anxious) personality disorder
    125*f*, 160*f*

B

Beck Depression Inventory (BDI) 54
behaviour 5–6
behaviour therapy 28, 28*f*
beliefs, abnormal *see* abnormal beliefs
benzodiazepines 23*f*
  abuse 158
  indications 23
  in pregnancy 168*f*
  side-effects 23
bereavement 94–95
  Parkes's stages 94*f*
  questions 220–221, 258
beta-amyloid plaques 173
Binswanger's disease 174–175
bipolar affective disorder 52, 60,
    137–138
  aetiology 137
  course and prognosis 138
  epidemiology 134*f*, 137
  management 137–138
    depressive symptoms 138
    drugs 137
    electroconvulsive therapy 138
    maintenance 138
    mania/hypomania 137
    psychotherapy 138
    treatment setting 137
  suicide risk 47*f*
bizarre delusions 68
blackouts 119
body dysmorphic disorder 99
body mass index (BMI) 127, 128*f*
borderline personality disorder 124*b*,
    125*f*, 160*f*
  management 160
brain-derived neurotrophic factor
    (BDNF) 13
breast-feeding, drugs and 168*f*
breathing-related sleep disorders 204
Briquet's syndrome (somatization
    disorder) 98
bulimia nervosa 127–128, 163–166
  aetiology 163–164

epidemiology 163, 164*f*
  management 165
  prognosis 166
  symptoms 128
  see also eating disorders
buprenorphine (Subutex) 24, 157
bupropion 15*f*, 189
buspirone 23

C

CADASIL 174–175
CAGE questionnaire 4, 122
cannabinoids 121*f*
capacity 38–39
carbamazepine 18
  side-effects and contraindications
    18–19, 19*f*
care coordinator 42
care programme approach 42
Care Quality Commission (CQC) 34*f*
case presentation 8–10, 9*f*, 10*b*
catatonia 71*f*
catatonic schizophrenia 71*f*, 72
Charles Bonnet syndrome 67
child abuse 192
  risk factors 192*f*
child/adolescent psychiatry 185–192
  acquired disorders 188–192
  adult disorders with childhood onset
    191–192
  assessment 185
  classification 186, 186*f*
  developmental disorders 187–188
  intellectual disability 186–187
  questions 230–231, 252, 253, 267
  see also specific disorders
childhood disintegrative disorder 188
chlordiazepoxide 23*f*
chlorpromazine 19*f*
  side-effects 144*f*
cholinesterase inhibitors 177
circadian rhythm sleep disorders 204
circumstantiality 59, 70*f*
citalopram 14*f*, 15*f*
classification 10–12
Clock Drawing Test 113*f*
clomipramine 13*b*, 14*f*, 15*f*
clonidine 189
closed questions 1
clozapine 19*f*
  side-effects 20, 21*b*, 144*f*
cognition 7, 103–104
cognitive analytic therapy 28, 162
cognitive behavioural therapy 28–29,
    30*f*, 161
cognitive disorders 103–114
  alcohol-related 119–120
  assessment 112–113, 113*f*, 114*f*
  definitions and clinical features
    103–105

differential diagnosis 110–112, 110*f*,
    111*f*
  questions 221–222, 260
  see also specific conditions
cognitive distortion 29*f*
cognitive impairment 106
  questions 243, 245
cognitive symptoms 51, 54
common law 39
community mental health nurses
    (CPNs) 41
community mental health teams 41–42
Community Treatment Order (TCO)
    35–36
compulsions *see* obsessive/compulsive
    disorders
compulsory admission 33–36, 35*f*
compulsory treatment order
    (CTO) 37
concentration, reduced 51, 58
concordance 183
conduct disorder 190
Conners rating scale (CRS-R) 185
consciousness 103, 104*f*
  impaired 106, 221–222, 260
consent to treatment 36–37
  capacity 38–39
conversion disorder *see* dissociation
convulsions, dissociative 93*f*
Cotard's syndrome 69*f*, 182*b*
counselling 25–26
counter-transference 27, 28*b*
court proceedings 199–200
  criminal responsibility 199–200
  fitness to plead 199
Creutzfeldt-Jakob disease 114*f*, 176
  neuropathology 175*f*
  new variant 114*f*, 176
criminal responsibility 199–200
cyclothymia 52, 60, 138–139
  aetiology 138–139
  epidemiology 134*f*, 139
  management 139

D

Da Costa's syndrome 99
dangerous severe personality disorder
    198*b*
day hospitals 42
declarative memory 104
defence mechanisms 27*f*
delirium 73, 106–107, 106*f*, 110, 178
  aetiology 178
  alcohol withdrawal 117–119
  course and prognosis 178
  differential diagnosis 108*f*, 111
  epidemiology 178
  management 178, 179*f*
  questions 228–229, 266
  see also dementia

delirium tremens 155b, 155f
 see also alcohol withdrawal
delusional disorder 73
delusional jealousy 69f, 197b
delusional perception
delusions 7, 51, 67–68, 75, 87f
 autochtonous 68
 bizarre 68
 classification 69f
 of control 69f
 grandiose 59, 69f
 of infidelity 69f
 of love 69f
 mood-congruent 59, 68
 persecutory 59, 69f
 of reference 69f
dementia 73, 107–110, 173–178
 aetiopathology 173–176
 alcohol-related 119–120
 behavioural and psychological
  symptoms 107
 clinical features 107–110, 109f
 course and prognosis 177–178
 CT appearances 114f
 differential diagnosis 108f, 111
 diseases causing 106–107
 epidemiology 173
 functional impairment 107
 legal issues 177
 management 176–177
  behavioural and psychological
   symptoms 177
  maintenance of cognitive function
   176–177
 memory impairment 107
 neurological symptoms 107
 neuropathology 175f
 prevalence 174f
 questions 228–229, 243, 244, 252,
  266
 treatment 24
 see also delirium; and specific types
denial 27f
dependent personality disorder 125f,
 160f
depersonalization 93b
depression 49–56, 60–61, 111–112,
 133–137
 aetiology 133–134, 134f
  acute stress 133–134
  chronic stress 134
  early life experience 133
  neurobiology 134
  personality 133
 biological (somatic) symptoms
  50–51
 bipolar *see* bipolar affective disorder
 cognitive symptoms 51, 54
 core symptoms 49–50
 course and prognosis 137
 differential diagnosis 51–53, 52f

diurnal variation 50
drugs causing 53f
 epidemiology 133, 134f
 examination 54
 genetics 133
 history 53–54
 ICD-10 classification 50
 investigations 54
 management 134–136, 135f
  antidepressants 135–136, 136f
  electroconvulsive therapy 136
  lifestyle advice 135
  psychotherapy 135
  treatment setting 134–135
 mood (affective) disorders 52, 52f
 older adults 181–182
 postnatal 169–170
 psychotic symptoms 51
 questions 217, 235, 236, 247, 257
 recurrent 52
 secondary 53
 suicide risk 47f, 51
depressive pseudodementia 181
derailment 69–70
derealization 6–7, 93
detoxification, alcohol 117–119, 119f,
 154–155, 155f
developmental disorders 187–188
 Asperger's syndrome 188, 188f
 autism 187–188, 188f
 childhood disintegrative disorder 188
 Rett's syndrome 188
dexamfetamine 24
Diagnostic Interview Schedule for
 Children (NIMH-DISC-IV) 185
dialectical behaviour therapy 31f, 161
diazepam 23f
differential diagnosis 8
 see also specific conditions
diminished responsibility 200
Diogenes' syndrome 182b
diphenhydramine (Nytol) 24
disinhibition 105f
disordered thought form 58–59, 68–70,
 70f
dissociation 93, 93f, 99
dissociative anaesthetics 121f
dissociative disorders 112
 questions 242
disulfiram (Antabuse) 24, 155
doctrine of necessity 39
donepezil 24, 177
Down's syndrome, neuropathological
 changes 174
Driver and Vehicle Licensing Authority
 (DVLA) 40, 177
driving, fitness for 40
 dementia 177
drug therapy 13–24
 questions 215, 252, 255
 see also specific drugs and categories

DSM-IV 10, 12
dyscalculia 193
dysexecutive syndrome 105f
dysfunctional assumptions 28–29
dysgnosia 105f
dyslexia 193
dysphasia 105f
dyspraxia 105f
dysthymia 52, 138–139
 aetiology 138–139
 epidemiology 134f, 139
 management 139
dystonia 6b, 21f

E

early wakening 50
eating disorders 127–132, 163–166
 assessment 128–129, 130f
 definitions and clinical features
  127–128
 differential diagnosis 129–131, 131f
 ICD-10 classification 128f
 medical complications 129f
 questions 224, 227–228, 247, 250,
  261, 267
 suicide risk 47f
 see also specific disorders
echolalia 70
echopraxia 71f
eclectic therapy 25b
ECT *see* electroconvulsive therapy
Ekbom's syndrome 69f
elderly *see* older adults
electroconvulsive therapy (ECT) 24
 contraindications 24
 history 24
 indications 24
  bipolar affective disorder 138
  depression 136
 mechanism of action 24
 older adults 181–182
 questions 215, 256
 side-effects 24
emergency detention order (EDO) 37
emotional disorders of
 childhood 190
emotional reasoning 29f
encopresis, non-organic 191
energy, increased 58
enuresis, non-organic 191
episodic memory 104–105
erotomania 69f
euphoria 57–58
European Convention on Human
 Rights (ECHR) 39
exhibitionism 211f
exposure therapy 28f
extracampine hallucinations 67
eye movement desensitization and
 reprocessing 31f

F

factitious disorder *see* Münchausen's syndrome
family history 3–4
family therapy 29
fantasy 27*f*
fat folder syndrome 97–98
fear 77–84
    questions 219, 240, 258
    see also anxiety disorders; phobia
fetishism 211*f*
first-rank symptoms 72*f*
fitness to plead 199
flight of ideas 58, 59, 70*f*
fluoxetine (Prozac) 13, 14*f*, 15*f*
flupentixol (Depixol) 19*f*
    side-effects 144*f*
fluvoxamine 15*f*
folie à deux 73
forensic history 4
forensic psychiatry 197–200
    court proceedings 199–200
    mental disorder and crime 197–198, 198*f*
    questions 231–232, 253, 268
    risk of violence 198–199, 199*f*
forensic sections 36, 36*f*
formulation 8–10, 9*f*, 10*b*
fortune telling 29*f*
free-floating anxiety *see* generalized anxiety disorder
Freud, Sigmund 26, 26*f*
frontotemporal dementia 109*f*, 114*f*, 175–176
    neuropathology 175*f*
fugue, dissociative 93*f*
functional hallucinations 67
functional symptoms 97, 98*b*

G

galantamine 24, 177
Ganser's syndrome 93*f*
gender identity 211
generalized anxiety disorder 77, 79*f*, 80
    questions 248
Gerstmann-Sträussler syndrome 176
Gilles de la Tourette's syndrome 191
grandiosity 58, 59, 69*f*
group therapy 29
guilt 51
gustatory hallucinations 67

H

hallucinations 7, 51, 66, 87*f*
    auditory 66–67
    classification 66*f*
    olfactory/gustatory 67
    somatic 67
    visual 67
    see also specific types
hallucinogens 121*f*
haloperidol 19*f*
    side-effects 144*f*
Hare Psychopathy Checklist – Revised (PCL-R) 198
hebephrenic schizophrenia 72
Heller's syndrome 188
history
    family 3–4
    past medical 3
    past psychiatric 3
    personal 4
    presenting complaint 3
histrionic personality disorder 125*f*, 160*f*
HIV-related dementia 176
home treatment teams 42
hopelessness 51
Hospital Anxiety and Depression Scale (HADS) 54
Human Rights Act (1998) 39
human rights legislation 39–40
humour 27*f*
Huntington's disease 114*f*, 176
    neuropathology 175*f*
hypersomnia 203–204, 204*f*
hypnagogic hallucinations 67
hypnotics *see* anxiolytics/hypnotics
hypochondriacal disorder 99
hypokalaemia 129*b*
hypomania *see* mania/hypomania
hypothalamic-pituitary-gonadal axis 127
hysteria 93–94

I

ICD-10 10, 11*f*
    depression 50
    eating disorders 128*f*
    obsessive/compulsive disorders 86*f*
    schizophrenia 72*f*
idiosyncratic word use 70
illusions 66
imipramine 14*f*, 15*f*, 189
impaired consciousness 106, 221–222, 260
in-patient units 43
Independent Mental Health Advocates (IMHA) 34*f*
infestation, delusions of 69*f*
inhalants 121*f*
insight 7
    impaired 58
insomnia 201–203
    assessment 202–203
    causes 203*f*
    management 203, 203*f*

intellectual disability 112, 193–196
    causes 195*f*
    children and adolescents 186–187
    classification and clinical features 194, 194*f*
    communication issues 196*f*
    and crime 198*f*
    definition and diagnosis 193
    epidemiology and aetiology 194
    management 194–196
        education, training and occupation 195
        help for families 195
        housing and social support 195
        medical care 195–196
        psychiatric care 196
    questions 231, 253, 268
intellectualization 27*f*
intelligence quotient (IQ) 193–194, 194*f*, 253
interpersonal therapy 29
interview 1–2
    closed questions 1
    current medication 3
    history *see* history
    open questions 1–2
    personal information 2
    premorbid personality 5
    presenting complaint 3
investigations 10
irritability 57–58
    questions 217–218, 238, 257
isocarboxazid 15*f*

J

jealousy, delusional 69*f*, 197*b*
judgement, impaired 58

K

Kiddie Schedule for Affective Disorders and Schizophrenia (K-SADS-P) 185
knight's move thinking 69–70
Korsakoff syndrome *see* Wernicke-Korsakoff syndrome
kuru 176

L

labelling 29*f*
lamotrigine 18
    side-effects and contraindications 18–19, 19*f*
lanugo hair 129
learning disability *see* intellectual disability
legal issues 33–40
    capacity 38–39
    common law 39

dementia 177
fitness to drive 40
human rights legislation 39–40
Mental Health Act (1983) (amended
    2007) 33–37
Mental Health (Care & Treatment)
    (Scotland) Act (2003) 37
Mental Health (Northern Ireland)
    Order (1986) 37–38
proxy decision making 38–39
questions 216, 256
Lewy body dementia 109f, 175
neuropathology 175f
libido, loss of 51
Lilliputian hallucinations 67
lithium 17–18
side-effects and contraindications
    18, 18f
lofepramine 14f
lofexidine 24
loosening of association 69–70, 70f
lorazepam 23f
low mood see depression

M

magnification 29f
malingering 99
mania/hypomania 57–64
assessment 62
biological symptoms 58
cognitive symptoms 58
diagnosis 62f
differential diagnosis 59–61, 59f
distinction between 60f
medical conditions and substance
    abuse 61, 61f
mood (affective) disorders 52, 52f,
    60–61
mood changes 57–58
older adults 182
psychotic symptoms 58–59
questions 217–218, 237, 238, 257
treatment 137
manic stupor 58
mannerisms 71f
medical conditions
and anxiety 81, 82f
and mania 61
and psychosis 73, 73f
medical history 3
medically unexplained physical
    symptoms 97–102
assessment 100–101, 101f
definitions and clinical features
    98–100
differential diagnosis 97b, 100
questions 221, 243, 259
memantine 24, 177
memory 104–105, 105f
impairment 107, 221–222, 260

loss see amnesia
menopause 167
Mental Capacity Act (2005) 38
Mental Health Act (1983) (amended
    2007) 33–37
civil sections 33–36, 35f
consent to treatment 36–37
definitions 33, 34f
forensic sections 36, 36f
Mental Health Act Managers 34–35, 34f
Mental Health (Care & Treatment)
    (Scotland) Act (2003) 37
Mental Health (Northern Ireland)
    Order (1986) 37–38
Mental Health Review Tribunal (MHRT)
    34f
mental health service provision 41–44
history 41
primary care 41
questions 216, 256
secondary care 41–43, 42f
mental retardation see intellectual
    disability
mental state examination 5–7
suicide 47–48
mentalization-based therapy 28, 31f,
    161
methadone 24
methylphenidate (Ritalin, Concerta,
    Equasym) 24, 189
mianserin 15f
mild cognitive impairment 111
milieu therapy 30
mind reading 29f
mindfulness-based cognitive therapy,
    28
Mini-Mental State Exam 113f, 177
Minnesota Multiphasic Personality
    Inventory 124
mirtazapine 13, 14f, 15, 15f
side-effects and contraindications 16
Misuse of Drugs Act (1971) 157f
mixed affective episode 57–58, 60
moclobemide 14f, 15f
side-effects and contraindications 16
modafinil 189
modelling therapy 28f
monoamine oxidase inhibitors 13, 15,
    15f
mechanism of action 14f
side-effects and contraindications
    16–17, 17f
mood 6
elevated see mania/hypomania
low see depression
mood (affective) disorders 52, 52f,
    60–61, 73, 107, 133–140
aetiology 134f
alcohol-related 120
and crime 198f
epidemiology 134f

questions 224–225, 262
see also specific disorders
mood stabilizers 17–19
history 17
indications 17–18
mechanism of action 17
in pregnancy 168f
side-effects and contraindications
    18–19
see also individual drugs
mood-congruent delusions 59, 68
motor disorders, dissociative 93f
multiple personality disorder 93f
Münchausen's syndrome 99
by proxy 100
mutism, elective 190–191

N

naltrexone (Nalorex) 24, 155
narcissistic personality disorder 125f,
    160f
narcolepsy 203–204
Nearest Relative (NR) 34f
necrophilia 211f
negative symptoms 70–71
neologisms 70
neurodevelopmental disorders 61
neurofibrillary tangles 173
neuroleptic malignant syndrome 22f
nightmares 205
nihilistic delusions see Cotard's
    syndrome
NOTCH3 174–175

O

obsessive-compulsive personality
    disorder 125f, 160f
questions 219–220, 241, 258
obsessive/compulsive disorders 6–7,
    85–90, 147
clinical features 85–86, 86f
course and prognosis 151
definitions 85–86
diagnosis 88f
differential diagnosis 86–88, 86f, 87f
ICD-10 classification 86f
questions 219–220, 241, 258
obstructive sleep apnoea syndrome 204
occupational record 4
olanzapine 19f
side-effects 144f
older adults, mental illness in 181–184
age-related physiological changes
    183, 183f
assessment 182–183
depression 181–182
epidemiology 181
late-onset schizophrenia 182
management 183

older adults, mental illness in
    (Continued)
    concordance 183
    polypharmacy 183
    psychosocial interventions 183
mania 182
prevalence 182f
questions 229–230, 252, 266
see also dementia; delirium
olfactory hallucinations 67
open questions 1–2
opiates 121f
    abuse 157–158
    questions 249
organic personality disorder 124
Othello syndrome 69f, 197b
out-patient clinics 42
over-generalization 29f
overvalued ideas 7, 68, 87f
oxazepam 23f

P

paediatric psychiatry see child/
    adolescent psychiatry
paedophilia 211f
palilalia 70
panic disorders 78, 79f, 81, 147
    course and prognosis 151
    questions 248
paranoid personality disorder 125f,
    160f
paranoid schizophrenia 72
paraphilias 210–211, 211f
parkinsonism 6b, 21f
Parkinson's disease
    with dementia 109f, 175
    neuropathology 175f
paroxetine 14f, 15f
perceptions 7
perceptual disturbance 59, 66–67, 107
persecutory delusions 59, 69f
perseveration 70, 105f
persistent somatoform pain disorder 99
personal alarms 1
personal history 4
    alcohol and substance abuse 4
    forensic history 4
    infancy/early childhood 4
    late childhood/adolescence 4
    occupational record 4
    relationships, marital and sexual
        history 4
    social circumstances 4
personal information 2
personality disorders 61, 73–74,
    123–126, 159–162
    aetiology 159
    assessment 124–126
    classification 124, 125f
    course and prognosis 162

and crime 197–198, 198f
definitions and clinical features 123
differential diagnosis 126
epidemiology 159, 160f
management 160–162
    crisis management 161
    drug therapy 161
    long-term 161–162
    psychotherapy 161
    short-term management 161
questions 223, 226–227, 246, 250,
    261, 264
suicide risk 47f
personality traits 123
personalization 29f
phenelzine 13, 14f, 15f
phobia 78–79
    agoraphobia 79
    social phobia 79
    see also anxiety; anxiety disorders
phobic anxiety disorder 190
physical examination 8
physical illness
    and depression 53, 53f
    suicide risk 46
Pick's bodies 175–176
polypharmacy 183
post-traumatic stress disorder 92–93
    course and prognosis 151
    questions 248
postnatal 'blues' 169
postnatal depression 169–170
Power of Attorney 38–39
pramipexole 15f
pregabalin 24
pregnancy 167–169
    indications for referral 168f
    medication during 168f
    pseudocyesis 168b
    puerperal disorders 169–171
    questions 228, 251, 265
premenstrual syndrome 167, 228
    questions 228, 265
premorbid personality 5
presenting complaint 3
primary care 41
prion protein 176
procedural memory 104
Prochaska-DiClemente transtheoretical
    model of change 249
prognosis 10
projection 27f
proxy decision making 38–39
pseudocyesis 168b
pseudohallucinations 66, 87f
psychiatric history 3
psychoanalysis 27
psychodynamic psychotherapy 26–28,
    162, 233
psychomotor excitation 58
psychomotor function 5–6, 71

psychomotor retardation 50–51
psychopathy 197–198
psychosexual disorders 207–212
    gender identity 211
    sexual dysfunction 207–210, 208f
    sexual preference (paraphilias)
        210–211
psychosis 65–76, 112
    alcohol-related 120
    assessment 74–75
    clinical features 65–71
    definitions 65–71
    diagnosis 74f
    early intervention 42–43
    medical conditions and substance
        abuse 73
    puerperal 170–171, 170f
    questions 218–219, 225, 238, 239,
        240, 257, 262
    see also specific disorders
psychosocial stress 91–92
psychostimulants 24
psychotherapy 25–32
    approaches to 25–30
    indications 30, 31f
        alcohol abuse 155
        anorexia nervosa 164, 165f
        anxiety disorders 150
        bipolar affective disorder 138
        depression 135
        personality disorders 161
        schizophrenia 144–145
    questions 215–216, 233, 255
    see also specific modalities
psychotic symptoms 51
psychotropic drugs see also specific types
puerperal disorders 169–171
    postnatal 'blues' 169
    postnatal depression 169–170
    psychosis 170–171, 170f
    questions 251

Q

quetiapine 19f
    side-effects 144f

R

rapport 2b
reaction-formation 27f
reboxetine 14f, 15f
refeeding syndrome 165f
rehabilitation units 43
relationships 4
relaxation therapy 28f
religious delusions 69f
repression 27f
residual schizophrenia 72
Responsible Clinician (RC) 34–35, 34f
Rett's syndrome 188

reversible inhibitor of monoamine oxidase A *see* RIMA
RIMA 15*f*
  side-effects and contraindications 16–17
risk assessment 8
risk factors for suicide 46, 46*f*, 47*f*
risperidone 19*f*
  side-effects 144*f*
rivastigmine 24, 177
rumination 87*f*
Russell's sign 129

S

schizoaffective disorder 52–53, 61, 73
schizoid personality disorder 125*f*, 160*f*
schizophrenia 61, 61*f*, 71–72, 141–146
  acute behavioural disturbance 145
  aetiology 141–143
    brain lesions 142
    expressed emotion 142–143
    life events 142
    neurotransmitter abnormalities 142
  course and prognosis 145
  and crime 198*f*
  differential diagnosis 72*f*
  epidemiology 141
  genetics 141–142, 142*f*
  history 141
  ICD-10 classification 72*f*
  late-onset 182
  management 143–145, 146*f*
    drugs 143–144, 144*f*
    physical health monitoring 144
    psychotherapy 144–145
    social inputs 145
    treatment setting 143
  motor symptoms 71*f*
  questions 225, 247, 262
  Schneider's first-rank symptoms 72*f*
  subtypes 72
  suicide risk 47*f*
  see also psychosis
schizophrenia-like psychotic disorders 72
schizophreniform disorders 61
schizotypal personality disorder 125*f*, 160*f*
school refusal 190*b*
scrapie 176
Second Opinion Approved Doctor (SOAD) 34*f*, 36–37
secondary care 41–43, 42*f*
  accommodation 43
  assertive outreach teams 42
  care programme approach 42
  community mental health teams 41–42
  day hospitals 42

early intervention in psychosis 42–43
  home treatment teams 42
  in-patient units 43
  out-patient clinics 42
  rehabilitation units 43
sectioning *see* compulsory admission
sedatives 121*f*
self-esteem
  elevated sense of 58
  poor 51
self-harm 45–48, 51
  assessment 45–48
  definition 45
  management 48
  questions 216–217, 234, 235, 256
  risk assessment 48
  see also specific conditions
self-help 25*b*
semantic memory 104–105
senile squalor 182*b*
sensory loss, dissociative 93*f*
separation anxiety disorder 190
serotonin reuptake inhibitors *see* SSRIs
serotonin syndrome 22*f*
serotonin-noradrenaline reuptake inhibitors *see* SNRIs
sertraline 14*f*, 15*f*
sexual abuse 4*b*
sexual dysfunction 207–210, 208*f*
  aetiology 209, 209*f*
  assessment 209–210
  clinical features 207
  differential diagnosis 209
  epidemiology 207–208, 208*f*
  frequency 209*f*
  management 210, 210*f*
  prognosis 210
sexual history 4
sexual masochism 211*f*
sexual preference disorders 210–211, 211*f*
sexual sadism 211*f*
short-term detention order (STDO) 37
sibling rivalry disorder 190
sleep disorders 107, 201–206
  breathing-related 204
  circadian rhythm 204
  decreased need for sleep 58
  definitions and classification 201–205
  early wakening 50
  hypersomnia and narcolepsy 203–204, 204*f*
  insomnia 201–203
  nightmares 205
  stages of sleep 202*f*
sleep terrors 204–205
sleepwalking 205
SNRIs 14*f*, 15*f*
social anxiety disorder 190
social circumstances 4

social phobia 79
  course and prognosis 151
sodium valproate *see* valproate
somatic delusions 69*f*
somatic hallucinations 67
somatization disorder (Briquet's syndrome) 27*f*, 98
somatoform autonomic dysfunction 99
somatoform disorders 124, 151–152
  aetiology 151
  course and prognosis 151
  epidemiology 151, 151*f*
  management 151–152, 152*f*
  questions 225–226, 263
somnambulism 205
speech 7
splitting 27*f*
SSRIs 13–15, 15*f*
  mechanism of action 14*f*
  in pregnancy 168*f*
  side-effects and contraindications 15–16, 16*f*
  see also individual drugs
stable cognitive impairment 111
stereotypies 71*f*
stimulants 121*f*
stress 91–96
  acute stress reaction 92
  bereavement 94–95
  definitions and clinical features 91–94
  and depression 133–134
  differential diagnosis 95, 95*f*
  nature of patient's reaction 92–94
  post-traumatic stress disorder 92–93
  psychosocial 91–92
  questions 220–221, 242, 258
stupor, dissociative 93*f*
subjective cognitive impairment 111
sublimation 27*f*
substance abuse 4, 115–122, 156–158
  aetiology 157
  and anxiety 81, 82*f*
  assessment 121–122
  and crime 198*f*
  definition and clinical features 115–116
  differential diagnosis 120–121
  drug effects 121*f*
  epidemiology 156
  management 24, 157–158
  and mania 61
  Misuse of Drugs Act (1971) 157*f*
  and psychosis 73, 73*f*
  questions 222–223, 226, 237, 239, 240, 245, 249, 260, 263
  see also alcohol abuse; and specific drugs
substance dependence 116
substance intoxication 116
substance withdrawal 116

suicidal intent 46–47, 51, 216–217, 256
suicide 45–48
  attempted 45
    management 48
  definition 45
  mental state examination 47–48
  planned 47
  questions 234
  risk factors 46, 46f, 47f
sulpiride 19f
superficial hallucinations 67
supportive psychotherapy 25–26
suppression 27f

T

tangentiality 59, 70f
tardive dyskinesia 6b, 21f
temazepam 23f, 203
therapeutic communities 162
therapy
  current 3
  drugs 13–24
  ECT 24
  psychological 25–32
  see also specific modalities

thoughts 7
  accelerated 58
  audible 66
  disordered form 58–59, 68–70, 70f
thought blocking 70
thought disturbance 107
  questions 240, 241
thought insertion 87f
tics 71f, 191
transference 27, 28b
transsexualism 211b
transvestism 211b
tranylcypromine 14f, 15f
traumatic stress 92
trazodone 15f, 177
  side-effects and contraindications 16
tricyclic antidepressants 13, 15, 15f
  contraindications 16, 16f
  mechanism of action 14f
  in pregnancy 168f
  side-effects 16, 16f, 181
  see also individual drugs

V

valproate 18, 18b
  side-effects and contraindications 18–19, 19f

vascular dementia 109f, 114f, 174–175
  neuropathology 175f
venlafaxine 14f, 15f
violence, risk of 198–199, 199f
visual hallucinations 67
voyeurism 211f

W

Wechsler Intelligence Scale 193–194
weight loss 50
  questions 224, 246, 261
Wernicke-Korsakoff syndrome 112, 119, 154
word salad 68–69

Y

Yerkes-Dodson law 77, 78f

Z

zaleplon 23f, 203
zolpidem 23f, 203
zoophilia 211f
zopiclone 23f, 203
zuclopenthixol (Clopixol) 19f
  side-effects 144f